NEW INSIGHTS INTO TOXICITY AND DRUG TESTING

Edited by **Sivakumar Gowder**

New Insights into Toxicity and Drug Testing
http://dx.doi.org/10.5772/55886
Edited by Sivakumar Gowder

Contributors

Ifeoma Obidike, Azad Mohammed, Michaela Reddy, Harvey Clewell, Thierry Lave, Melvin Andersen, Ray Greek, Abdelmigid, Nasir Mohamad, Peter Ward, David La, J. Eric McDuffie, Sandra Snook, Elsa Dias, Carina Menezes, Elisabete Valério, Jose M Fuentes, Jacob John Van Tonder, Mary Gulumian, Vanessa Steenkamp

Published by InTech

Janeza Trdine 9, 51000 Rijeka, Croatia

Publishing Process Manager Ana Pantar
Technical Editor InTech DTP team
Cover InTech Design team

Additional hard copies can be obtained from orders@intechopen.com

New Insights into Toxicity and Drug Testing, Edited by Sivakumar Gowder
p. cm.
ISBN 978-953-51-0946-4

For EU product safety concerns:
IN TECH d.o.o., Prolaz Marije Krucifikse Kozulić 3, 51000 Rijeka, Croatia,
info@intechopen.com or visit our website at intechopen.com.

Meet the editor

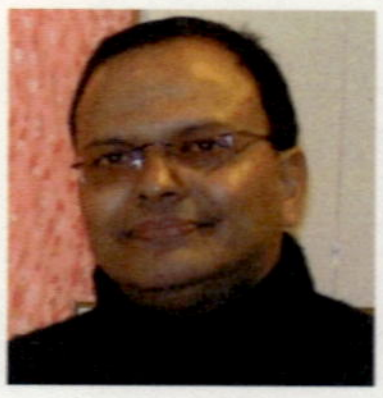

Dr Sivakumar Gowder got his academic training and carried out his research in institutions of high academic ranking in India and US. He earned his PhD from the University of Madras, India and continued his research at AIIMS, India. He then moved to the US to continue his research at the UT Southwestern Medical Center, LSU Medical Center, and University of Pittsburgh School of Medicine. Currently, he is working as an Associate Professor of Pharmacology at the Qassim University, KSA. Sivakumar received several prizes / awards during his academic career. He has developed his own methods / techniques relevant to his research projects. Currently, he serves as an author / editor for books; an editor in chief for an international journal; an editorial member; and a reviewer for many journals and is a fellow of various international organizations. Sivakumar has also served as an invited speaker and a chairperson for international conferences.

Contents

Preface

In this book, the section on Toxicity reveals the emerging technologies (profiling technologies, 3D cultures etc.) to evaluate hepatotoxicity of candidate drugs; suitability of kidney Vero cell line in evaluating toxicity of microcystins; suitability of aquatic larva to evaluate environmental toxicants and advanced level techniques (next generation sequencing etc.) to screen the safety of medicinal plants. Chapters in the section on Drug testing and Development reveal reductionist approach of using animal models in drug development, especially in toxicity testing; the role of renal transporters in the safety assessment of drugs; role of autophagy in Parkinson's diseases and the clinical importance of Methadone Maintenance Therapy. In this section, there are also interesting discussions on the emerging role of physiologically based pharmacokinetic modeling in the pharmaceutical industry throughout the drug development. This book is a significant resource for scientists and physicians who are directly dealing with drugs / medicines and human life. It is my privilege to present this book to the scientific community.

I extend my gratitude towards my mother, my late father and my brothers for introducing me to higher education. My thanks to higher authorities, and colleagues of Qassim University for their motivation to carry out this project. I am continuously indebted to my wife Anitha for her encouragement and technical support for this book project. I also acknowledge the interest and commitment from the Senior Commissioning Editor of InTech Ms Ana Pantar and the Publishing Process Manager Ms Sandra Bakic whose patience and focus were of immense support in this project. Finally, I express deep and sincere gratitude to all the authors for their valuable contributions and scholarly cooperation for timely completion of this book.

Dr Sivakumar Joghi Thatha Gowder
Qassim University – College of Pharmacy
Kingdom of Saudi Arabia

Section 1

Toxicity

Chapter 1

Pre-Clinical Assessment of the Potential Intrinsic Hepatotoxicity of Candidate Drugs

Jacob John van Tonder, Vanessa Steenkamp and Mary Gulumian

Additional information is available at the end of the chapter

http://dx.doi.org/10.5772/54792

1. Introduction

1.1. The cost of new drugs and need to streamline drug development

Innovation is fundamental to discovering new drugs for the variety of human conditions that exist. It is also one of the key requirements for any pharmaceutical organization that wishes to gain a competitive edge. The pharmaceutical industry is profit-driven because it has to fund its own drug innovation, which highlights why research and development (R&D) forms the backbone of this industry. According to the CEO of the Pharmaceutical Research and Manufacturers of America (PhRMA), John Castellani, member companies of PhRMA spent a record US$ 67.4 billion on R&D in 2011. This is approximately 20% of generated revenue, which is 5 times more than the average manufacturing firm invests into R&D [1]. The pharmaceutical sector was responsible for 20% of all R&D expenditures by U.S. businesses in 2011 [2]. The aforesaid figures do not describe global R&D expenditures, but serve to give some indication of the astronomical contributions that are annually devoted by the pharmaceutical industry to drug development.

Substantial fiscal investments are made against the backdrop of enormous investment risks. It is estimated that only 5 of every 10 000 compounds explored will make it to clinical trials [1]. Although the likelihood that an investigational new drug in clinical testing reaches the market has increased over the past couple of decades to 16%, the probability is still low. Furthermore, of those that do get approved, only 2 or 3 out of every 10 drugs recover their full pecuniary investment [1]. The stakes are incredible and the strain on the industry as a whole is overt. In 2011 the world's largest research-based pharmaceutical company, Pfizer, closed its R&D centre located in the U.K. owing to financial viability concerns. In an attempt to dissuade some of the financial pressures, many companies have opted for mergers to either maintain existing pipelines or acquire new development opportunities [3].

A fairly regular citation estimates the out-of-pocket, pre-approval cost per drug developed to be more than US$ 800 million [4]. Estimations reported in peer-reviewed literature ranges from US$ 391 million [5] to US$ 1.8 billion [6]. Evident from literature is the fact that the estimates increase over time, in other words, the cost of developing drugs is escalating, which implies ever-increasing financial pressures on industry.

Two of the most prominent concerns for the pharmaceutical industry are patent expirations and attrition rates. Patent expirations result in decreased revenue generation and, as stated, this industry is profit-driven, meaning that diminished earnings cripple the R&D of an organization. Not only does this predict deterioration for a pharmaceutical company, but decreased R&D output also slows the production of new drugs. This also has a major impact on healthcare. It is estimated that in the U.S. a new case of Alzheimer's develops every 68 seconds [7]. Using these figures, more than 460 000 new cases of Alzheimer's will develop each year the approval of an effective new drug is delayed. Whereas patent expirations prune generated revenues, attrition rates affect the opposite side of the equation, needlessly raising the cost of developing new drugs. Attrition rates are high (Figure 1). A chemical entity that reaches phase I clinical trials has a 71% chance of reaching phase II clinical trials. Those chemical entities that do reach phase II trials have only a 31% chance of entering phase III trials. Further compounding the issue are rising failure rates in phase III trials [4]. Attrition drives development costs for two reasons: 1) monetary investments into failed ventures are lost and 2) failing development programs occupy resources and time that could otherwise be spent on drug candidates that would eventually succeed to be approved for marketing.

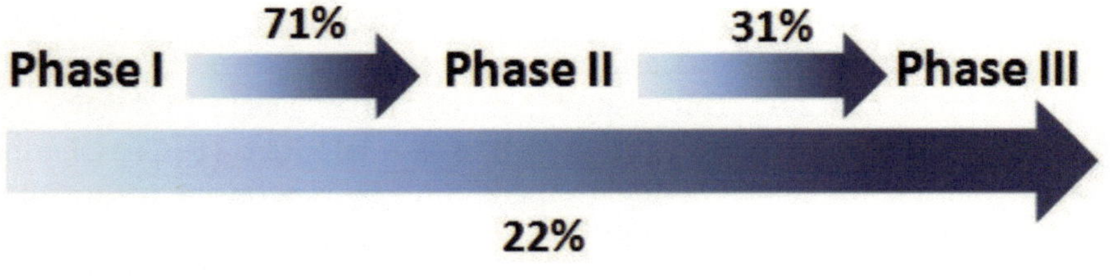

Figure 1. The probability that a chemical entity under development will progress from one clinical phase to the next. Candidate drugs have only a 22% chance of completing clinical development prior to review by regulatory authorities [4].

Together, patent expirations and drug attrition add enormous strain on new drug development, in a cumulative way inhibiting productivity and output of the entire R&D process. An article recently published by Forbes offers some perspective on the impact of attrition on development costs [8]. According to this article, AstraZeneca has been plagued by development failures, which escalated their average cost to develop a new drug to US$ 12 billion. In comparison, for Eli Lilly the average cost of developing a new drugs is estimated at only US$ 4.5 billion. The difference in development cost between the two companies can be attributed to the difference in approval rates of new drug i.e. less failures [8].

The average times, from the start of a particular phase to entering the next phase, are 4.3 years for pre-clinical development and 1.0, 2.2 and 2.8 years for phase I, II and III trials, respectively. Regulatory perusal adds another 1.5 years to the entire process [4]. Collectively, the duration of drug development from initiation of clinical testing until drug approval is estimated at 7.5 years [4]. Including pre-clinical development, it takes, on average, 10 - 15 years to develop a new drug from its discovery to regulatory approval [1,4] (Figure 2). A study that investigated the reduction in costs associated with drug development with improved productivity of the process reported that a 5% reduction in total development time will decrease development costs by 3.5% [9]. Although this may not sound like much, 3.5% of US$ 1 billion is a substantial saving. The study also emphasized the reduction in costs if decisions to terminate unproductive development programs are shifted to earlier phases of the discovery process. For example, the study estimated that if a company manages to shift a quarter of its decisions to terminate from phase II to phase I, it would save US$ 22 million [9]. Again, it relates back to why attrition drives development costs. Making the decision to terminate (a development program) earlier would stop further investment into unfruitful programs and free resources to promote approval ratings.

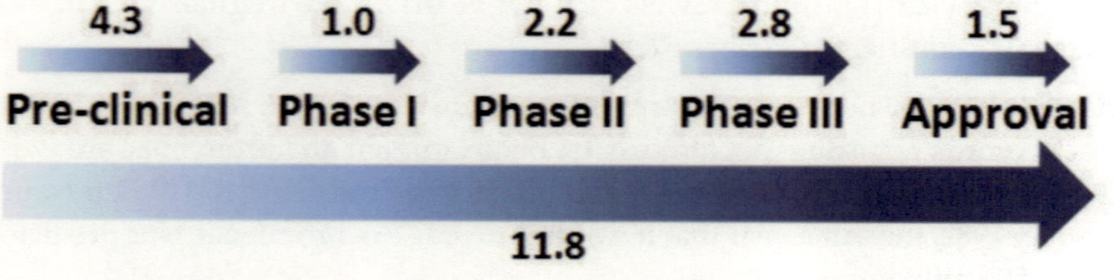

Figure 2. Average duration (in years) of different phases of drug development [4]. Reducing phase duration will reduce associated development costs.

Industry continuously struggles to bring new drugs to the market, despite the process being overextended, costly and particularly uncertain of success. Over the last decade, overall drug development time has increased by 20% and the rate of approval of new chemical entities has dropped by 30% [10]. There is a mounting need to nurture output from the drug development process. Minor restructuring and streamlining of this process is required to increase its productivity and alleviate some of the financial pressures that drug developers experience. One area in particular where pruning of this process is overdue is the early pre-clinical detection / prediction of potential hepatotoxic chemical entities.

2. Attrition due to hepatotoxicity

Drug-induced liver injury (DILI) is a challenge for both the pharmaceutical industry and regulatory authorities. The most severe adverse effect that DILI may lead to is acute liver failure, resulting in either death or liver transplant. Of all the cases of acute liver failure in the U.S., between 13% and 50% can be attributed to DILI [11,12]. Without a doubt there is great concern for the safety of consumers exposed to drugs that may cause DILI because patients have only one liver. For this reason, government and the public put pressure on regulatory authorities to establish safer drugs [13]. However, if regulatory authorities unnecessarily raise safety standards without scientific evidence, this will discourage drug development because of attrition, which is predominantly unwanted when considering the current scenario where fewer antimicrobials are being developed alongside increased antibiotic resistance.

A prevailing issue in drug development is the attrition of new drug candidates. Between 1995 and 2005, a total of 34 drugs were withdrawn from various markets (Table 1) and the reason for withdrawal in the majority of cases was hepatotoxicity [14]. Hepatotoxicity is the leading cause of drug withdrawals from the marketplace [15-17]. Examples include the monoamine oxidase inhibitor, iproniazid, the anti-diabetic drug, troglitazone, and the anti-inflammatory analgesic, bromfenac, all of which induced idiosyncratic liver injury. Iproniazid, the first monoamine oxidase inhibitor released in the 1950's, was probably the most hepatotoxic drug ever marketed [16]. Troglitazone was available on the U.S. market from March 1997. By February 2000, 83 patients had developed liver failure, of which 70% died. Of the 26 survivors, 6 required liver transplants [18]. While on the market, troglitazone accrued approximately US $ 700 million per year [14]. Withdrawals of lucrative drugs like troglitazone diminish return on investments and threaten further R&D.

Of all classes of drugs, non-steroidal anti-inflammatory drugs (NSAIDs) have had one of the worst track records regarding hepatotoxicity. Benoxaprofen and bromfenac are two NSAIDs that were withdrawn from public use after reports of hepatotoxicity [16,19]. Benoxaprofen was withdrawn in 1982, the same year that it was approved [16]. Bromfenac was predicted to earn around US$ 500 million per year [14].

Although diclofenac is widely used to treat rheumatoid disorders, approximately 250 cases of diclofenac-induced hepatotoxicity have been reported. In perspective, DILI caused by diclofenac has an incidence of 1-2 per every million prescriptions [20,21], being high enough that a considerable amount of literature has been generated warning against diclofenac-induced hepatotoxicity. Between 1982 and 2001 in France, more than 27 000 cases of NSAID-induced liver injuries were reported. Clometacin, and silundac were the NSAIDs with the highest risk of DILI. Over the same peroid approximately 2100 cases of NSAID-induced liver injuries were reported in Spain, with the main culprits being droxicam, silundac and nimesulide [22]. Acetaminophen (a.k.a. paracetamol) must be the most notorious of all the NSAIDs, if not all drugs, when it comes to DILI. Its mechanism of hepatotoxicity is better understood than its therapeutic mechanism of action. Fortunately, acetaminophen has a substantial therapeutic index and copious amounts need to be administered before the liver will not be able to manage its onslaught anymore [23].

Troglitazone was available on the U.S. market for three years before withdrawal, during which time it was used by almost 2 million patients, realising some return on investment [18]. Ximelagatran, on the other hand, was in the very late stages of development when its fate was sealed. In fact, AstraZeneca had already applied at the EMEA for marketing approval when the company withdrew all applications due to concerns over the hepatotoxic potential of the drug [24]. Although this drug did reach the market in France, the U.S. FDA was not prepared to grant approval and the drug was never marketed in the U.S. [25]. Ximelagatran, which was the first orally available thrombin inhibitor that would have replaced the troublesome warfarin as an oral anticoagulant, serves as a good example where huge investments were made to get the drug to market, but a return on investment was never realised. This example emphasizes the necessity for improved methodologies to predict intrinsic hepatotoxicity more accurately during the initial phases of the drug development process.

Alpidem	Ebrotidine	Troglitazone
Bendazac	Fipexide	Temafloxacin
Benoxaprofen	Iproniazid	Tolcapone
Bromfenac	Nevazodone	Tolrestat
Clormezanone	Pemoline	Trovafloxacin
Dilevalol	Perhexilene	Ximelagatran

Table 1. Drugs that have been withdrawn from international marketplaces between 1995 and 2005 due to associated hepatotoxicity.

Examples of other drugs that were never marketed in the U.S. because of hepatotoxicity include drugs such as ibufenac, perhexilene and dilevalol. There are also drugs for which the use / application has been limited because of possible DILI. These include the drugs isoniazid, pemoline, tolcapone and trovafloxacin [15]. A big question that remains a challenge for regulatory authorities is how rare or mild does hepatotoxicity have to be for a drug to be approved and to remain on the market? [13] Undoubtedly, DILI has a sizeable influence on drug development output. Pre- and post-marketing attrition as a result of DILI causes further financial stresses for those in the industry. Limiting attrition to the early phases of drug development can only be beneficial. Both the pharmaceutical industry and regulatory authorities agree that there is a great need for improved methodologies and strategies to accurately assess the hepatotoxic potential of compounds, earlier in the drug development process [13,26].

3. Safety pharmacology and current practices used to detect hepatotoxicity

Distinct from pharmacology proper, which examines the desired effects and kinetics of a particular drug, safety pharmacology identifies and characterises secondary adverse pharmacological and toxicological effects of potential drugs, mainly through the use of established animal models [27]. Regulatory authorities require that certain minimal safety pharmacology examinations be completed before a new investigation drug application will be approved. These international regulatory guidelines were compiled by the International Committee for Harmonization (ICH) in the documentation covering topic S7. The ICH S7A and ICH S7B guidelines have been in effect since 2000 and 2001, respectively [27].

At present, the attention of pre-clinical safety pharmacology investigations is drawn to three physiological systems: the cardiovascular system, the respiratory system and the central nervous system (for compounds that may cross the blood-brain barrier). Effects on the cardiovascular system are of great concern because 1) it is a system often found to be affected and 2) due to its redundancy (organisms relevant to drug development have only one heart). Like the heart, the respiratory system is of concern because it is essential to the immediate survival of the organism.

Hepatic safety does not form part of the core battery of pre-clinical tests performed for initial safety pharmacology. The EMEA have published draft guidance on the non-clinical assessment of hepatotoxic potential [28]. This draft amounted to a clinical white paper [29], however, no regulations are set in place yet. This initial draft may demonstrate the future intent of regulatory authorities. If this is the case, not only is it worthwhile for the pharmaceutical companies to consider improved pre-clinical evaluation of hepatotoxic potential for their own profit, but it may soon be required as part of their investigational drug applications before first-in-human trials.

Currently, *in vivo* screening for hepatotoxicity during both the pre-clinical animal testing and clinical phases of the development process forms the basis of hepatic safety testing. However, from an extensive study on available literature, Biowisdom, a healthcare intelligence company, estimates that between 38% and 51% of compounds showing liver effects in humans do not present similar effects in animal studies including both rodents and non-rodents [30]. The mainstay clinical chemistry can be used to detect certain types of hepatic injury. For example, the aminotransferases, alanine aminotransferase (ALT) and aspartate aminotransferase (AST), can be used to identify hepatocellular injury, whereas levels of bilirubin and alkaline phosphatase can be used to assess hepatobiliary health [28,31]. Of the two aminotransferases ALT is by and large superior at predicting hepatocellular injury for two reasons: 1) ALT is a more sensitive signal than AST because it is found in higher concentrations in the cytosol of hepatocytes and 2) ALT is also more specific to the liver than AST as AST is normally also present in the blood, skeletal muscle and heart [32]. The ratio of ALT/AST has been found useful to differentiate, to some degree, between different types of liver injury. An ALT/AST ratio >2:1 may be indicative of an alcoholic type liver injury, whereas a ration of 1:1 could point to non-alcoholic steatohepatitis a.k.a. NASH [33]. Logistic regression analysis on 784 reports of DILI received by the Swedish Adverse Drug Reaction Advisory Committee between 1970 and 2004 found that, in combination, an AST/ALT ratio > 1 and bilirubin > 2 × upper limit of normal (ULN) had a higher positive predictive value than either AST in combination with bilirubin or ALT in combination with bilirubin [34]. The "Rezulin rule" was coined to describe the fact that the more marked any ALT elevations and the frequency of such elevations during clinical trials, the more significant post-approval hepatotoxicity appears to become [35]. Rezulin was the marketing name of troglitazone.

Elevations of > 3 × ULN are considered a sensitive signal of a potential hepatotoxic test compound. Data from 28 clinical trials (phases II - IV) conducted by GlaxoSmithKline between 1995 and 2005 found elevations in ALT of > 3 × ULN at baseline to be rare, with a prevalence of 6.265% [36]. A study of Merck clinical trial databases, reported that elevations of ALT or AST > 3 × ULN had an 83% sensitivity to detect serious liver disease [Senior, 2003]. ALT > 3 × ULN has proved a useful threshold for screening for clinically significant DILI from various hepatotoxic substances. This includes drugs that have been withdrawn from the market due to hepatotoxicity, such as troglitazone and bromfenac [15]. However, this is not a very specific signal as increases in aminotransferase levels can also be induced by drugs that do not cause DILI such as aspirin, statins and heparin [17]. Indeed, the Merck study showed that the predictive power of elevations of ALT or AST > 3 × ULN, was only 11% [37]. A separate manuscript also reported high sensitivity and specificity when using ALT > 3 × ULN, but again with very low predictive power (only 6%) [38]. Serum ALT or AST levels are therefore a sensitive screen for possible hepatotoxic side-effects, but not definitive enough to terminate a drug development program.

Even though it was originally not intended as such, the most successful predictor of hepatotoxicity is "Hy's law", which is based on the original observations made by Dr. Hyman Zimmerman. It was described by Dr. Zimmerman as "clinical jaundice" and its modern application has proved valuable in being able to predict idiosyncratic hepatotoxicities brought about by drugs / potential drugs such as troglitazone and dilevalol. A more recent description is a state of drug-induced jaundice caused by hepatocellular injury, without any significant obstructive component [17,35]. Therefore, Hy's Law is met when:

1. There exists the possibility that a drug (or potential drug) can induce hepatocellular damage as evident from elevations in serum aminotransferase levels of ≥ 3 × ULN and

2. These elevations are accompanied by elevations in total bilirubin of ≥ 2 × ULN with no evidence of intra- or extra-hepatic obstruction (elevated ALP) or Gilbert's syndrome.

It is worth noting that Dr. Zimmerman himself placed some weight on the degree of jaundice as it often served to predict a negative outcome [35]. Hy's Law is, however, not exclusive to DILI and if it is met, it is of utmost importance that any other condition(s) that may also cause these symptoms be excluded before any conclusions are drawn about a potential intrinsic hepatotoxin. Such conditions may include viral hepatitis, hypotension or congestive heart failure [17]. Obviously, the possibility of DILI caused by concomitant drugs should also be excluded.

The incidence of idiosyncratic DILI is generally 1 per 10 000 or less. This makes it exceptionally difficult to detect idiosyncratic hepatotoxicity due to an investigational drug during clinical testing, even if several thousands of subjects are studied [39]. Generally, an investigational drug does not get administered to more than 2000 subjects [33], which makes it unlikely to detect a single incidence in 10 000. Although it portrays the role of the key predictor of the hepatotoxic potential of an investigational drug during drug development, Hy's Law falls short of constituting a "gold standard"' and validation of Hy's Law is much needed, chiefly with regards to its sensitivity and specificity [35]. Moreover, for the purposes of detecting potential intrinsic hepatotoxins as early as possible during drug development, the foremost drawback of Hy's law is that it requires *in vivo* testing of the investigational drug. Hy's Law is therefore not a realistic approach for traditional *in vitro* testing, the type of testing that can be applied prior to vast resources being invested into *in vivo* testing.

4. Methodologies applicable to the early pre-clinical assessment of potential intrinsic hepatotoxicity

The ultimate goal of research into this field is to establish an *in vitro* model or tier of *in vitro* tests that is valid and able to accurately predict DILI during lead optimisation before any hepatotoxic chemical entity under development unnecessarily progresses into *in vivo* studies. Currently, this is still desired as more than 90% of candidate drugs that enter the clinical phases of drug development still fail to complete development due to inadequate safety, pharmacokinetics or efficacy [40]. The following sections will focus mainly on *in vitro* methods as these can be conducted at the lowest expense and at higher throughput than conventional animal studies.

4.1. Cell-based models

4.1.1. Cell cultures

Cell-based models are increasingly used as there is a growing pressure to reduce, refine and replace the use of animals from organisations such as the European Centre for the Validation of Alternative Methods (ECVAM). The three basic types of cells used for *in vitro* toxicity testing are transformed cell lines, primary cells and pluripotent cells. The latter will be discussed in more detail later in the manuscript. The advantages of using transformed cell lines include unlimited supply, no genetic variation, which aids reproducibility and predictive power of an outcome, as well as access to the collective knowledge gained from global research conducted on the geno- and phenotype of the cell line in question. The HepG2 cell line, was one of 20 cell lines of human origin that was used in one of the first international attempts to try and predict *in vivo* toxicity through *in vitro* techniques during the Multicentre Evaluation of *In Vitro* Cytotoxicity (MEIC) program, initiated by the Scandanavian Society of Cell Toxicology in 1989. The program was based on two main assumptions: 1) there exists some "basal cytotoxicity" that can be quantified, and 2) *in vitro* methods can be used to model some type of "general toxicity", which is related to the *basal cytotoxicity* concept [41]. *Basal cytotoxicity* was defined as "the toxicity of a chemical to basic cellular functions and structures, common to all human cells". Although the study lacked some systemic focus, results from the MEIC study conducted on 50 reference chemicals, demonstrated that *in vitro* cytotoxicity assays were able to predict lethal human blood concentrations just as well as rodent LD_{50} values were able to [42].

The use of immortalized human hepatocytes cell lines, like HepG2 cells, were proposed to overcome limitations of primary human hepatocytes including the scarce availability of fresh human liver samples, complicated isolation procedures, short life-span, inter-donor variability, and cost. HepG2 cells display morphological features similar to that of liver parenchymal cells and maintain many functions of *in vivo* hepatocytes, expressing receptors for insulin, transferrin, epidermal growth factor and low density lipoprotein [43]. These cells also express a plethora of cellular products (www.atcc.org). The HepG2 cell line has been used extensively in research as a model to study cytotoxicity [41], liver lipid metabolism [44], mitochondrial homeostasis [45,46], oxidative stress [46], gluconeogenesis and glucose uptake [47], to mention just a few. The applications are very broad and there is a vast collective knowledge about how these cells behave and respond under specified conditions or when exposed to various stressors. This must be one of the greatest advantages when using these cells, especially in mechanistic studies. However, it is believed that observations made with these cells cannot be extrapolated to humans as they do not behave as native hepatocytes would because of discrepancies in drug biotranformation [48]. HepG2 cells are known to express low levels of cytochrome P450 (CYP) enzymes compared to primary hepatocytes [49,50].

The chief advantage that primary cell cultures have over most perpetual cell lines is that they are the closest *in vitro* representation of the *in vivo* cell type under scrutiny. Hence, primary hepatocytes are considered the "gold standard" used for predictive toxicology [51]. Unlike transformed cell lines, primary cultures have a limited growth and life-span and fresh stock needs to be sourced regularly. This is problematic in itself as human hepatocytes are scarce and availability sporadic [52]. Another drawback of using primary cultures is the occurrence of donor-to-donor variability that is introduced into the results, which will decrease the power of predicting a specific outcome. Although primary hepatocytes initially express higher levels of metabolic enzymes than transformed cell lines like HepG2 cells [49], in culture their liver-specific function decrease over time [52].

Two techniques have received attention over the years to try and improve the life-span of primary hepatocytes in culture. These are sandwich culturing techniques and special medium formulations. Sandwich culturing techniques address the conformational / spatial discrepancies between the 2D *in vitro* and 3D *in vivo* microenvironments. Hepatocytes are seeded on top of a layer of either collagen I or matrigel, which mimics *in vivo* extracellular matrix. An additional overlay of extracellular matrix is then layered on top of the seeded hepatocytes [51,53]. Additives to medium formulations attempt to imitate endogenous signalling found in the *in vivo* milieu. Serum and corticosteroids are known to affect cultured hepatocyte morphology. Contradictory to the general thought that adding serum to medium is good for cells, adding serum to medium that is used for culturing primary hepatocytes will cause the cells to rapidly deteriorate and lose cytoplasmic integrity and bile canaliculi-like structures. The corticosteroid, dexamethasone, has also proven helpful in improving primary hepatocyte life-span when in culture [51]. Culturing primary hepatocytes in a sandwich conformation with extracellular matrix, no serum and dexamethasone allows the conservation of liver-specific functionality for several weeks [51].

The problems of low levels of enzyme expression in HepG2 cells and limited life-span of primary hepatocytes was overcome with the emergence of the HepaRG cell line. These cells express higher levels of CYP's than HepG2 cells and respond acutely to induction of these enzymes [50]. HepaRG cells maintain hepatic functions of primary hepatocytes and express normal levels of liver-specific genes while lacking the inter-donor variability observed with primary hepatocytes [50,54]. A lot of literature praises HepaRG for the increased metabolic activity, which allows the *in vitro* study of drug metabolism using a theoretically unlimited supply of cells. This is certainly a remarkable advancement for *in vitro* drug metabolism and pharmacokinetic (DMPK) studies. However, this is a fairly new cell line (first described in 2002 [55]) and the accrued collective knowledge of this cell line is dwarfed by that of the HepG2 cell line. A recent study compared the whole genome expression profiles of HepG2, HepaRG (differentiated and undifferentiated) and primary human hepatocytes to that of human liver tissues [56]. It was found that in terms of correlation with human liver tissues, the cell cultures ranked: primary human hepatocytes > HepaRG > HepG2, which boasts well for the future of the HepaRG cell line for use in predictive toxicology.

4.1.2. Outcomes and detection methods

Researchers at Pfizer postulate that the poor predictive power of conventional cytotoxicity assays is related to the endpoint being measured [57]. Cytotoxicity endpoint assays only assess the final extreme from a series of pathological events that lead to cellular death. Assays that target such late events are likely to fail in detecting more subtle types of toxicity that develop after chronic, low-dose exposure to manifest as non-lethal, but definite adverse, complications [46]. In addition to this, the liver is the only organ in mammals that can fully regenerate after injury [58], making testing for adaptive changes even more relevant and applicable. An example of this scenario of subtle toxicity can be found in troglitazone, which exerts sub-acute hepatotoxicity by acting on a sub-cellular level, disrupting mitochondrial homeostasis. The mechanism of toxicity of troglitazone was investigated by means of *in vitro* models [45,59,60], which emphasizes the role that cell-based test systems can play during early drug development. It is substantially easier to utilize cell-based *in vitro* models to examine sub-cellular events, compared to higher levels of biological organization i.e. whole organisms. Cells are the first level of organization where all the lifeless constituents that comprise a cell, functions together as an entity, and the first level where disrupted interplay between sub-cellular components can be evaluated. Cell-based models are more than suitable for the task at hand, but what is being evaluated using these models is critical to the success of such attempts. Rather than cell death / survival endpoints, some adaptive / pre-lethal mechanistic endpoints that can be considered include mitochondrial homeostasis [45,46,61,62], generation of reactive oxygen species (ROS) [46], lipid peroxidation [62], Ca^{2+} signalling [62] and inhibition of enzymes and transporters [63], especially bile acid transporters [63] (Figure 3).

An important tool that was used in the MEIC study, and remains relevant to current methodologies, is that of mathematical modelling. In the MEIC study, researchers employed partial least squares regression [42]. Mathematical modelling provides a way in which researchers can combine data from different endpoint assays, thereby allowing them to piece together underlying associations and correlations observed when drugs (or groups of drugs) affect normal cellular function. Previous research illustrated how mathematical modelling of multiparametric data can aid prediction [64]. Seventeen compounds (7 known hepatotoxins and 10 "unknowns") were subjected to testing using 6 separate endpoint assays monitored with a fluorescent plate reader. The data was then used to develop 5 prediction models. Modelling techniques included logistic regression, support vector machines (using several different kernel functions), decision tree, quadratic discriminant analysis and neural networks. Discriminant analysis was found to yield the best positive and negative predictive values [64]. In addition, the study highlighted the significance of adequate sample size and careful consideration and defining of positive and negative test values in the training data set. It is important to realise that the task of predicting DILI from *in vitro* studies does not only depend on the parameters that are measured but also on how the acquired data is reduced and utilised to reach the critical "go" / "no-go" decision.

http://dx.doi.org/10.5772/54792

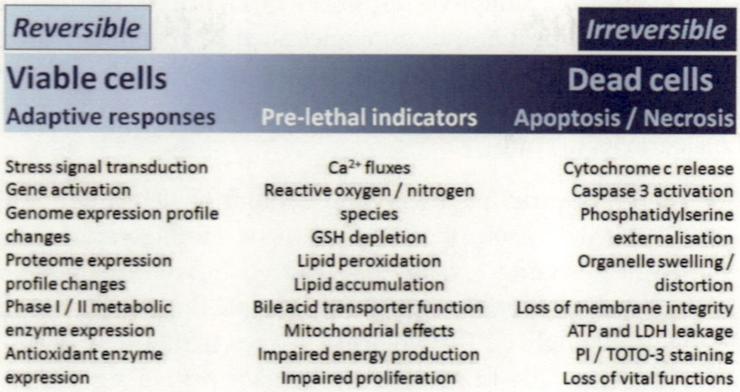

Figure 3. Sequenced outcomes that can be considered for endpoint assays in pre-clinical *in vitro* assays. Endpoint assays examining adaptive and pre-lethal outcomes can be detected early in the progression towards cellular death and detect subtle types of toxicity, which late stage endpoint assays fail to do.

As with the study by Flynn and Ferguson [64], high content screening (HCS), which is based on automated microscopy, also employs fluorescent probes. HCS is one cell-based methodology that has shown promising results in predicting DILI. This methodology has three key strengths: 1) the ability to simultaneously examine multiple parameters of cellular function, 2) all parameters can be examined in individual cells, and 3) it has the potential for high-throughput screening since it is based on a microplate format. Combined, these features culminate in powerful technology. Testing more than 240 drugs using an HCS platform, researchers at Pfizer demonstrated that this methodology had overall sensitivity and specificity of 90% and 98%, respectively, for predicting *in vivo* hepatotoxicity [46]. When employing the HCS platform the sensitivity of predicting severely hepatotoxic drugs was 100%, and 80% for moderately hepatotoxic drugs. This is a noteworthy improvement over the conventional cytotoxicity assays that showed scores of 20% and 24% for the same predictions [46]. The authors again stressed the value of chronic, sub-lethal exposure conditions to allow cellular phenomena to manifest. Recently, a similar study on 61 hepatotoxic and 12 non-hepatotoxic drugs / compounds examined the same parameters (nuclear morphology, plasma membrane integrity, mitochondrial membrane potential, and Ca^{2+} fluxes) with the added parameter of lipid peroxidation, where scores of >90% for both sensitivity and specificity were reported [62].

Another fluorescence detection method that has a potential role in early pre-clinical assessment of intrinsic hepatotoxicity is flow cytometry. Essentially, this method of detection can analyse the same parameters as fluorometry and fluorescence microscopy. It has not been explored in as much detail as HCS, but initial reports are positive [65]. There is room for research comparing these different methods of detection and the verdict is still out on which platform outperforms the rest.

4.2. Profiling technologies

Virtually all responses to toxic insults are accompanied by differential gene expression [66]. Differential gene expression is likely to be accompanied by differential transcription and differential protein expression (adaptive responses in Figure 3). On this conceptual basis, researchers have tried to use profiling technologies such as genomics / transcriptomics and proteomics to discern between compounds that may or may not induce liver injury and even between subsets of chemical entities that cause different types of hepatotoxicity like necrosis, steatosis and cholestasis [67].

The sensitivity of genomics experiments is high enough to detect subtle changes in gene expression profiles. For this reason, it is argued to be more sensitive than conventional methodologies aimed at detecting toxicity [68]. Indeed this was demonstrated in rats exposed to sub-toxic doses of acetaminophen, where subtle changes in gene expression profile were observed although no histological changes manifested [69]. This boasts well for toxicogenomics as being able to identify the most sensitive signals of potential hepatotoxicity. The authors did however emphasise the weight of demarcating toxic events, sub-toxic / adverse events, and adaptive responses as this will have great influence on the outcomes of toxicogenomic studies. The ability to detect responses at a molecular level that are not necessarily revealed at phenotypic level makes it possible to address questions about linearity of the dose-response curve at low exposure levels and allows for more accurate determination of inflection points along to dose-response curve and threshold exposure levels [68]. These determinants can play pivotal roles in safety pharmacology when selecting dosages for clinical studies. Regarding the predictive power of genomics, Zhang *et al.* [70] were able to achieve 83% accuracy in predicting human DILI using data obtained from rats. Rats that met Hy's law were found to express a gene expression signature, which led to an 83% accuracy [70]. Unfortunately, toxicogenomics using cell cultures and toxicogenomics using rodents do not correlate as well as one would hope. Following acetaminophen exposure, *in vitro* toxicogenomics using primary hepatocytes yielded results comparable to that of *in vivo* toxicogenomics regarding acute cellular toxicity. However, *in vivo* toxicogenomics revealed genetic expression changes due to an inflammatory response, which *in vitro* toxicogenomics failed to detect [71]. This unearths the stubborn dilemma of inter-dependent physiological systems within an organism, which is very difficult to recreate experimentally.

Unlike the genome, the proteome is a dynamic entity that changes as gene activation and epigenetic factors alter protein expression due to endogenous and exogenous signals and factors. Studying the proteome allows the surveillance of current cellular events, which can only be deduced from genomics data. This is probably the greatest disadvantage of toxicogenomics compared to toxicoproteomics; there are many splice variants, post-translational modifications and subcellular localizations of the final products originating from genes [72,73] implying that some degree of extrapolation is necessary when predicting cellular events from genomics data. When studying the proteome, differential expression such as this can be detected and this may in fact form part of the solution, rather than part of the problem.

Studying the proteome provides a direct description of cellular functions [74]. Thus far, toxicoproteomic attempts to predict DILI have demonstrated limited efficacy when performed *in vitro* [75]. Toxicoproteomics performed on *in vitro* cultures have the key advantage that biologically significant alterations can be monitored without relying on whole animals [76].

Exposing HepG2 cells to three model hepatotoxins that are known to cause necrotic, steatotic or cholestatic liver injury, researchers were only able to distinguish cholestatic injury from untreated controls [75]. The study failed to successfully discern necrotic and steatotic events, however, the ability to detect adverse cholestatic events in HepG2 cells is noteworthy, as these cells are not known to form biliary structures in a monolayer but rather present as parenchymal cells [43]. This implies that morphological studies would not have been able to detect this event and further suggests that native morphological features may not be required in order to detect / predict certain types of toxicity when utilising *in vitro* proteomic approaches.

Perhaps a more integrated approach would eventually prove more fruitful. Researchers conducted a study in which they characterised methapyrilene-induced hepatotoxicity in rats employing three profiling technologies simultaneously: genomics, proteomics and metabolomics [77]. The report demonstrated the possibility and great value of these technologies when used in an integrative manner, where responses to the toxic insult could be followed from genetic expression changes, to protein up- / down-regulation, through to changes in the metabolite profile, which gave a very good indication of where and how the chemical entity may exert its biochemical action(s). Conducting this type of study on a substantial number of compounds, both hepatotoxic and not, will yield a vast amount of data on how hepatocytes react toward challenges with different types of chemical entities and provide insight into which responses should raise concern and which are harmless. It may also deliver further understanding of the mechanisms by which hepatocyte injury occurs.

One major drawback of all the profiling technologies is that most of the current research has been carried out *in vivo*, which is predominantly unwanted in the drug development scenario. The ultimate goal of predictive toxicology would be to develop techniques that can be used *in vitro*. However, it should also be noted that it is highly unlikely that animal studies will be avoided altogether, at least not for the foreseeable future, which leaves room for *in vivo* profiling technologies as adjuvants to conventional safety pharmacology testing. In fact, it may help justify the use of animals for safety pharmacology testing. It is not impossible to employ these technologies using *in vitro* platforms, but more research is necessary to develop and establish effective methodologies and biomarkers.

4.3. Emerging technologies

The main reason for a lack of *in vitro* predictive power is the difference in phenotype between perpetual hepatocyte monolayers and native *in vivo* hepatocytes. The traditional approach to circumvent this problem was the use of primary hepatocytes, which are considered to be the "gold standard" for *in vitro* hepatotoxicity studies. Two emerging technologies that may offer alternative solutions are hepatocytes differentiated from stem cells and 3D culturing techniques.

4.3.1. Stem cell technologies

As all physiological processes take place in a cellular setting, the highest quality of cells should be used to determine safety and efficacy. This led to the use of stem cells. Stem cells are classified as embryonic or adult, which is distinguished by developmental status. Where adult stem cells are multipotent (yield the cell type from the tissue from which they originate), embryonic stem cells are pluripotent (can give rise to differentiated cell lineages of all three germ layers). Stem cells that originate from embryos have a normal diploid karyotype and do not exhibit donor-dependent variability. The advantage of these cells compared to primary cells are that they can be maintained in culture for a longer period of time and can be grown up in large scale, producing high volumes.

The implementation of murine embryonic cells to predictably identify human developmental toxins, allowing for early identification of toxicity or candidate compounds in the discovery pipeline was initiated by ECVAM. Mouse hepatocyte-like cells, which were established from embryonic stem cells were the first to be used in hepatotoxicity models. The efficacy of cell differentiation and maturation was improved, where the cells generated alpha fetoprotein and albumin [78]. Cell characteristics included: 70% expressed the phenotypical marker albumin, they metabolized ammonia, lidocaine and diazepamat nearly two-thirds the rate of primary mouse hepatocytes. However, the difference in metabolism between humans and mice is considerable leading to interspecies extrapolation problems. Subsequently hepatocyte-like cells were differentiated from hESC [79]. These cells contained liver-related characteristics such as; expression of α-fetoprotein, production of albumin, hepatocyte nuclear factor 4α and induction of CYP450 enzymes, stored glycogen and showed uptake of idocyanine green. This was followed by more differentiated hepatocyte-like cells which additionally express functional glutathione transferase activity at levels comparable to human hepatocytes [80].

The advantages of stem cells in relation to transformed/tumour or primary cells are that the former possesses normal growth, genetic transformation and genetic composition as well as uniform physiology and pharmacology [81]. Since stem/progenitor cells can differentiate into clinically relevant cell types, but still maintain functional similarities to their *in vivo* counterparts, they allow for safer drugs to be introduced into clinical trials and the market place. Other advantages of stem cells include; the availability of cell types which were not previously available and the ability to investigate cellular renewal, regeneration, expansion as well as differentiation [82]. Stem cells can also be genetically modified using reporter gene construct, thereby providing specific disease models [83].

As with all technologies, there are still hurdles to overcome with stem cell technology. Many clinically relevant cell types cannot be efficiently differentiated, purified and isolated [82]. Human stem cells that reproducibly deliver hepatocytes with predictive pharmacology results for high-throughput safety screens are limited. Although progress has been made in the differentiation protocols, scaling cell growth and plating for cell-based assays, as well as refining of these protocols in order to ensure homogeneous preparations will continue. Currently, panels of human embryonic stem cells which reflect the wide variation in the population are not available.

Although these hurdles exist, stem cells hold the potential for investigation into metabolic competence, biotransformation capacity and transformation of exogenous compounds. Also, the ability to determine human inter-individual differences due to genetic polymorphisms.

4.3.2. 3D culturing techniques

Although 2D techniques have the advantages of being relatively inexpensive, reproducible, robust and convenient, they have the chief disadvantage of loss of much of the functionality of native hepatocytes [84], which raises the question of the relevance of such a model in predicting DILI. Three-dimensional culturing of hepatocytes is an attempt to imitate an *in vivo* environment in order to obtain more innate hepatocyte-like cells, thus producing a more relevant model to study hepatotoxicity whilst using an *in vitro* platform.

The sandwich configuration of 3D culturing is frequently used when propagating primary hepatocytes as it has been shown that maintaining these cells in this configuration prolongs their *in vitro* life-span by promoting cellular junctions, cell-cell and cell-matrix interactions, and maintaining differentiation [85-87]. After seeding a sandwich culture of primary hepatocytes, the cells require a recuperation period of > 40 h. During this period a number of morphological changes occurs as the hepatocytes acclimatise to their new environment, one of which is the formation of bile canaliculi [63,88]. The latter highlights a particular role that 3D culturing techniques may play in predicting cholestatic type DILI. Cholestatic DILI has been problematic to detect or predict using *in vitro* systems because most cell lines do not produce the native biliary structures when propagated in monolayer configuration. HepaRG cells, differentiated using dimethyl sulphoxide and glucocorticosteroids, have been reported to form biliary-like structures when grown in 2D format [52]. Building on the work of Liu *et al.* [89], Ansede *et al.* [63] demonstrated that it is possible to determine whether drugs may induce cholestasis using primary rat hepatocytes in the sandwich culture configuration. Deuterated taurocholic acid was used, which is easily discernable from endogenous sodium taurocholate using liquid chromatography/tandem mass spectrometry, to monitor bile acid transport. The effect of Ca^{2+} on hepatocyte tight junction integrity was exploited in order to discern between hepatic uptake and efflux of deuterated taurocholic acid. Using this approach the researchers were able to determine total and intracellular bile acid accumulation, biliary excretion index and *in vitro* biliary clearance.

A manuscript that unmistakeably illustrates the important role that 3D culturing techniques can play in drug development is Lee *et al.* [90]. Using sandwich-cultured rat primary hepatocytes, the authors were able to elucidate the hepatoprotective effect of dexamethasone on tabectedin-induced hepatotoxicity. At the time of the study, trabectedin was a promising new antineoplastic agent showing activity against various cancers at nanomolar concentrations and which had already reached phase II clinical trials, but was found to have dose-limiting hepatotoxic side-effects. The report highlights the fact that experiments using primary rat hepatocytes cultured in a monolayer configuration were unable to replicate the known hepatoprotective effect of dexamethasone against trabectedin-induced toxicity. The reason for this was the lack of hepatobiliary functionality of the hepatocytes in monolayer configuration, and explains why the sandwich configuration was able to show that dexamethasone protected hepatocytes by restoring normal hepatobiliary function. This demonstrates that 3D culturing techniques hold the key to predicting different subtypes of DILI such as hepatocellular necrosis and cholestatic injury. Whether or not similar experiments would prove successful when using HepaRG cells is still to be determined.

It is difficult for nutrients to reach, and for waste products to be removed from hepatocytes in a traditional sandwich configuration because the cells are entrapped in a thick extracellular matrix. The perfusion sandwich culture [91] and entrapment between ultra-thin porous silicon membranes technologies [92] were developed to surmount these complications. In addition to maintaining hepatobiliary function, both these methods claim added predictive capabilities for DILI as demonstrated through increased sensitivity to acetaminophen toxicity due to preserved metabolic enzyme functionality. Still, even with these improved methods, the life-span of these primary hepatocytes remains limited, which restricts the use of such methods on a large scale.

Other 3D culturing methods are mainly based on bio-artificial liver bioreactors that are aimed at developing extracorporeal liver support systems for patients with acute liver failure. In the past, such bioreactors were based on adult hepatocytes and proved unsuccessful because the hepatocytes failed to proliferate [93]. The latest of these that are being explored for its use in drug toxicity testing is the four-compartment perfusion model. Cells are contained in one of the four compartments, the remaining three compartments comprises three independent but interwoven artificial capillary bundles that form the capillary bed in which the cells are housed. Cells are derived from hESCs and currently research is being carried out to obtain the optimal protocol for differentiating these cells into mature hepatocytes that closely resemble innate hepatocytes. This research project is headed by the EU Vitrocellomics project [94].

Anchorage-free 3D culturing methods result in the formation of small hepatocyte aggregates known as spheroids. There are different ways to induce the formation of spheroids including continuously-stirred bioreactors [94], the rocked suspension technique [95] and rotating wall bioreactors [96]. Initial experimentation demonstrated that, between spheroids and monolayers, there was indeed differential toxicity induced by 7 day methotrexate exposure. It was thought that this was due to preservation of hepatocyte functionality, but could also have been due to lack of the test compound to penetrate the spheroidal structure [97]. More than a decade later it is well known that liver-specific functions like albumin and urea synthesis and metabolic activities are maintained for prolonged periods of up to 21 days [94]. In time, spheroids deposit an extracellular matrix consisting of laminin, fribronectin and collagen, which encapsulates each individual spheroid. These structures also preserve histotypical cytarchitechture, intercellular contacts (gap junctions) and biliary canaliculi [98]. Moreover, when hepatocytes grown under these conditions are encapsulated in alginate polymers, albumin and urea synthesis doubles and phase I and II metabolic activities are also elevated. This may be attributed to the bulk added to the extracellular matrix, provided by the alginate polymers, which protects the hepatocytes from shear stresses under hydrodynamical conditions [94]. A setback of this technique is the difficulty of obtaining spheroids that are of a specific mean diameter (100 μm) and batches of spheroids that are all similar in size. This is necessary as necrotic cell death may occur at the centre of spheroids if the diameter of these

http://dx.doi.org/10.5772/54792

aggregates exceeds approximately 300 μm. The reason for this is lack of oxygen perfusion to cells located in the central region of spheroids that are too large in size [99].

Recently researchers attempted to predict hepatotoxicity employing hepatocyte spheroids developed from an immortalised cell line, a HepG2 derivative (C3A), instead of primary hepatocytes [96]. The study emphasizes the value of proper dosing during toxicity testing. In the study spheroids were not exposed to a set concentration of drug in the culture medium for individual experiments. Rather, the concentration of drug in the culture medium was adjusted with each experiment to mimic *in vivo* dosing practices where the amount of drug was altered according to the amount of protein present in the bioreactor i.e. dosages were reported as mg drug / mg protein. Using this approach the researchers were able to obtain more accurate predictions of lethal human blood concentrations compared to conventional 2D culturing techniques.

5. Future directions

It would be fair to say that 2D culturing techniques have predominated since the inception of research on artificially cultured cells and as such numerous ways have been developed to analyse cells in the 2D format. Amongst others, this is one of the key advantages that 2D culturing techniques have over 3D culturing techniques, demonstrated by the multiple parameters that can be simultaneously assessed using HCS. Currently, this is not possible when using 3D cultures as all cells are not in the same pane and cannot be examined individually. On the other hand, the relevance of 2D culture models is questionable when compared to 3D models that more closely resemble their native counterparts. Various reports have shown that 3D culturing methods are superior to 2D cultures in detecting or predicting certain types of DILI, especially cholestatic injury as 2D models do not express the necessary morphology to study this. Profiling technologies may be able to breach the chasm between 2D and 3D culture models because it is applicable to both scenarios and have been shown to distinguish cholestatic hepatotoxins even when applied to 2D cultures.

The proteome represents current events on a cellular level and 3D cultures are better depictions of innate hepatocytes. Therefore, proteomic investigations that are based on 3D cultures, dosed using *in vivo* practices (mg drug/ mg protein), and are similar in size to the large DILI prediction studies that have been conducted on 2D cultures may prove exceedingly valuable in providing researchers with a set of protein biomarkers that can successfully predict DILI in humans. A substantial amount of research is necessary into this field of interest.

What is missing from current literature is the assessment of 3D cultures to express / secrete biomarkers that are currently used in the clinical setting, i.e. ALT, AST, ALP and bilirubin, and how these respond following challenge with various drugs. Research into this area may uncover possible accurate extrapolations that can be validated for use in predicting DILI. For instance, it is possible that 3D cultures secrete sufficient quantities of ALT and bilirubin to be measured in the surrounding culture medium. Maybe these markers will fluctuate in a way similar to what would occur in the *in vivo* setting and it may therefore be possible to assess the criteria for, and apply, Hy's law on an *in vivo*-like *in vitro* system.

The *in vitro* technologies necessary to shift the detection and prediction of candidate drugs that may cause DILI from the clinical phases of drug development to the early pre-clinical phase, is available at present. There are various types of *in vitro* technologies available and each has its own unique advantages and disadvantages. For this reason, different approaches may be able to identify and predict certain types of DILI better than others and *vice versa*. Therefore, an integrated approach based on multiple models may be a step in the right direction if an *in vitro* platform is desired. Cultures of hepatocyte spheroids may be convenient in this scenario. At the end of an experiment, individual spheroids from the same bioreactor can be examined using different technologies (some can be used for profiling, others for microscopic evaluation, and still others for fluorescent analyses following digestion), which would make the results truly comparable in that all the spheroids would be subjected to the exact same conditions.

Work is necessary to incorporate the available methods into a standard set of tests, comprising of different tiers, which generate data that can be interpreted as a whole, to aid the critical 'go' / 'no-go' decision (the earlier, the better). Such a set of experiments will greatly improve lead prioritization before astronomical amounts of funds are invested into a particular potential drug. In the long run this will increase the productivity of the entire drug development process by alleviating some of the financial pressures and improving time-scales from drug discovery to marketing as less time is spent on candidates that will eventually fail in the clinical phases. Finally, it should aid regulatory authorities in granting approval and provide safer drugs for consumers.

Abbreviations

European Centre for the Validation of Alternative Methods (ECVAM); Drug metabolism and pharmacokinetic (DMPK); Drug-induced liver injury (DILI); High content screening (HCS); International Committee for Harmonization (ICH); Multicentre evaluation of *in vitro* cytotoxicity program (MEIC); Non-steroidal anti-inflammatory drugs (NSAIDs); Pharmaceutical Research and Manufacturers of America (PhRMA); Research and development (R&D);

Author details

Jacob John van Tonder[1], Vanessa Steenkamp[1] and Mary Gulumian[2,3]

1 Department of Pharmacology, Faculty of Health Sciences, University of Pretoria, Pretoria, South Africa

2 Toxicology and Biochemistry Section, National Institute for Occupational Health, Johannesburg, South Africa

http://dx.doi.org/10.5772/54792

3 Department of Haematology and Molecular Medicine, Faculty of Health Sciences, University of the Witwatersrand, Johannesburg, South Africa

References

[1] Castellani JJ. Problems and possibilities in the pharmaceutical industry. Vital Speeches of the Day 2011 September; 77(9): 324-327.

[2] Castellani JJ. Pharmaceutical industry critics: How dare they? Vital Speeches of the Day 2012 June; 78(6): 175-178.

[3] Curtis MJ, Pugsley MK. Attrition in the drug discovery process: lessoms to be learned from the safety pharmacology paradigm. Expert Review of Clinical Pharmacology 2012; 5(3): 237-240. DOI: 10.1586/ecp.12.22

[4] DiMasi JA, Hansen RW, Grabowski HG. The price of innovation: new estimates of drug development costs. Journal of Health Economics 2003; 22: 151-185.

[5] DiMasi JA. Cost of innovation in the pharmaceutical industry. Journal of Health Economics 1991; 10: 107-142.

[6] Paul SM, Mytelka DS, Dunwiddie CT, Persinger CC, Munos BH, Lindborg SR, *et al*. How to improve R&D productivity: The pharmaceutical industry's grand challenge. Nature Reviews Drug Discovery 2010; 9: 203-214.

[7] LaFerla FM. Preclinical success against Alzheimer's disease with an old drug. The New England Journal of Medicine 2012; 367: 570-572.

[8] Herper M. Strategies: The truly staggering cost of inventing new drugs. 2012 http://www.forbes.com/forbes/2012/0312/strategies-pharmaceuticals-lilly-stagger-cost-inventing-new-drugs.html (accessed 15 August 2012).

[9] DiMasi JA. The value of improving the productivity of the drug development process: Faster times and Better decisions. Pharmacoeconomics 2002; 20(Suppl 3): 1-10.

[10] Valentin J-P, Hammond T. Safety and secondary pharmacology: Successes, threats, challenges and opportunities. Journal of Pharmacological and Toxicological Methods 2008; 58: 77-87. DOI: 10.1016/j.vascn.2008.05.007

[11] Park BK, Kitteringham NR, Powell H, Pirmohamed M. Advances in molecular toxicology - towards understanding idiosyncratic drug toxicity. Toxicology 2000; 153: 39-60.

[12] Ostapowicz G, Fontana RJ, SchiødFV, Larson A, Davern TJ, Han SH, *et al*. Results of a prospective study of acute liver failure at 17 tertiary care centres in the United States. Annals of Internal Medicine 2002; 137: 947-954.

[13] Spilker B. Impact of hepatotoxicity on the pharmaceutical industry. FDA-PhRMA-AALSD Conference, Virginia, February 2001. http://www.fda.gov/Drugs/ScienceResearch/ResearchAreas/ucm091365.htm (accessed on 22 August 2012).

[14] Need AC, Motulsky AG, Goldstein DB. Priorities and standards in pharmacogenetic research. Nature Genetics 2005; 37(7): 671-681.

[15] CDER-PhRMA-AASLD Conference 2000. Clinical White Paper. November 2000. http://www.fda.gov/downloads/Drugs/ScienceResearch/ResearchAreas/ucm091457.pdf (accessed 17 August 2012).

[16] Temple R. Drug induced liver injury: A national and global problem. FDA-PhRMA-AALSD Conference, Virginia, February 2001. http://www.fda.gov/Drugs/ScienceResearch/ResearchAreas/ucm091365.htm (accessed on 22 August 2012).

[17] Temple R. Hy's law: predicting serious hepatotoxicity. Pharmacoepidemiology and Drug Safety 2006; 15: 241-243.

[18] Faich GA, Moseley RH. Troglitazone (Rezulin) and hepatic injury. Pharmacoepidemiology and Drug Safety 2001; 10: 537-547. DOI: 10.1002/pds.652

[19] Moses PL, Schroeder B, Alkhatib O, Ferrentino N, Suppan T, Lidofsky SD. Severe hepatotoxicity associated with bromfenac sodium. The American Journal of Gastroenterology 1999; 94(5): 1393-1396.

[20] Purcell P, Henry D, Melville G. Diclofenac hepatitis. Gut 1991; 32(11): 1381-1385.

[21] Bulsterli UA. Diclofenac-induced liver injury: a paradigm of idiosyncratic drug toxicity. Toxicology and Applied Pharmacology 2003; 192(3): 307-322. DOI: 10.1016/S0041-008X(03)00368-5

[22] Lapeyre-Mestre M, Rueda de Castro AM, Bareille M-P, Garcia Del Poza J,Alvarez Requejo A, Arias LM, *et al.* Non-steroidal anti-inflammatory drug-related hepatic damage in France and Spain: Analysis from national spontaneous reporting systems. Fundamemtal and Clinical Pharmacology 2006; 20(4): 391-395.

[23] Muñiz AE, Rose SR, Liner SR, Foster RL. Unsuspected acetaminophen toxicity in a 58-day-old infant. Pediatric Emergency Care 2004; 20(12): 824-828.

[24] European Medicines Agency. Press release: AstraZeneca withdraws its application for Ximelagatran 36-mg film-coated tablets. 2006. http://www.ema.europa.eu/docs/en_GB/document_library/Press_release/2010/02/WC500074073.pdf (accessed on 21 August 2012).

[25] Vaughan C. Ximelagatran (Exanta): an alternative to warfarin? BUMC Proceedings 2005; 18: 76-80.

[26] Hughes B. Industry concern over EU hepatotoxicity guidance. Nature Reviews Drug Discovery 2008; 7: 719. DOI: 10.1038/nrd2677

[27] Kinter LB, Valentin J-P. Safety pharmacology and risk assessment. Fundamental and Clinical Pharmacology 2002; 16: 175-182.

[28] European Medicines Agency. Non-clinical guideline on drug-induced hepatotoxicity. 2008 http://www.emea.europa.eu/docs/en_GB/document_library/Scientific_guideline/2009/09/WC500003355.pdf (accessed 16 August 2012).

[29] European Medicine Agency. Reflection paper on the non-clinical ecvaluation of drug-induced liver injury (DILI). 2010 http://www.ema.europa.eu/docs/en_GB/document_library/Scientific_guideline/2010/07/WC500094591.pdf (accessed on 20 August 2012).

[30] Spanhaak S, Cook D, Barnes J, Reynolds J. Species concordance for liver injury: From the Safety Intelligence Program Board. 2008. http://www.biowisdom.com/downloads/SIP_Board_Species_Concordance.pdf (accessed 21 August 2012).

[31] KaplowitzN. Drug-induced liver injury. Clinical Infectious Diseases 2004; 38(Suppl 2): S44-S48.

[32] Green RM, Flamm S. AGA technical review on the evaluation of liver chemistry tests. Gastroenterology 2002; 123: 1367-1384.

[33] Hunt CM, Papay JI, Edwards RI, Theodore D, Alpers DH, Dollery C, *et al.* Monitoring liver safety in drug development: The GSK experience. Regulatory Toxicology and Pharmacology 2007; 49: 90-100.

[34] Björsson E, Olsson R. Outcome and prognostic markers in severe drug-induced liver disease. Hepatology 2005; 42(2): 481-489.

[35] Lewis JH. 'Hy's law,' the 'Rezulin Rule,' and other predictors of severe drug-induced hepatotoxicity: putting risk-benefit into perspective. Pharmacoepidemiology and Drug Safety 2006; 15(4): 221-229.

[36] Weil JG, Bains C, Linke A, Clark DW, Stirnadel HA, Hunt CM. Background incidence of liver chemistry abnormalities in a clinical trial population without underlying liver disease. Regulatory Toxicology and Pharmacology 2008; 52: 85-88. DOI: 10.1016/j.yrtph.2008.06.001

[37] Senior JR. Serum transaminase elevations alone lack specificity for detecting rare serious liver disease. Hepatology 2003; 38(Suppl 1): 701A.

[38] Senior JR. Monitoring for hepatotoxicity: What is the predictive value of liver "function" tests? Clinical Pharmacology and Therapeutics 2009; 85(3): 331-334. DOI: 10.1038/clpt.2008.262

[39] U.S. Food and Drug Administration. Guidance for industry. Drug-induced liver injury: Premarketing clinical evaluation. July 2009. http://www.fda.gov/downloads/Drugs/.../Guidances/UCM174090.pdf (accessed 16 August 2012).

[40] Kola I, Landis J. Can the pharmaceutical industry reduce attrition rates? Nature Reviews drug Discovery 2004; 3: 711-716.

[41] Bondesson I, Ekwall B, Hellberg S, Romert L, Stenberg K, Walum E. MEIC - A new international multicenter project to evaluate the relevance to human toxicity of in vitro cytotoxicity tests. Cell Biology and Toxicology 1989; 5: 331-347.

[42] Ekwall B, Barile FA, Castano A, Clemedson C, Clothier RH, Dierickx P, *et al*. MEIC evaluation of acute systemic toxicity: Part IV. The prediction of human toxicity by rodent LD50 values and results from 61 in vitro methods. Alternatives to Laboratory Animals 1998; 26(Suppl 2): 617-658.

[43] Iwasa F, Galbraith RA, Sassa S. Effects of dimethyl sulphoxide on the synthesis of plasma proteins in the human hepatoma HepG2. Biochemical Journal 1988; 253: 927-930.

[44] Gebhardt R. Inhibition of cholesterol biosynthesis in HepG2 cells by artichoke extracts is reinforced by glucosidase pretreatment. Phytotherapy Research 2002; 16(4): 368-372.

[45] Tirmenstein MA, Hu CX, Gales TL, Maleeff BE, Narayanan PK, Kurali E, *et al*. Effects of troglitazone on HepG2 viability and mitochondrial function. Toxicological Sciences 2002; 69(1): 131-138. DOI: 10.1093/toxsci/69.1.131

[46] O'Brien PJ, Irwin W, Diaz D, Howard-Cofield E, Kresja CM, Slaughter MR, *et al*. High concordance of drug-induced human hepatotoxicity with in vitro cytotoxicity measured in a novel cell-based model using high content screening. Archives of Toxicology 2006; 80: 580-604. DOI: 10.1007/s00204-006-0091-3

[47] Yamashita R, Saito T, Satoh S, Aoki K, Kaburagi Y, Sekihara H. Effects of dehydroepiandrosterone on gluconeogenic enzymes and glucose uptake in human hepatoma cell line, HepG2. Endocrine Journal 2005; 52(6): 727-733.

[48] Anene-Nzelu C, Wang Y, Yu H, Liang LH. Liver tissue model for drug toxicity screening. Journal of Mechanics in Medicine and Biology 2011; 11(2): 369-390.

[49] Westerink WMA, Schoonen WGEJ. Cytochrome P450 enzyme levels in HepG2 cells and cryopreserved primary human hepatocytes and their induction in HepG2 cells. Toxicology In Vitro 2007; 21: 1581-1591.

[50] Gerets HHJ, Tilmant K, Gerin B, Chanteux H, Depelchin BO, Dhalliun S, *et al*. Characterization of primary human hepatocytes, HepG2 cells, and HepaRG cells at the mRNA level and CYP activity in response to inducers and their predictivity for the detection of human hepatotoxins. Cell Biology and Toxicology 2012; 28: 69-87.

[51] Hewitt NJ, Gómez-Lechón MJ, Houston JB, Hallifax D, Brown HS, Maurel P, *et al*. Primary hepatocytes: Current understanding of the regulation of metabolic enzymes and transporter proteins, and pharmaceutical practice for the use of hepatocytes in metabolism, enzyme induction, transporter, clearance, and hepatotoxicity studies. Drug Metabolism Reviews 2007; 39: 159-234.

[52] Giullouzu A, Corlu A, Aninat C, Glaise D, Morel F, Guguen-Guilouzu C. The human hepatoma HepaRG cells: A highly differentiated model for studies of liver metabolism

and toxicity of xenobiotics. Chemico-Biological Interactions 2007; 168: 66-73. DOI: 10.1016/j.cbi.2006.12.003

[53] Richert L, Binda D, Hamilton G, Viollon-Abadie C, Alexandre E, Bigot-Lasserre D, *et al*. Evaluation of the effect of culture configuration on morphology, survival time, antioxidant status and metabolic capacities of cultured rat hepatocytes. Toxicology in Vitro 2002; 16(1): 89-99.

[54] Anthérieu S, Chesné C, Li R, Camus S, Lahoz A, Picazo L, *et al*. Stable expression, activity and inducibility of cytochromes P450 in differentiated HepaRG cells. Drug Metabolism and Disposition 2010; 38: 516-525.

[55] Gripon P, Rumin S, Urban S, Le Seyec J, Glaise D, Cannie I, *et al*. Infection of a human hepatoma cell line by hepatitis B virus. Proceedings of the National Academy of Sciences 2002; 26: 15655-15660.

[56] Hart SN, Li Y, Nakamoto K, Subileau E, Steen D, Zhong X. A comparison of whole genome gene expression profiles of HepaRG and HepG2 cells to primary human hepatocytes and human liver tissues. Drug Metabolism and Disposition 2010; 38: 988-994.

[57] Xu JJ, Diaz D, O'Brien P. Applications of cytotoxicity assays and pre-lethal mechanistic assays for assessment of human hepatotoxicity potential. Chemico-Biological Interactions 2004; 150: 115-128.

[58] Beyer TA, Xu W, Teupser D, auf dem Keller U, Bugnon P, Hildt E, *et al*. Impaired liver regeneration in Nrf2 knockout mice: role of ROS-mediated insulin/IGF-1 resistance. EMBO Journal 2008; 27: 212-223.

[59] Bova MP, Tam D, McMahon G, Mattson MN. Troglitazone produces a rapid drop of mitochondrial membrane potential in liver HepG2 cells. Toxicology Letters 2005; 155(1): 41-50. DOI: 10.1016/j.toxlet.2004.08.009

[60] Masubuchi Y, Kano S, Horie T. Mitochondrial permeability transition as a potential determinant of hepatotoxicity of antidiabetic thiazolidinediones. Toxicology 2006; 222(3): 233-239. DOI: 10.1016/j.tox.2006.02.017

[61] Labbe G, Pessayre D, Fromenty B. Drug-induced liver injury through mitochondrial dysfunction: Mechanisms and detection during preclinical safety studies. Fundamental and Clinical Pharmacology 2008; 22: 335-353.

[62] Tolosa L, Pinto S, Monato MT, Lahoz A, Castell JV, O'Connor JE, *et al*. Development of a multiparametric cell-based protocol to screen and classify the hepatotoxicity potential of drugs. Toxicological Sciences 2012; 127(1): 187-198.

[63] Ansede JH, Smith WR, Perry CH, St. Claire III RL, Brouwer KR. An in vitro assay to assess transporter-based cholestatic hepatotoxicity using sandwich-cultured rat hepatocytes. Drug Metabolism and Disposition 2010; 38: 276-280.

[64] Flynn TJ, Ferguson MS. Multiendpoint mechanistic profiling of hepatotoxicants in HepG2/C3A human hepatoma cells and novel statistical approaches for development

of a prediction model for acute hepatotoxicity. Toxicology in Vitro 2008; 22(6): 1618-1631.

[65] Zanese M, Suter L, Roth A, De GiorgiF, Ichas F. High-throughput flow cytometry for predicting drug-induced hepatotoxicity. In: Clinical Flow Cytometry - Emerging Applications. InTech 2012 ISBN 978-953-51-0575-6.

[66] Nuwaysir EF, Bittner M, Trent J, Barrett JC, Afshari CA. Microarrays and toxicology: The advent of toxicogenomics. Molecular Carcinogenesis 1999; 24: 153-159.

[67] Van Summeren A, Renes J, Bouwman FG, Noben J-P, van Delft JHM, Kleinjans JCS, *et al*. Proteomics investigations of drug-induced hepatotoxicity in HepG2 cells. Toxicological Sciences 2011; 120(1): 109-122.

[68] Daston GP. Gene expression, dose-response, and phenotypic anchoring: Applications for toxicogenomics in risk assessment. Toxicological Sciences 2008; 105(2): 233-234.

[69] Heinloth AN, Irwin RD, Boorman GA, Nettesheim P, Fannin RD, Sieber SO, *et al*. Gene expression profiling of rat livers reveals indicators of potential adverse effects. Toxicological Sciences 2004; 80: 193-202.

[70] Zhang M, Chen M, Tong W. Is toxicogenomics a more reliable and sensitive biomarker than conventional indicators from rats to predict drug-induced liver injury in humans. Chemical Research in Toxicology 2012; 25: 122-129.

[71] Tachibana S, Shimomura A, Inadera H. Toxicity monitoring with primary cultured hepatocytes underestimates the acetaminophen-induced inflammatory responses of the mouse liver. Tohoku Journal of Experimental Medicine 2011; 225: 263-272.

[72] Brunet S, Thibault P, Gagnon E, Kearney P, Bergeron JJ, Desjardins M. Organelle proteomics: Looking at less to see more. Trends in Cell Biology 2003; 13: 629-638. DOI: 10.1016/j.tcb.2003.10.006

[73] Wetmore BA, Merrick BA. Toxicoproteomics: Proteomics applied to toxicology and pathology. Toxicologic Pathology 2004; 32: 619-642.

[74] Tyers M, Mann M. From genomics to proteomics. Nature 2003; 422: 193-197.

[75] Van Summeren A, Renes J, van Delft JHM, Kleinjans JCS, Mariman ECM. Proteomics in the search for mechanisms and biomarkers of drug-induced hepatotoxicity. Toxicology in Vitro 2012; 26: 373-385. DOI: 10.1016/j.tiv.2012.01.012

[76] Amacher DE. The discovery and development of proteomic safety biomarkers for the detection of drug-induced liver toxicity. Toxicology and Applied Pharmacology 2010; 245: 134-142. DOI: 10.1016/j.taap.2010.02.011

[77] Craig A, Sidaway J, Holmes E, Orton T, Jackson D, Rowlinson R, *et al*. Systems toxicology: Integrated genomic, proteomic and metabonomic analysis of methapyrilene induced hepatotoxicity in the rat. Journal of Proteome Research 2006; 5: 1586-1601.

[78] Gouon-Evans V, Boussemart L, Gadue P, Nierhoff D, Koehler CI, Kubo A, *et al*. BMP-4 is required for hepatic specification of mouse embryonic stem cell–derived definitive endoderm. Nature Biotechnology 2006; 24: 1402-1411.

[79] Hay DC, Zhao D, Ross A, Mandalam R, Lebkowski J, Cui W. Direct differentiation of human embryonic stem cells to hepatocyte-like cells exhibiting functional activities. Cloning Stem Cells 2007; 9: 51-62.

[80] Söderdahl T, Küppers-Munther B, Heins N, Edsbagge J, Björquist P, Cotgreave I, *et al*. Glutathione transferases in hepatocyte-like cells derived from human embryonic stem cells. Toicology in Vitro 2007; 21: 929-937.

[81] McNeish J. Embryonic stem cells in drug discovery. Nature Reviews Drug Discovery 2004; 3: 70-80.

[82] McNeish JD. Stem cells as screening tools in drug discovery. Current Opinion in Pharmacology 2007; 7: 515-520.

[83] Friedeich Ben-Nun I, Benvenisty N. Human embryonic stem cells as a cellular model for human disorders. Molecular and Cellular Endocrinology 2006; 252: 154-159.

[84] Meng Q. Three-dimensional culture of hepatocytes for prediction of drug-induced hepatotoxicity. Expert Opinion on Drug Metabolism and Toxicology 2010; 6(6): 733-746.

[85] Dunn JC, Tompkins RG, Yarmush ML. Long-term in vitro function of adult hepatocytes in a collagen sandwich configuration.Biotechnology Progress 1991; 7: 237-245.

[86] Tuschl G, Mueller SO. Effects of cell culture conditions on primary rat hepatocyte cell morphology and differential gene expression. Toxicology 2006; 218: 205-215.

[87] Dash A, Inman W, Hoffmaster K, Sevidal S, Kelly J, Obach RS, *et al*. Liver tissue engineering in the evaluation of drug safety. Expert Opinion on Drug Metabolism and Toxicology 2009; 5(10): 1159-1174.

[88] Mathijs K, Kienhuis AS, Brauers KJ, Jennen DG, Lahoz A, Kleinjans JC, *et al*. Assessing the metabolic competence of sandwich-cultured mouse primary hepatocytes. Drug Metabolism and Disposition 2009; 37: 1305-1311.

[89] Liu X, Lecluyse EL, Brouwer KR, Lightfoot RM, Lee JI, Brouwer KLR. Use of Ca^{2+} modulation to evaluate biliary excretion in sandwich-cultured rat hepatocytes. Journal of Pharmacology and Experimental Therapeutics 1999; 289: 1592-1599.

[90] Lee JK, Leslie EM, Zamek-Gliszczynski MJ, Brouwer KLR. Modulation of trabectedin (ET-743) hepatobiliary dispositionby miltudrug resistance-associated proteins (Mrps) may prevent hepatotoxicity. Toxicology and Applied Pharmacology 2008; 228(1): 17-23.

[91] Xia L, Ng S, Han R, Tuo X, Xiao G, Leo HL, *et al*. Laminar-flow immediate-overlay hepatocyte sandwich perfusion system for drug hepatotoxicity testing. Biomaterials 2009; 30(30): 5927-5936.

[92] Zhang S, Xia L, Kan CH, Xiao G, Ong SM, Toh YC, *et al.* Microfabricated silicon nitride membranes for hepatocyte sandwich culture. Biomaterials 2008; 29(29): 3993-4002.

[93] Monga SPS, Hout MS, Baun MJ, Micsenyi A, Muller P, Tummalapalli L, *et al.* Mouse fetal liver cells in artificial capillary beds in three-dimensional four-compartment bioreactors. The American Journal of Pathology 2005; 167(5): 1279-1292.

[94] Mandenius C-F, Andersson TB, Alves PM, Batzl-Hartmann C, Bjorquist P, Carrondo MJT, *et al.* Toward preclinical predictive drug testing for metabolism and hepatotoxicity by using *in vitro* models derived from human embryonic stem cells and human cell lines - A report on the Vitrocellomics EU-project. Alternatives to Laboratory Animals 2011; 39: 147-171.

[95] Luebke-Wheeler JL, Nedredal G, Yee L, Amiot BP, Nyberg SL. E-Cadherin protects primary hepatocyte spheroids from cell death by a caspase-independent mechanism. Cell Transplantation 2009; 18: 1281-1287.

[96] Fey SJ, Wrzesinski K. Determination of drug toxicity using 3D spheroids constructed from an immortal human hepatocyte cell line. Toxicological Sciences 2012; 127(2): 403-411.

[97] Walker TM, Rhodes PC, Westmoreland C. The differential cytotoxicity of methotrexate in rat hepatocyte monolayer and spheroid cultures. Toxicology in Vitro 2000; 14: 475-485.

[98] LeCluyse EL, Witek RP, Andersen ME, Powers MJ. Organotypic liver culture models: Meeting current challenges in toxicity testing. Critical Reviews in Toxicology 2012; 42(6): 501-548.

[99] Glicklis R, Merchuk JC, Cohen S. Modeling mass transfer in hepatocyte spheroids via cell viability, spheroid size and hepatocellular functions. Biotechnology and Bioengineering 2004; 86(6): 672-680.

Chapter 2

The Kidney Vero-E6 Cell Line: A Suitable Model to Study the Toxicity of Microcystins

Carina Menezes, Elisabete Valério and Elsa Dias

Additional information is available at the end of the chapter

http://dx.doi.org/10.5772/54463

1. Introduction

Microcystins (MCs) are toxins produced by cyanobacteria from water environments that can induce acute and chronic effects on humans and animals, after ingestion/contact with contaminated water [1]. This group of cyclic heptapeptides comprises approximately 80 variants, being microcystin-LR (MCLR) the most frequent and toxic variant [1]. MCs are mainly known for their hepatotoxicity due to their inhibitory activity of serine/threonine phosphatases PP1 and PP2A [2]. This inhibition interferes with hepatocyte homeostasis and structure, leading to the collapse of liver tissue organization, liver necrosis and hemorrhage (Figure 1), which can culminate, in severe cases, in the death of the intoxicated individuals [3, 4].

It has been reported that microcystins cross cell membranes through the transmembrane solute carriers transport family OAPT (Organic Anion Polypeptide Transporters), in particular the OATP1B1, OATP1B2, OATP1B3 and OATP1A2 [7, 8]. They are responsible for the sodium-independent uptake of large amphipathic endogenous and exogenous organic anions into cells and across the blood-brain barrier [9, 10]. The knowledge on the mechanism(s) of OATP-mediated transport is still scarce [9] however, the available information suggests that, in a general way, OATPs act as organic anion exchangers [11], functioning in a rocker-switch type of mechanism and translocating the substrate through a central positively charged pore [9].

Some OATPs are expressed ubiquitously, whereas others are expressed in a tissue-specific way [10]. In fact, the organotropism of MC is due to the selective uptake of microcystins by the OATPs that are primarily expressed in liver [8], such as those mentioned above. For this reason, the study of the toxicological properties of microcystins has been conducted mainly in liver cells *in vivo* and cultured hepatic cells *in vitro*. However, OATP expression in other organs has also been reported, like the case of OATP1A2 in the kidneys [7, 8, 10, 12] and an increasing number of studies have been showing that MCLR can indeed induce nephrotoxicity [13, 14, 15]. In fact, although MCLR is mostly accumulated in the liver and excreted by biliary route, a fraction of the toxin (9%) is filtrated in the kidneys and eliminated through the urine [16], which makes the kidneys a potential target for MCLR toxicity. In figure 2 is depicted the toxicokinetics of microcystins.

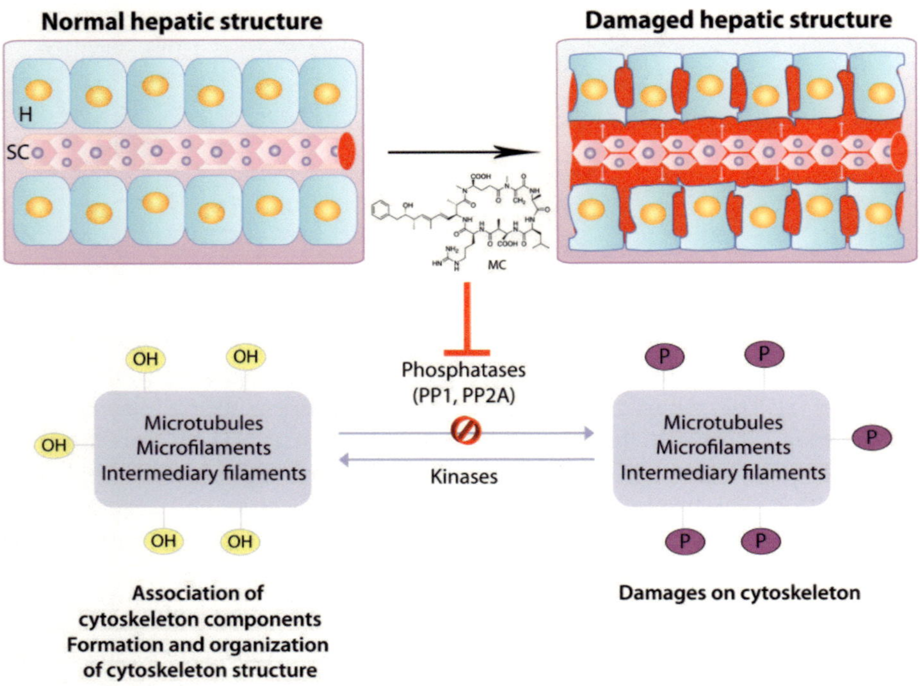

Figure 1. Representation of the effects of microcystins in cytoskeleton, namely the changes of the hepatocytes and sinusoidal capillary structure, and intrahepatic bleeding, mediated by the inhibition of protein phosphatases PP1 and PP2A (partially adapted from [5] and [6]). Legend: **H** – hepatocyte; **SC** – Sinusoidal capillary; **MC** – microcystins; **OH** – hydroxyl group; **P** – phosphate group; **PP1** – protein phosphatase 1; **PP2** – protein phosphatase 2.

Established cell lines have been considered, for a long time, as unsuitable to study the toxic effects of MCs. This was due to the observation that, comparing with primary cell lines, high amounts of MCs were required to elicit toxicity in permanent cell lines [17, 18, 19]. A proposed explanation was the fact that established cell lines lose their OATPs, which render them unable to uptake the toxin [19, 20]. Despite this fact, an increasing number of studies have demonstrated that MCs clearly induce toxic effects on several mammalian cell lines, in particular in the human hepatoma HepG2 cell line [21-24]. Indeed, it was already demonstrated that OATP transport system is preserved in the HepG2 cells [25].

http://dx.doi.org/10.5772/54463

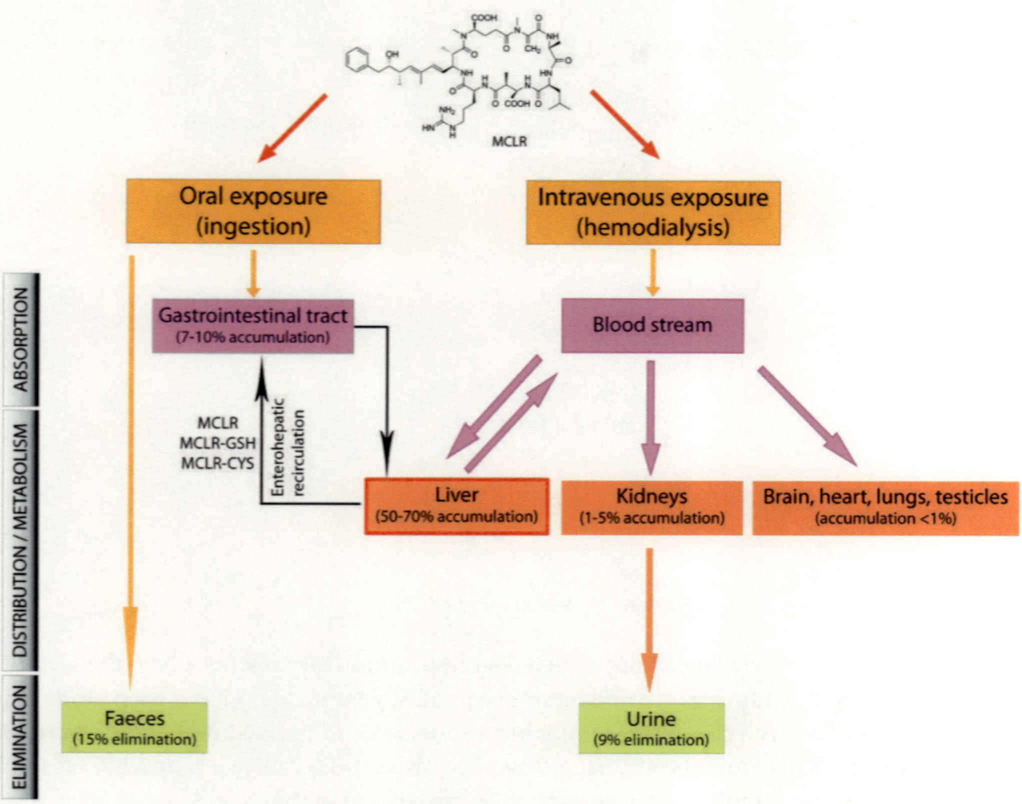

Figure 2. Schematic representation of MCLR absorption, distribution, metabolization and excretion (ADME) processes. Legend: **MCLR** – microcystin-LR; **MCLR-GSH** – microcystin-LR conjugated with glutathione; **MCLR-CYS** – microcystin-LR conjugated with cysteine.

When we started our work on MCLR toxicity in mammalian cell lines we evaluated the effects of *Microcystis aeruginosa* extracts containing MCLR in the cell viability of AML12 (*Mus musculus* hepatocytes, ATCC-CRL 2254), HepG2 (human hepatoma, ATCC-CRL 10741) and Vero-E6 (african green monkey *Cercopithecus aethiops* kidney epithelial cells, ATCC-CRL 1586) cell lines. Surprisingly, we observed that the dose-response curve of cell viability decrease induced by MCLR was quite similar in Vero-E6 and in liver-derived cell lines [26]. Since then, we have been demonstrated that MCLR induces a multiplicity of effects on Vero cells within a wide range of concentrations [26-30], according to a dose-effect relationship (Figure 3).

To our knowledge no previous study reported the expression of OATPs in Vero cell line, neither if an alternative transport system is involved in the microcystin uptake by kidney cells. The elucidation of this issue would be obviously an important contribution to the knowledge of microcystins toxicokinetics in the kidney and, consequently, an important stimulus to the investigation of microcystins toxicity in the kidneys.

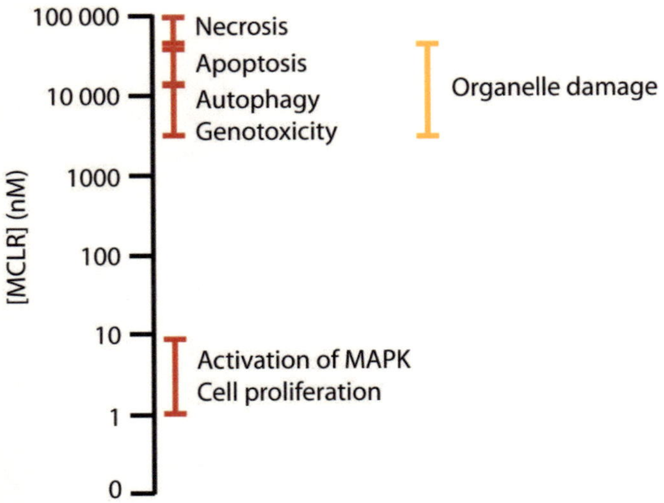

Figure 3. Dose-effect relationship of MCLR on Vero-E6 cell line.

The studies of MCs effects on cell lines often lead to contradictory results, given the fact that distinct MC toxicity endpoints (mainly cytotoxicity and genotoxicity) have been studied in diverse cell lines (and cell clones) under distinct exposure conditions (different doses-ranges, time of exposure, MCs variants, etc). In our work with Vero-E6 cells we tested MCLR (both pure toxin and from cyanobacterial extracts of *M. aeruginosa*) within a wide range of concentrations (1 nM- 200 μM), using several endpoints and methodologies (cytotoxicity, morphology, genotoxicity, protein expression). In this chapter we will summarize our results and discuss the utility of Vero-E6 cell line to evaluate the toxicological properties of MCLR.

2. Effects of MCLR in Vero-E6 cell line

2.1. Cell viability

In our studies with Vero-E6 cell line we have consistently observed that MCLR induces a concentration-dependent decrease of cell viability [26, 27, 29, 30]. This was achieved using distinct cell viability assays (MTT, Neutral Red and LDH release) and distinct toxin sources (commercially available MCLR and *M. aeruginosa* extracts). We observed that the most sensitive methods for cytotoxicity evaluation were MTT and Neutral Red assays [26, 27, 29] and that the response of pure toxin and cyanobacterial extracts was quite similar with cytotoxic thresholds within 22-50 μM of MCLR (Table 1). The MCLR-induced loss of Vero-E6 viability was attributed to apoptosis and necrosis [29, 30] as widely described for various cell types *in vitro* and *in vivo* [18, 31, 32].

http://dx.doi.org/10.5772/54463

2.2. Cellular organelles

In Vero-E6 cell line, exposure to MCLR (within the micromolar concentrations range) affected several cellular organelles in a concentration-dependent form (Table 1, Figure 3). In our articles, we proposed that at lower MCLR concentrations, autophagy is triggered as a survival mechanism of Vero cells, in an attempt to eliminate the toxin or/and the MCLR-induced cellular damages [29, 30]. Also, we reported the vacuolization of the Golgi apparatus and cytoplasm, effects also previously described in MCLR-exposed hepatocytes [17, 18]. The disorganization of the microfilaments and microtubules, which is one of the most commonly described cytotoxic effects of MCLR in hepatic cells [34-36], was also triggered by MCLR in Vero cells [29, 30]. The observation that MCLR induced the destructuring of the endoplasmic reticulum (ER) suggested that this organelle is involved in MCLR toxicity in Vero cell line [29, 30]. The involvement of the ER in MCLR-mediated toxicity was also previously reported in mouse kidney and liver [37]. At higher concentrations, MCLR induced the disruption of the plasma membrane, lysosomes and mitochondria of Vero cells [29, 30]. So far, studies that have used other cell types proposed mitochondria as a major target of MCLR toxicity [38-42]. However, studies with Vero cells show that mitochondria, although involved in MCLR-induced toxicity, may not be the pivotal intracellular target of the toxin [29, 30].

2.3. Genotoxicity

Based on its tumour promoter activity MCLR is classified by the International Agency for Research on Cancer as a potential human carcinogen (class 2B) [43]. In addition, some epidemiologic studies have associated the increase of human hepatocarcinoma [44, 45] and colorectal [46] cancers with the ingestion of water frequently contaminated with microcystins. However it is still unclear if, besides a tumor promoter, MCLR can also act as a tumor initiator. In fact, the potential genotoxicity of MCLR is still a matter of some controversy within the scientific community, with several authors reporting apparently contradictory results.

The hypothesis of MCLR being a genotoxic compound was mainly supported by the evidence that this toxin induces DNA damage in liver cells *in vivo*, in cultured hepatocytes and in some non-liver cell lines (revised in [47]). This data was obtained by the Comet assay, which measures DNA strand breaks that constitute primary DNA lesions with relevance for the formation of gene and chromosome mutations [48]. Several mutagenicity studies excluded the hypothesis of MCLR being a mutagen [49, 50], which was further supported by the fact that MCLR do not form adducts with DNA that would represent a pre-mutagenic lesion [51]. On the other hand, some authors reported that MCLR-induced DNA damage was a consequence of early apoptosis due to oxidative stress and not a real genotoxic effect [52]. This hypothesis was supported by the discovery that MCLR induces the formation of 8-oxo-dG, a marker of oxidative DNA damage in liver cells [51].

Chromosome damage (aneugenesis/clastogenesis) has been suggested for microcystins by an increase of the micronucleus (MN) frequency in mouse erythrocytes [49] and in the human TK6 cell line [53]. However, no effect on the micronucleus frequency has been reported for other cell types [50, 54-56] neither chromosome aberrations have been described so far [54, 57].

Some authors have also proposed that MCLR might interfere with DNA repair processes, namely the repair of gamma radiation and ultra-violet-induced DNA damage [52, 54, 57], thus increasing the genotoxic potency of those agents and contributing to their carcinogenesis.

Effects		Pure MCLR	Cyanobacteria extract w/ MCLR	Methods	References
		Toxin concentration that elicited effect at 24 h (extension of effect)			
Cytotoxicity (cell viability decrease)		25 – 200 μM (52-82%)	22-175 μM (55-58%)	MTT assay	[27]
		–	30 μM - 150 μM (35-67%)	MTT assay	[29]
		–	30 μM - 150 μM (26-79%)	Neutral Red assay	[29]
		50 -100 μM (48-66%)	50 -100 μM (80-82%)	Neutral Red assay	[30]
		200 μM (55%)	88-175 μM (38-29%)	LDH release	[27]
Cellular organelles damages and /or changes	Autophagosome induction	–	5-12 μM	TEM (Immuno)fluorescence microscopy Tunnel assay	[29, 30]
	Endoplasmic reticulum		5-50 μM		
	Cytoskeleton damages		12-50 μM		
	Lysosome rupture		20-50 μM		
	Mitochondria damages				
Apoptosis			20-50 μM (13-27%)		
Necrosis			12-100 μM (10-25%)		
Genotoxicity		Within micromolar range	20 and 40 μM (3.4 and 4.1 fold)	Micronucleus assay	[26, 58]
ERK1/2 activation		5-5000 nM (2.8–4 fold)	5-5000 nM (1.7–3.7 fold)	Western Blot	[28]
Cell proliferation		1– 10 nM (1.5-2.1 fold)	-	BrdU incorporation assay	

Table 1. Effects induced by pure MCLR and toxic *M. aeruginosa* extracts in Vero-E6 cell line: effective toxin concentrations, effect extension and methods used in their evaluation.

In our early studies with the Vero-E6 cell line we demonstrated that cyanobacterial extracts from a MCLR-producer cyanobacterial strain increased the frequency of micronuclei at non-cytotoxic concentrations [26]. Afterwards, we confirmed this observation using pure MCLR [58, submitted for publication]. In this study, we found that MCLR induces the micronucleation of Vero-E6 and human hepatoma HepG2 cell lines. In order to disclose the mechanism underlying micronuclei formation we used the centromere labelling Fluorescent in situ Hybridization technique in HepG2 exposed cells to MCLR (since there are no commercial centomere probes for monkey cells) and we observed that MCLR induced both centromere-positive and centromere-negative micronuclei [58]. Our data, together with those from other works, suggests that MCLR genotoxicity occurs indirectly by both clastogenic and aneugenic mechanisms: the first, possibly through oxidative stress; the second, perhaps through damages on the mitotic spindle, induced by the inhibition of PP1/PP2A. Since clastogenesis and aneugenesis have been associated with human cancer development [59] it can be hypothesized that both underlie the carcinogenic activity of MCLR. Moreover, the confirmation of genotoxic activity of MCLR *in vivo* is of major importance for regulatory purposes because a safe level could not be applied to clastogens conversely to aneugens [59, 60]. This is fundamental for the prevention of the risk of exposure of human populations to water contaminated with toxic cyanobacteria.

In figure 4 we summarize the proposed effects/mechanisms of MCLR genotoxicity, based on the previous reports from other authors and our own contribution.

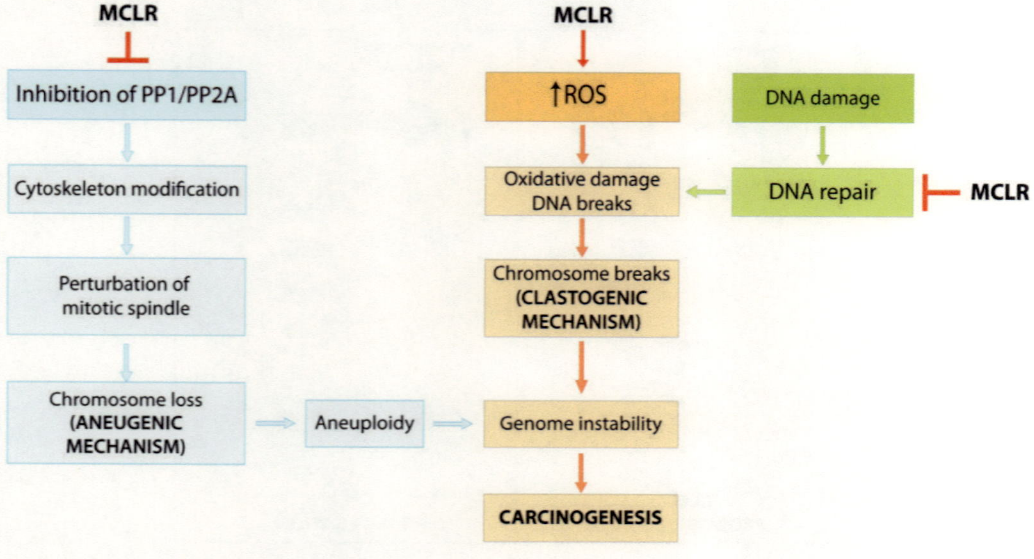

Figure 4. Representation of possible mechanisms of genotoxicity induced by MCLR. Legend: **MCLR** – microcystin-LR; **PP1** – protein phosphatase 1; **PP2** – protein phosphatase 2; **ROS** – reactive oxygen species.

2.4. Cell proliferation

It is generally assumed that MCLR is a potent tumor promoter. This assumption is based on rodent carcinogenicity studies which revealed that MCLR is able to induce cellular transformation of rat liver [61] and mouse skin [62] of animals previously exposed to a genotoxic agent. However, the mechanisms underlying MCLR-induced tumor promotion are still unknown. It has been suggested that this activity is mediated by the inhibition of serine/threonine phosphatase PP1 and PP2A, given their role on the regulation of cellular division and proliferation, namely through the activation of Mitogen-Activated Protein Kinases (MAPK) [63]. MAPKs are involved in signaling pathways that regulate many cellular processes through phosphorylation cascades, in particular the Ras-Raf-MEK1/2-ERK1/2 cascade, with a key role in cellular proliferation and being regulated by several types of phosphatases including the serine/threonine phosphatases PP1 and PP2A [64]. The Ras-Raf-MEK1/2-ERK1/2 cascade is activated by growth factors and mitogenic agents (Figure 5). They bind to tyrosine kinase membrane receptors (RTK), which activate the membrane G-protein GTPase, the recruitment and activation of Raf protein and the subsequent phosphorylation cascade of ERK1/2 pathway [65]. The activated (phosphorylated) forms of ERK1/2 are translocated to the cell nucleus, inducing the activation of transcription factors such as c-Fos and c-Jun thus triggering cell proliferation [64]. The fact that Ras-Raf-MEK-ERK cascade is regulated by several types of phosphatases including the protein serine/threonine phosphatases PP2A [64, 66] supports the hypothesis that, by inhibiting PP2A, MCLR deregulates the ERK1/2 pathway and promotes cell proliferation (Figure 5).

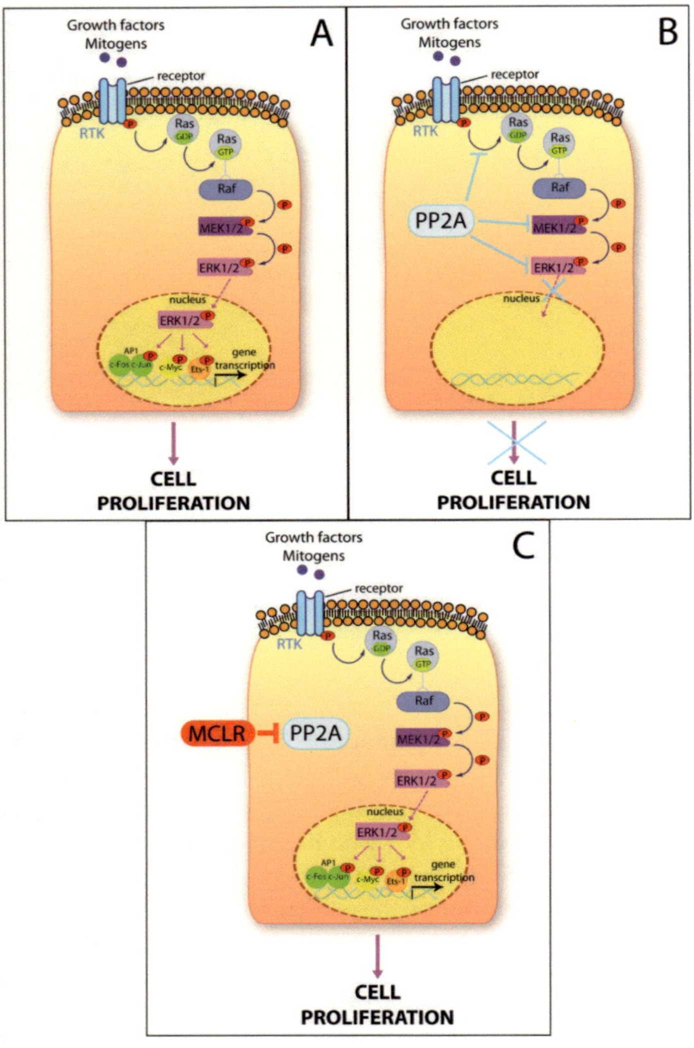

Figure 5. The role of protein phosphatase PP2A in the regulation of the signaling pathway Ras-Raf-MEK1/2-ERK1/2. Partly based on Kolch [67] and Junttila et al [64]. Legend: **RTK** (*tyrosine kinase receptor*); **Ras** (GTPase); **Raf** (*MAP kinase kinase kinase*); **GDP** (guanosine diphosphate); **GTP** (guanosine triphosphate); **P** (phosphate group); **MEK** (*MAP kinase kinase*); **ERK** (*extracellular-signal-regulated kinase*); **AP1** (*activator protein-1*); **c-Fos, c-Jun, c-Myc, ETS-1** (transcription factors); **PP2A** (type 2A protein phosphatase).↓ Activation, ⊥ Inhibition.

http://dx.doi.org/10.5772/54463

Few studies support this hypothesis: (1) Li et al [68] reported the activation of proto-oncogenes c-jun, c-fos and c-myc by a cyanobacterial extract containing microcystins in rat liver, kidney and testis; (2) Zhu et al [69] demonstrated that MCLR induces the transformation of immortalized colorectal crypt cells through the constitutive activation of AKT and MAPK (p38 and JNK) cascades. Our team has evaluated the effect of MCLR in Vero-E6 cell line proliferation through the BrdU incorporation assay that evaluates the G1/S transition in cell cycle [28]. We showed that MCLR (1 to 10 nM) induces a significant increase in Vero cells proliferation with a maximum of 2.2 fold increase at 5 nM [28]. We further analyzed the expression of MAPK (ERK1/2, JNK and p38) by Western-blot and concluded that MCLR stimulates Vero cells proliferation by the activation of the ERK1/2 signaling pathway [28]. These results emphasize the importance to confirm the impact of MCLR on tumor promotion *in vivo*, in particular at kidney level.

3. Comparison of MCLR-induced toxicity in kidney cell lines

The effects of microcystins in kidney cell lines, namely in Vero cells, have been barely evaluated. Thompson et al [70] reported that cyanobacteria extracts containing up to 10 μM of MCLR did not interfere with the morphology and LDH release of Vero cells. Chong et al. [21] also did not found changes in Vero cells viability (evaluated by the MTT assay) after exposure to concentrations up to 37.5 μM of pure MCLR during 24–96 h. Grabow et al. [71] described cytopathogenic effects (rounding and disintegration of cells) of Vero cells induced by *M. aeruginosa* extracts containing 500 μM of MCLR. The results from our studies show a higher sensitivity of Vero-E6 cell line to MCLR than those previously reported data for Vero cells (Table 1).

Additionally, in a previous study we also observed that MCLR induce cytotoxic effects in the Madin-Darbin canine kidney cell line (MDCK – ATCC CCL-34) [72]. However, the sensitivity of this cell line was lower than that of Vero cells. In fact, while significant reduction of Vero cells viability occurs above 25 μM of MCLR (Table 1), only 30% decrease in MDCK cell viability was observed after exposure to 100 μM of MCLR, using the Neutral Red Assay [72].

Effects of MCLR on cell morphology and ultrastructure were previously evaluated in the rat renal epithelial cell line NRK-52E (ATCC-CRL 1571) in studies developed in 1990's decade. Wickstrom et al. [73] found that MCLR affects the cytoskeleton components namely the microtubules, intermediate filaments and microfilaments in a similar way to that observed in hepatocytes. However, the renal cell line required a 100-fold higher concentration (more than 100 μM) and prolonged time of exposure comparing to primary hepatocytes [73]. Reports from Khan et al. [17, 74] also demonstrated the collapse and condensation of cystoskeleton elements induced by MCLR (133 μM) on NRK-52E cell line.

The differences reported in the above mentioned distinct studies might be explained by differences in experimental design, such as the use of toxins from different sources (pure or crude extracts), applied in different dosages and tested by different endpoints of toxicity. Besides, the use of different clones of Vero cells (often not mentioned in the papers) may also justify the distinct sensitivities observed among several authors. Further studies would also be required to conclude if the effects of MCLR on kidney cells could be species-dependent.

Overall, the cytotoxic, morphological and ultrastructural effects of MCLR on Vero-E6 cell line reported by us are quite similar to those reported for other cell lines. However, we observed these effects at lower concentrations, which might suggest an eventual higher sensitivity of Vero-E6 cell line comparing to other kidney cell lines.

4. Is Vero-E6 cell line a suitable model to study toxicological properties of microcystins?

The assessment of kidney injury/dysfunction *in vivo* presents some complexity given the fact that the kidney is constituted by over 20 different cell types exhibiting distinct morphologies and functions and, consequently, diverse responses to toxic compounds [75, 76]. For this reason, *in vitro* models are useful tools to assess specific nephrotoxic effects on specific cell types [75]. Renal epithelial cell lines, in particular, present some advantages: there are several well characterized commercially available clones, they are easy to grow and manipulate and some of them retain basic functions of their original ancestors from kidney *in vivo* [76]. Specific biochemical, morphological and functional markers such as transepithelial resistance and transport, might therefore be used as endpoints of nephrotoxicity *in vitro* [75-77].

Vero-E6 monkey kidney cell line has been widely used on toxicology, virology and pharmacology research, as well as, on the production of vaccines and diagnostic reagents [78]. In particular, these cells have been used as model for assays to evaluate the toxicity of compounds of different nature, either chemical or microbial toxins. The chemical substances tested include carbamazepine [79]; triclosan [80]; lead nitrate [81]; pentachlorophenol and rotenone [82], where the Vero cell line revealed to be one of the most sensitive model used in these studies. These cells have also been validated as a cellular model for other microbial toxins such as diphtheria toxin, a polypeptide with 535 a.a. [83] and Shiga-like toxins, a protein of enterohemorrhagic *Escherichia coli* [84]. The sensitivity of Vero cell line to another cyanobacterial toxin, cylindrospermopsin, was also reported although, such as MCs, the mechanism of toxin uptake by this cell line remains to clarify [85, 86].

In our studies on the effects of MCLR on Vero-E6 cell line we did not evaluate any specific nephrotoxicity marker. Instead, we evaluated the basal toxicity of MCLR, that is, the effects that might be common to all cell types [87].

Using diverse methodologies including standard methods to evaluate cytotoxicity (Neutral Red, MTT and Lactate Dehydrogenase release) and genotoxicity (Micronucleus and Comet assay) we observed that MCLR induces a multiplicity of effects on Vero-E6 cells at distinct levels: cellular morphology/ultrastructure, cell viability/death, MAPK expression and genotoxicity (as referred in section 2). The type and extension of these effects were highly dependent of toxin concentration and, generally, a dose-response relation could be established: for a dose range of 1-10 nM, MCLR stimulates cell proliferation through the activation of the mitogen

http://dx.doi.org/10.5772/54463

activated protein kinase ERK1/2 signalling pathway; however, within the μM range, MCLR triggers a variety of effects in almost all cell compartments, from genotoxicity (induction of micronuclei) and autophagy to apoptotic and necrotic cell death. Therefore, MCLR induces a dual effect on the Vero-E6 cell line: at low doses it stimulates the cell growth but at high doses it induces a decrease in viability and cell death (Figure 6).

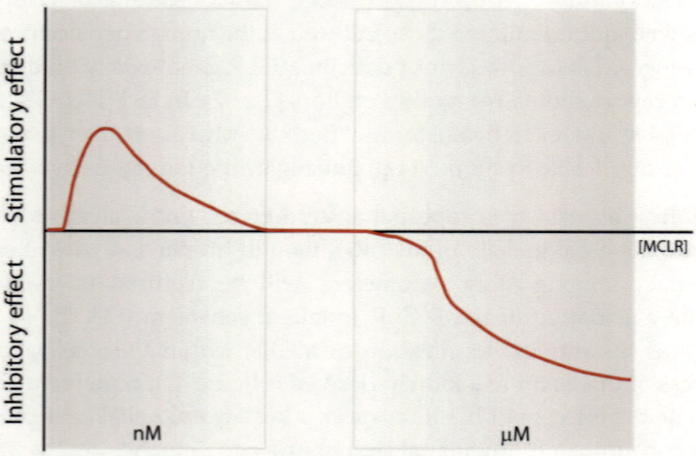

Figure 6. Hormetic dose-response curves of MCLR on the growth of Vero-E6 cells.

This duality of low-dose growth stimulation *vs* high-dose growth inhibition was commented by Li et al [88] as a characteristic hormetic dose-response phenomenon, such as they observed for the low-dose PP2A stimulation *vs* high-dose PP2A inhibition by MCLR. However, additional experiments would be required to support the hypothesis of MCLR exhibiting a hormesis dose-response relation.

Another aspect we would like to underline is that we can attribute with high certainty the observed responses of Vero-E6 cell line to MCLR exposure. The results obtained with toxic cyanobacterial extracts are often questioned due to the uncertainty of cyanobacteria extracts composition and the putative interference between cyanotoxins and other cyanobacterial bioactive compounds [89]. In our studies, we tested two sources of MCLR: cyanobacterial extracts from MCLR-producers (strains of *Microcystis aeruginosa* LMECYA 7, LMECYA 110 and LMECYA 113) [90] and commercially available pure MCLR. We have included in our experiments two types of controls: culture medium when using pure toxin and a cyanobacterial extract from a non toxic *Microcystis aeruginosa* strain (LMECYA 127) when using the toxic cyanobacterial extract. All the strains of *M. aeruginosa* were phylogenetically close related [91] and the ability (or inability) to produce MCLR was previously tested by several analytical methodologies [92]. According to our results on cytotoxicity, genotoxicity and ERK1/2 (MAPK) activation, all toxin solutions induced statistically significant responses in relation to respective controls. Besides, the type and extension of effects were quite similar irrespectively of the toxin source (Table 1) and the results were repeatable after performing independent experiments. In this sense we conclude that the observed effects were induced specifically by MCLR.

Usually it is assumed that high amounts of MCLR are required to elicit any effect on cell lines comparing to primary cells [19]. This is true, but it also depends on the effects that are being evaluated. In fact, cytotoxic MCLR concentrations for Vero cells were found within the range of micromolar (μg/mL). However, the lowest concentration that elicited an effect (cell proliferation) on Vero-E6 cell line was 1 nM (μg/L) [28]. Many of the effects induced by MCLR in Vero-E6 cell line were quite similar to those induced in the human hepatoma cell line (HepG2) at similar dose-ranges. This applies to our data on MCLR genotoxicity on distinct cell models [58] as well as on reported data from other authors [22, 47]. In fact, HepG2 cell line has been considered a suitable model to evaluate the effects of MCLR on liver-derived cells, which similarly might be applicable to Vero-E6 cell line regarding kidney-derived cells.

Considering all these aspects, we propose that Vero-E6 cell line is an appropriate *in vitro* cell model to evaluate the basal toxicity of MCLR, although proper assessment of the specificity, sensitivity, accuracy, among other parameters, will be required to validate this model. Additionally, the elucidation of the MCLR uptake mechanism (OATPs or other transport system), as well as the immunolocalization of MCLR within Vero cells, could be used to confirm the access of this toxin to a kidney-derived cell line. Ultimately, further experiments aiming at evaluate the effects of MCLR on specific kidney epithelial cells properties/nephrotoxic endpoints constitute a fundamental step in order to demonstrate the utility of Vero-E6 cell line as an *in vitro* model to investigate the nephrotoxic mechanisms of MCLR.

5. Concluding remarks

Despite the gaps in knowledge regarding the toxicological properties of microcystins, an increasing number of recent publications emphasize the need to carefully evaluate their effects on other organs besides the liver, particularly their carcinogenicity. The adverse effects of MCLR in distinct organs is an important issue for risk assessment, because the guideline value for MC in drinking water (1 nM) is still a provisional value, based on limited toxicological data [93].

The exposure to low doses of MCLR corresponds to the most realistic kidney intoxication scenario, considering that it is not the main target organ of this toxin. However, the role of kidneys in toxin elimination might lead to the exposure of kidney cells to a low internal dose that can be biologically effective in the induction of nephrotoxic effects. Besides, the chronic adverse effects of microcystins on kidneys, specially the potential tumorigenic/carcinogenic effects, may assume a particular importance in populations exposed to water persistently contaminated with toxic cyanobacteria.

Although further studies will be required to recognize the epithelial monkey kidney-derived Vero-E6 cell line as a nephrotoxicity model, we propose that Vero-E6 cell line constitutes a valuable in vitro model to evaluate the basal toxicity of MCLR and to study the mechanisms of MCLR toxicity.

http://dx.doi.org/10.5772/54463

In figure 7 we summarize the effects induced by MCLR on Vero-E6 cell line.

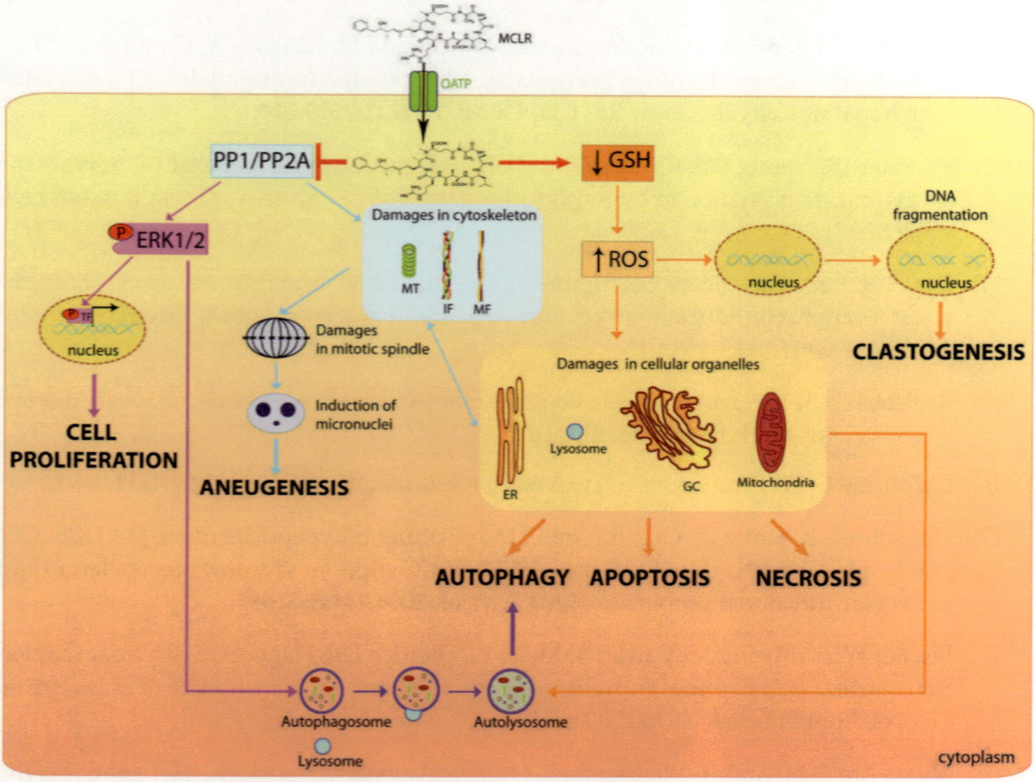

Figure 7. Effects and mechanisms of toxicity of MCLR on Vero-E6 cell model. Legend: **OATP** (organic anion transporters polypeptide); **PP1/PP2A** (protein phosphatases PP1 and PP2A); **P** (phosphate group); **ERK1/2** (extracellular-signal-regulated kinase); **TF** (transcription factors); **MT** (microtubules); **IF** (intermediary filaments); **MF** (microfilaments); **GSH** (reduced glutathione); **ROS** (reactive oxygen species); **ER** (endoplasmic reticulum); **GC** (golgi complex). ↓ Activation, ⊥ Inhibition.

Author details

Carina Menezes, Elisabete Valério and Elsa Dias*

*Address all correspondence to: elsa.dias@insa.min-saude.pt

Biology and Ecotoxicology Laboratory, Environmental Health Department, National Health Institute Dr. Ricardo Jorge, Lisbon, Portugal

References

[1] Funari E, Testai E. Human health risk assessment related to cyanotoxins exposure. Critical Rev Toxicol 2008;38:97-125.

[2] Yoshizawa I, Matsushima R, Watanabe MF, Harada H, Ichihara A, Carmichael WW, Fujiki H. Inhibition of protein phosphatases by microcystis and nodularin associated with hepatotoxicity. J Cancer Res Clin Oncol. 1990;116:609-614.

[3] Falconer IR, Yeung DS. Cytoskeletal changes in hepatocytes induced by microcystis toxins and their relation to hyperphosphorilation of cell proteins. Chem Biol Interact. 1992; 81:181-196.

[4] Duy TN, Lam PKS, Shaw GR, Connell DW. Toxicology and risk assessment of freshwater cyanobacterial (blue-green algal) toxins in water. Reviews Environ Contam Toxicol. 2000;163:113-186.

[5] Boelsterli UA. Mechanistic toxicology: the molecular basis of how chemicals disrupt biological targets. Informa Healthcare USA, Inc., New York. 2009. pp.233.

[6] Carmichael WW. The toxins of cyanobacteria. Scient American. 1994;270:11, 64-70.

[7] Hagenbuch B, Meier PJ. Organic anion transporting polypeptides of the OATP/SLC21 family: phylogenetic classification as OATP/SLCO superfamily, new nomenclature and molecular/functional properties. Eur J Physiol. 2004;447:653–665.

[8] Fischer WL, Altheimer S, Cattori V, Meier PJ, Dietrich DR, Hagenbuch B. Organic anion transporting polypeptides expressed in liver and brain mediate uptake of microcystin. Toxicol Appl Pharmacol. 2005;203:257-263.

[9] Meier-Abt F, Mokrab Y, Mizuguchi K. Organic Anion Transporting Polypeptides of the OATP/SLCO Superfamily: Identification of New Members in Non-mammalian Species, Comparative Modeling and a Potential Transport Mode. J. Membrane Biol. 2005;208:213–227.

[10] Obaidat A, Roth M, Hagenbuch B. The Expression and Function of Organic Anion Transporting Polypeptides in Normal Tissues and in Cancer. Annu Rev Pharmacol Toxicol. 2012;52:135-151.

[11] Leuthold S, Hagenbuch B, Mohebbi N, Wagner CA, Meier PJ, Stieger B. Mechanisms of pH-gradient driven transport mediated by organic anion polypeptide transporters. Am J Physiol Cell Physiol. 2009;296:C570–C582.

[12] Hagenbuch B, Meier PJ. The superfamily of organic anion transporting polypeptides. Biochem Biophys Acta. 2003;1609:1–18.

[13] Andrinolo D, Sedan D, Telese L, Aura C, Masera S, Giannuzzi L, Marra CA, Alaniz MJT. Hepatic recovery after damage produced by sub-chronic intoxication with the cyanotoxin microcystin LR. Toxicon. 2008;51:457-467.

[14] Milutinović A, Sedmark B, Horvat-ŽnidarŠić I, Šuput D. Renal injuries induced by chronic intoxication with microcystins. Cell Mol Biol Lett. 2002;7: 139-141.

[15] Milutinović A, Živin M, Zorc-Plesković R, Sedmark B. Šuput D. Nephrotoxic effects of chronic administration of microcystins-LR and –YR. Toxicon. 2003;42:281-288.

[16] Robinson NA, Pace JG, Matson CF, Miura GA, Lawrence WB. Tissue distribution, excretion and hepatic biotransformation of microcystin-LR in mice. J Pharmacol Exp Therap. 1990;256:176-182.

[17] Khan SA, Ghosh S, Wickstrom M, Miller LA, Hess R, Haschek WM, Beasley VR. Comparative Pathology of Microcystin-LR in Cultured Hepatocytes, Fibroblasts, and Renal Epithelial Cells. Nat Toxins. 1995;3:119-128.

[18] McDermott CM, Nho CW, Howard W, Holtons B. The cyanobacterial toxin, Microcystin-LR, can induce apoptosis in a variety of cell types. Toxicon 1998;36(12):1981-1996.

[19] Boaru DA, Dragoş N, Schrimer K. Microcystin-LR induced cellular effects in mammalian and fish primary hepatocyte cultures cell lines: A comparative study. Toxicology. 2006;218:134-148.

[20] Boyer JL, Hagenbuch B, Ananthanarayanan M, Suchy F, Stieger B, Meier PJ. Phylogenic and ontogenic expression of hepatocellular bile acid transport. PNAS. 1993;90:435–438.

[21] Chong MWK, Gu K D, Lam PKS, Yang M, Fong WF. Study on the cytotoxicity of microcystin-LR on cultured cells. Chemosph. 2000;41:143-147.

[22] Nong Q, Komatsu M, Izumo K, Indo H, Xu B, Aoyama K, Majima H, Horiuchi M, Morimoto K, Takeuchi T. Involvement of reactive oxygen species in Microcystin-LR-induced cytogenotoxocity. Free Rad Res. 2007;41(12):1396-1337.

[23] Žegura B, Sedmak B, Filipič M. Microcystin-LR induces oxidative DNA damage in human hepatoma cell line HepG2. Toxicon. 2003;41:41-48.

[24] Žegura B, Zajc I, Lah T, Filipič M. Patterns of microcystin-LR induced alteration of the expression of genes involved in response to DNA damage and apoptosis. Toxicon. 2008;51:615-623.

[25] Kullak-Ublick GA, Beuers U, Paumgartner G. Molecular and Functional Characterization of Bile Acid Transport in Human Hepatoblastoma HepG2 Cells. Hepatology. 1996;23:1053-1060.

[26] Dias E, Pereira P, Batoréu MCC, Jordan P, Silva MJ. Cytotoxic and genotoxic effects of microcystins in mammalian cell lines. In: Moestrup, Ø. et al. (eds), Proceedings of the 12th International Conference on Harmful Algae, 4-8 September 2006, Copenhagen, Denmark. Paris: ISSHA and IOC- UNESCO; 2008.

[27] Dias E, Andrade M, Alverca E, Pereira P. Batoréu MCC, Jordan P, Silva MJ. Comparative study of the cytotoxic effect of microcistin-LR and purified extracts from Microcystis aeruginosa on a kidney cell line. Toxicon. 2009;53:487-495.

[28] Dias E, Matos P, Pereira P, Batoréu MCC, Silva MJ, Jordan P. Microcystin-LR activates the ERK1/2 kinases and stimulates the proliferation of the monkey kidney derived cell line Vero-E6. Toxicology in Vitro. 2010;24:1689-1695.

[29] Alverca E, Andrade M, Dias E, Sam Bento F, Batoréu MCC, Jordan P, Silva MJ, Pereira P. Morphological and ultrastructural effects of microcystin-LR from *Microcystis aeruginosa* extract on a kidney cell line. Toxicon. 2009;54:283-294.

[30] Menezes C, Alverca A, Dias E, Sam Bento F, Pereira P. Involvement of endoplasmic reticulum and autophagy in microcystin-LR toxicity in Vero-E6 and HepG2 cell lines . Toxicology in vitro. 2013;27:138–148.

[31] Hooser S. Fulminant Hepatocyte Apoptosis In Vivo Following Microcystin-LR Administration to Rats. Toxicol Pathol. 2000;28(5):726-733.

[32] Mankiewicz J, Tarczynska M, Fladmark KE, Doskeland SO, Walter Z, Zalewski M. Apoptotic effect of cyanobacterial extract on rat hepatocytes and human lymphocytes. Environ Toxicol. 2001;16:225-233.

[33] Li L, Xie P, Chen J. Biochemical and ultrastructural changes of the liver and kidney of the phytoplanktivorours silver carp feeding naturally on toxic Microcystis blooms in Taihu Lake, China. Toxicon. 2007;49:1042-1053.

[34] MacKintosh C, Beattie KA, Klumpp S, Cohen P, Codd GA. Cyanobacterial microcystin-LR is a potent and specific inhibitor of protein phosphatases 1 and 2A from both mammals and higher plants. FEBS. 1990;264(2):187-192.

[35] Toivola DM, Goldman RD, Garrod D, Ericksson JE. Protein phosphatases maintain the organization and structural interactions of hepatic keratin intermediate filaments. J Cell Sci. 1997;110:23-33.

[36] Batista T, Sousa G, Suput JS, Rahmani R, Šuput D. Microcystin-LR causes the colapse of actin filaments in primary human hepatocytes. Aquatic Toxic. 2003;65:85-91.

[37] Qin W, Xu X, Zhang X, Wang Y, Meng X, Miao A, Yang L. Endoplasmic reticulum stress in murine liver and kidney exposed to microcystin-LR. Toxicon. 2010;56:1334–1341.

[38] Ding W, Shen H, Ong C. Microcystic Cyanobacteria Causes Mitochondrial Membrane Potential Alteration and Reactive Oxygen Species Formation in Primary Cultured Rat Hepatocytes. Environ Health Persp. 1998;106(7):409-413.

[39] Ding W, Shen H, Ong C. Critical role of reactive oxygen species and mitochondrial permeability transition in microcystin-induced rapid apoptosis in rat hepatocytes. Hepatology. 2000;2:547-555.

[40] Ding W, Shen H, Ong C. Calpain activation after mitochondrial permeability transition in microcystin-induced cell death in rat hepatocytes. Bioch Bioph Res Communic. 2002;291:321-331.

[41] Weng D, Lu Y, Wei Y, Liu Y, Shen P. The role of ROS in microcystin-LR-induced hepatocytes apoptosis and liver injury in mice. Toxicology. 2007;232:15-23.

[42] Žegura B, Lah T, Filipič M. The role of reactive oxygen species in microcystin-LR induced DNA damage. Toxicology. 2004;200:59-68.

[43] IARC Monographs on the Evaluation of Carcinogenic Risks to Humans. Ingested Nitrate and Nitrite, and Cyanobacterial Peptide Toxins. Lyon, France. 2010;94:329-412.

[44] Ueno Y, Nagata S, Tsutsumi T, Hasegawa A, Watanabe MF, Park HD, Chen GC, Chen G, Yu, SZ. Detection of microcystins, a blue-green algal hepatotoxins, in drinking water sampled in Haimen and Fusui, endemic areas of primary liver cancer in China, by highly sensitive immunoassay. Carcinogenesis. 1996;17:1317-1321.

[45] Yu SZ. Primary prevention of hepatocellular carcinoma. J Gastroenterol Hepatol. 1995;10:674-82.

[46] Zhou L, Yu H, Chen K. Relationship between microcystin in drinking water and colorectal cancer. Biomed Environ Sci. 2002;15:166-71.

[47] Žegura B, Štraser A, Filipič M. Genotoxicity and potential carcinogenicity of cyanobacterial toxins – a review. Mut Res. 2011;727:16–41.

[48] Collins AR. The comet assay for DNA damage and repair. Principles, applications and limitations, Mol Biotechnol. 2004;26:249–261.

[49] Ding WX, Shen HM, Zhu HG, Lee BL, Ong CN. Genotoxicity of microcystic cyanobacterial extract of a water source in China. Mutat Res. 1999;442:69-77.

[50] Žegura B, Gajski G, Štraser A, Garaj-Vrhovac V, Filipič M. Microcystin-LR induced DNA damage in human peripheral blood lymphocytes. Mut Res. 2011;726:116–122.

[51] Bouaïcha N, Maatouk I, Plessis MJ, Périn F. Genotoxic potential of microcystin-LR and nodularin *in vitro* in primary cultured rat hepatocytes and *in vivo* rat liver. Environ Toxicol. 2005;20:341-347.

[52] Lankoff A, Krzowski L, Glab J, Banasik A, Lisowska H, Kuszwski T, Gozdz S, Wojcik A. DNA damage and repair in human peripheral blood lymphocytes following treatment with microcystin-LR. Mut Res. 2004;559:131-142.

[53] Zhan L, Sakamoto H, Sakuraba M, Wu S, Zhang S, Suzuki T, Hayashi M, Honma M. Genotoxicity of microcystin-LR in human lymphoblastoid TK6 cells. Mut Res. 2004;557:1-6.

[54] Lankoff A, Bialczyki J, Dziga D, Carmichael WW, Lisowska H, Wojcik A. Inhibition of nucleotide excision repair by microcystin-LR in CHO-K1 cells. Toxicon 2006;48: 957-965.

[55] Fessard V, Le Hegarat L, Mourot A. Comparison of the genotoxic results obtained from the in vitro cytokinesis-block micronucleous assay with various toxins inhibitors of protein phosphatases: okadaic acid, nodularin and microcystin-LR. In: Proceedings of Sixth International Conference on Toxic Cyanobacteria, 21-27 June 2004, Bergen, Norway. 2004;68-69.

[56] Abramsson-Zetterberg L, Sundh UB, Mattsson R. Cyanobacterial extracts amd microcystin-LR are inactive in the micronucleous assay in vivo and in vitro. Mutat Res. 2010;699:5-10.

[57] Lankoff A, Bialczyki J, Dziga D, Carmichael WW, Gradzka I, Lisowska H, Kuszewski T, Gozdz S, Piorun I, Wojcik A. The repair of gamma-radiation-induced DNA damage is inhibited by microcystin-LR, the PP1 and PP2A phosphatase inhibitor. Mutagenesis. 2006;21:83-90.

[58] Dias E, Louro H, Santos T, Antunes S, Pereira P, Silva MJ. Genotoxicity of Microcystin-LR in distinct biological models: cell lines, mouse blood cells and human lymphocytes. Environmental and molecular mutagenesis, submitted for publication.

[59] Kirsch-Volders M, Vanhauwaert A, De Boeck M, Decordier I. Importance of detecting numerical versus structural chromosome aberrations. Mut Res. 2002;504:137-148.

[60] Iarmarcovai G, Botta A, Orsière T. Number of centromeric signals in micronuclei and mechansims of aneuploidy. Toxicol Lett. 2006;166:1-10.

[61] Nishiwaki-Matsushima R, Ohta T, Nishiwaki S, Suganuma M, Kohyama K, Ishikawa T, Carmichael WW, Fujiki H. Liver tumor promotion by the cyanobacterial cyclic peptide toxin microcystin-LR. J Cancer Res Clin Oncol. 1992;118:420–424.

[62] Falconer IR. Tumour promotion and liver injury caused by oral consumption of cyanobacteria. Environ Toxicol Water Qual. 1991;6:177–184.

[63] Gehringer MM. Microcystin-LR and okadaic acid-induced cellular effects: a dualistic response. FEBS Lett. 2004;557:1–8.

[64] Junttila MR, Li SP, Westermarck J.Phosphatase-mediated crosstalk between MAPK signalling pathways in the regulation of cell survival. FASEB J. 2008;22:954–965.

[65] McKay MM, Morrison DK. Integrating signals from RTKs to ERK/MAPK. Oncogene 2007;26:3113-3121.

[66] Raman M, Chen W, Cobb MH. Differential regulation and properties of MAPKs. Oncogene. 2007;26:3100-3112.

[67] Kolch W. Meaningful relationships: the regulation of the Ras/Raf/MEK/ERK pathway by protein interactions. Biochem J. 2000;351:289–305.

[68] Li H, Xie P, Li G, Hao L, Xiong Q. In vivo study on the effects of microcystin extracts on the expression profiles of proto-oncogenes (c-fos, c-jun and c-myc) in liver, kidney and testis of male Wistar rats injected i.v. with toxins. Toxicon. 2009;53:169–175.

[69] Zhu Y, Zhong X, Zheng S, Ge Z, Du Q, Zhang S. Transformation of immortalized colorectal crypt cells by microcystin involving constitutive activation of Akt and MAPK cascade. Carcinogenesis. 2005;26:1207–1214.

[70] Thompson WL, Allen MB, Bostian KA. The effects of microcystin on monolayers of primary rat hepatocytes. In: Gopalakrisnakonef, P., Tan, C.K. (Eds.), Progress in venom and toxin research. National University of Singapore, Singapore, 1987;725–731.

[71] Grabow W, Randt W, Prozesky O, Scott W. Microcystis aeruginosa toxin: cell culture toxicity, hemolysis and mutagenicity assays. Appl Environ Microbiol. 1982;43(6):1425–1433.

[72] Menezes C. Comparative study of the cytotoxic effects of Microcystin-LR in mammalian cell lines. Universidade de Lisboa, 2009. Available from: http://repositorio.ul.pt/handle/10451/1488

[73] Wickstrom ML, Khan SA, Haschek WM, Wyman JF, Eriksson JE, Schaeffer DJ, Beasle VR. Alterations in Microtubules, Intermediate Filaments and Microfilaments Induced by Microcystin-LR in Cultured Cells. Toxicol Pathol 1995;23:326-337.

[74] Khan, S.A,. Wickstrom, M.L, Haschek, W.M., Schaeffer, D.J., Ghosh, S., Beasley, V.R. 1996.Microcystin-LR and kinetics of cytoskeletal reorganization in hepatocytes, kidney cells and fibroblasts. Nat. Toxins 4: 206-214.

[75] Raju S, Kavimani S, Uma MRV, Sriramulu RK. Nephrotoxicants and Nephrotoxicity Testing: An Outline Of *In Vitro* Alternatives. J Pharm Sci Res. 2011;3:1110-1116.

[76] Prieto P. Barriers, nephrotoxicology and chronic testing in vitro. ATLA. 2002;30:101-105.

[77] Hawksworth GM, Bach PH, Nagelkerke JF, Dekant W, Diezi JE, Harpur E, Lock EA, MacDonald C, Morin PP, Pfaller W, Rutten AAJJL, Ryan MP, Toutain HJ, Trevisan A. Nephrotoxicity testing *in vitro*. The report and recommendations of ECVAM workshop 10. ATLA 1995;23:713-727.

[78] Matskevich AA, Jung JS, Schümann M, Cascallo M, Moelling K. Vero Cells as a Model to Study the Effects of Adenoviral Gene Delivery Vectors on the RNAi System in Context of Viral Infection. J Innate Immun. 2009;1:389–394.

[79] Jos A, Repetto G, Rios JC, Hazen MJ, Molero ML, del Peso A, Salguero M, Fernández-Freire P, Pérez-Martín JM, Cameán A. Ecotoxicological evaluation of carbamazepine using six different model systems with eighteen endpoints. Toxicology in Vitro. 2003;17:525–532.

[80] Jirasripongpun K, Wongarethornkul T, Mulliganavin S. Risk Assessment of Triclosan Using Animal Cell Lines. Kasetsart J Nat Sci. 2008;42(2):353-359.

[81] Romero D, Gómez-Zapata M, Luna A, García-Fernández AJ. Morphological characterization of renal cell lines (BGM and VERO) exposed to low doses of lead nitrate. Histol Histopathol, 2004;19:69-76.

[82] Freire PF, Peropadre A, Pérez Martín JM, Herrero O, Hazen MJ. An integrated cellular model to evaluate cytotoxic effects in mammalian cell lines. Toxicology in Vitro. 2009;23:1553–1558.

[83] Kumar S, Kanwar S, Bansal V, Sehgal R. Standardization and validation of Vero cell assay for potency estimation of diphtheria antitoxin serum. Biologicals. 2009;37(5):297–305.

[84] Lindgren SW, Samuel JE, Schmitt CK, O'Brien AD. The specific activities of Shiga-Like toxin type II (SLT-II) and SLT-II-related toxins of enterohemorrhagic *Escherichia coli* differ when measured by Vero cell cytotoxicity but not by mouse lethality. Infect Immun. 1994;62(2):623-631.

[85] Froscio SM, Fanok S, Humpage AR. Cytotoxicity Screening for the Cyanobacterial Toxin Cylindrospermopsin. J ToxicolEnviron Health, Part A: Current Issues. 2009;72(5): 345-349.

[86] Froscio SM, Cannon E, Lau HM, Humpage AR. Limited uptake of the cyanobacterial toxin cylindrospermopsin by Vero cells. Toxicon. 2009;54:862–868.

[87] Ekwall B, Silano V, Paganuzzi-Stammati A, Zucco F. Toxicity Tests with Mammalian Cell Cultures. In: Bourdeau P. (ed.) Short-term Toxicity Tests for Non-genotoxic Effects. New York: John Wiley & Sons Ltd; 1990. p75-98.

[88] Li T, Huang P, Liang J, Fu W, Guo Z, Xu L. Microcystin-LR (MCLR) Induces a Compensation of PP2A Activity Mediated by α4 Protein in HEK293 Cells. Int J Biol Sci. 2011;7:740-752.

[89] Falconer IR. Cyanobacterial toxins present in Microcystis aeruginosa extracts – More than microcystins!. Toxicon. 2007;50:585–588.

[90] Paulino S, Sam-Bento F, Churro C, Alverca E, Dias E, Valério E, Pereira P. The Estela Sousa e Silva Algal Culture Collection: a resource of biological and toxicological interest. Hydrobiologia. 2009;636:489–492.

[91] Valério E, Chambel L, Paulino S, Faria N, Pereira P, Tenreiro R. Molecular identification, typing and traceability of cyanobacteria from freshwater reservoirs. Microbiology. 2009;155:642–656.

[92] Valério E, Chambel L, Paulino S, Faria N, Pereira P, Tenreiro R. Multiplex PCR for detection of microcystins-producing cyanobacteria from freshwater samples. Environ Toxicol. 2010;25(3):251–260.

[93] WHO. Guidelines for Drinking Water Quality, third ed. Incorporating the First and Second Addenda, vol. 1, Recommendations. World Health Organization, Geneva. 2008.

Chapter 3

Why are Early Life Stages of Aquatic Organisms more Sensitive to Toxicants than Adults?

Azad Mohammed

Additional information is available at the end of the chapter

http://dx.doi.org/10.5772/55187

1. Introduction

1.1. The selection of a suitable test species

Toxicity tests are designed to determine the specific concentrations of chemicals that induce a measured effect on a target organism. However, the potency of any toxicant can be influenced by the characteristics of the chemical, as well as environmental (temperature, ph, water chemistry, salinity) and species (life stage, sensitivity, pre-exposure) specific factors. Environmental factors can either modify the toxicant itself or the immediate environment of an organism, increasing or decreasing the effects of the toxicants. Species specific factors can alter the organism/toxicant interaction by modifying the rate of uptake, distribution, elimination and detoxification pathways. Therefore when conducting toxicity tests, it is important to have controlled environmental conditions and select suitable test species to ensure reliable, relevant, reproducible, defensible and ecologically significant results. The selection of a suitable test species can be based on several criteria:

- the species should be widely available
- they should be easily maintained under laboratory conditions and provide sufficient numbers of an appropriate size and age
- the genetics, genetic composition and history of the organisms should be known
- they should the most sensitive species in the environment.
- should be recreationally, ecologically and commercially important
- organisms should be in good physiological condition
- it should be indigenous or representative of the eco-region being studies

Since the first toxicity tests were performed over 60 years ago, fish and invertebrates continue to be the most popular test species because there exist a significant knowledge base on their physiology, biochemistry, behavior, reproduction, life cycle and ecological importance. However there continues to be an ongoing debate as to whether certain life stages are more sensitive to toxicants than others. The general assumption in toxicology has been to utilize the 'most sensitive' life stage which toxicologists assume to be the earliest life stages for a given species. Selecting the most sensitive life stage provides a quick, relatively easy and sensitive toxicity test with the added advantage of having a low cost and test duration. In fact, many standardized test protocols often specify the preferred life stage to be used for testing. For example, US Environmental Protection Agency (US EPA) [EPA-600/4-80/001, EPA-812-R-02-012], and American Society for Testing and Materials (ASTM) [ASTM E1192-97(2008), ASTM E1267-03(2008) and ASTM E724-98(2004)] test protocols recommend the use of early life stages; first instar of daphnia, juvenile mysids, juvenile fish or embryos of mollusks as the most suitable for toxicity tests. The choice of early life stages has been based on the premise that they are the most susceptible to toxicants and that toxicity data using the most vulnerable life stage would offer protection to all life stages in the natural environment.

2. Early life stages in toxicity tests

Numerous studies have reported that the early life stages of fish and invertebrates were more sensitive to toxicants than the adult organisms (Herkovits et al. 1997, Schmieder et al. 2000, Hutchinson et al. 1998, Mohammed et al. 2009). Schmieder et al. (2000) reported that for medake, embryo-larval stages showed 50% mortality when 2,3,7,8-Tetrachlorodibenzo-*p*-dioxin (TCDD) residues in the eggs were 1396 pg/g, however, for adults 50% mortality occurred when the whole body concentration of 2,3,7,8-TCDD residue was 2400 pg/g. Using data from the European Centre for Ecotoxicology and Toxicology of Chemicals (ECETOC) Acute Toxicity (EAT) data base, Hutchinson et al. (1998) analysed the EC50 data from partial and full life cycle studies and reported that the sensitivity of aquatic invertebrate larvae were greater than or equal to juveniles for 66% of the substances tested, while the sensitivity of juveniles was greater than or equal to the adults' for 54% of the substances tested. Hutchinson et al. (1998) also reported that for fish, NOEC data indicated that larvae were more sensitive than embryos for 68% of substances, while the sensitivity of fish larvae was greater than or equal to that of juveniles for 83% of the substances tested. Based on fish EC50 data, juveniles were more sensitive than adults to 92% of the substances tested (Hutchinson et al. 1998). For fishes, it has been reported that the larvae are more sensitivity than embryos, and embryos are more sensitive than adults (larvae > embryos > adults). However, for invertebrates such as molluscs, embryos may sometimes appear to be more sensitive than larvae. Therefore, in scales of relative sensitivity, the position of specific life stages may vary depending on species.

http://dx.doi.org/10.5772/55187

3. Early life stages as the most sensitive stage

Variations in sensitivity between life stages have been reported for organisms such as *Callosobruchus maculatas, Metamysidopsis insularis* and *Danio rerio*. Macova et al. (2008) reported that juvenile *D. rerio* exposed to 2-phenoxyethanol had a significantly lower LC50 (338.22 +/- 15.22 mg/L) than embryonic stages (486.35 +/- 25.53 mg/L) indicating a higher larval sensitivity. Fisher et al. (1994) showed that veliger larva had similar sensitivity to Bayer 73 and 3-trifluoromethyl-4-nitrophenol (TFM), whereas plantigrades and adults were less sensitive. Hardersen and Wratten (2000) found that the most susceptible life stage of *Xanthocnemis zealandica* following exposure to azinphos-methyl and carbaryl, was instar 7, while the least susceptible were instars 2 and 13. Lotufo and Fleeger (1997) also reported significant differences in sensitivity of nauplii, copepodites, and adults of *Schizopera knabeni* following exposure to phenanthrene. However, Borlongan et al. (1998) showed that for *Cerithidea cingulata* (a brackish water pond snail) sensitivity typically increased as the snail grew and matured.

Other studies have reported that early life stages such as first instar of daphnia, juvenile mysids, juvenile fish and embryos are more susceptible than adults following exposure to toxicants such as heavy metal (Bodar et al. 1989; Gopalakrishnan 2008; Hoang and Klaine 2007; Green et al. 1986; Verriopoulos and Morai'tou-Apostolopoulou 1982). For example, George et al. (1996) reported that the larva (yolk sac stage) of *Scophthalmus maximus* was more sensitive than other larval stages (larval and posthatch larval stages) following exposure to cadmium. Green et al. (1986) also reported that for the crustacean *Asellus aquaticus* exposed to cadmium, the juveniles (96 hr LC50 = 80 μg Cd/L) were more sensitive than the embryos (96 hr LC50 = >2,000 μg Cd/L). Ringwood (1990) reported that older larval of the bivalve *Isognomon californicum* were approximately 10 times more sensitive than adults while embryos and early larval stages were more than 50 times more sensitive than adults. Kennedy et al. (2006) also reported that adult *Dreissena polymorpha* had a 48 hr LC50 of 1,214 μg Cu/L which was several orders of magnitude higher than the 24hr LC50 (13 μg Cu/L) for earlier life stages (72-h old trochophores). Verriopoulos and Morai'tou-apostolopoulou (1982) also reported that the most sensitive life stage of *Tisbe holothuriae* to both copper and cadmium was the one-day-old nauplius which had a 48h LC50 of 0.3142 mg Cu/L and 0.5384 mg Cd/L, while the five-days-old nauplii had a 48h LC50 of 0.3415 mg Cu/L and 0.645 mg Cd/L, and the ten-days-old nauplii showed a 48h LC50 of 0.5289 mg Cu/L and 0.9061 mg Cd/L. The most resistance stage was the ten-days-old copepodids but generally, the resistance of *Tisbe holothuriae* to copper and cadmium progressively increased with larval age.

4. Probable causes for variations in sensitivity between life stages

The apparent variability in sensitivity between early life stages and adults may be due to several factors; surface area/volume ratio (particularly with young fish); the greater likelihood that juveniles may have accumulated less fat than adults thus having less capacity to store lipophilic substances; greater uptake of toxicant from the environment; under developed homeostatic mechanism to deal with the toxicants; immature immune systems and under developed organs (liver and kidney) which has an important role in detoxification and elimination of toxicants.

There are various ideas that seek to explain why early life stages are more sensitive than adults. These often take into consideration specific behavioral, morphological, physiological and biochemical characteristics which may be different between life stages. Some of the main ideas include:

1. Organ systems may become sensitive to the effects of toxicant at certain periods during early development but once developed, they may no longer be vulnerable (Ozoh 1979, Bentivena and Piatkowski 1998).

2. The time taken for toxicants to reach target sites may be shorter in early life stages, because of their smaller size when compared to later stages and adults.

3. Most embryo and larval forms may have poorly developed organs such as gills, liver and kidneys. They also have permeable skin which, in early life stages, is the primary means of ionic regulation. The skin presents a larger surface area for the uptake of toxicants, resulting in increased susceptibility of the larva when compared to the adults.

4. In crustaceans research has shown that metals can concentrate in the body covering thus reducing their entry into the body. The completion of body covering diminishes the entry of metal into the body, thereby increasing the resistance of older forms.

5. Some toxicants may be sequestered in fat tissue or specific proteins preventing them from reaching target organs.

The increased susceptibility of early life stages may also be related to other factors such as; differential rates of absorption/uptake distribution or detoxification. Organisms have also evolved intricate regulatory (physiological, immunological and biochemical) mechanisms which allow them to survive, grow and reproduce. Some of these mechanisms are also important in the elimination, detoxification or reduction of the effects of toxicant. For example, kidneys and liver may be involved in the elimination of toxicants, while various proteins and enzymes such as Metallothioneins and Mixed Function Oxygenases are induced following exposure to metals and hydrocarbons. It is often suggested that the difference in the development of these mechanism and immature detoxification pathways in early life stages can also be a basis for the apparent increased sensitivity of juveniles exposed to toxicants. A few specific factors for increased sensitivity will me discussed below.

4.1. Avoidance strategies

The higher sensitivity of early life stages may be explained by behavioral, morphological, physiological or biochemical changes. Free swimming species are able to avoid toxicants, while some sessile species such as bivalves may close their valves to avoid contact with the toxicants. Disruption in behavioral responses may include:

1. impaired feeding ability resulting in poor diet, which can cause reduced growth and longevity;
2. altered predator - avoidance behavior;
3. impaired schooling leading to increased mortality and/or altered reproductive function,
4. movement away from the source of the toxicant, or
5. as in the case of bivalves, closure of the valves for varying periods of time in order to reduce exposure (Weis, 2005).

Behavioral responses can have greater impacts on earlier life stages, which show significantly less physiological and morphological development than adults. Kennedy et al. (2006) showed that adult *Dreissena polymorpha* (unlike the free swimming larva or early life stages) closed their valves when exposed to copper at 777 ± 40 μg Cu/L, while exposure to 99 ± 9 μg Cu/L caused partial valve closure and/or retraction of siphons. It has been suggested that they may possess chemoreceptors which can detect elevated levels of Copper which triggers closure of the valves. Scott et al. (2003) also reported that exposure of *Oncorhynchus mykiss* to 2 μg Cd/L for 7 days eliminated normal antipredator behaviors whereas exposures of shorter duration or lower concentration had no effect on normal behavior.

4.2. Morphological characteristics

Avoidance strategies undoubtedly result in decreased exposure, but it is unlikely that chemical avoidance alone can account for the difference in sensitivity between adults and early life stages. In some species such as *I. californicum, A. aquaticus* and *D. rerio,* embryos have been shown to be less sensitive than other life stages. In this instance, embryonic membranes can act as a physical barrier which reduces exposure and consequently reduces toxicity. Eggs of *I. californicum* contain a single membrane about 2μm thick which is shed about 8hr post fertilization. Similarly in fish the chorionic membranes in embryos may act as an effective barrier to toxicants, lowering the sensitivity of the embryo when compared to larval forms. In some fish and isopods species, the embryos may be encased in several layers of membranes. The membrane not only forms a physical barrier, but may also bind metals, effectively reducing their passage to the embryos, as does the chorion in fish eggs (Beattie and Pascoe 1978). Plhalová et al. (2010) reported that exposure of the embryonic stage of *D. rerio* to terbutryn gave a 144hr LC50 of 8.04±1.05 mg/L while for the juvenile stage the 96hr LC50 was 5.71±0.46 mg/L which suggested that juvenile stages were more sensitive to terbutryn than the embryonic stages. Green et al (1986) also showed that the embryos of *Asellus aquaticus* (L) were more resistant to the effects of cadmium than the early juveniles. The eggs of *A. aquaticus* possess four membranes which are successively shed as the embryo passes through the various stages of development (Holditch and Tolba 1981). When the last membrane is shed, they reported that the sensitivity may increase by as much as 20 times (Beattie and Pascoe 1978). However, the membrane barrier may only be effective at certain concentrations above which the capacity to bind or adsorb metals is exceeded and reducing its effectiveness to lower toxicity. Green et al. (1986) showed that when embryos of *Asellus aquaticus* were exposed to 1,750 μg Cd/L, the last embryonic membranes offered little or no protection and embryos responded in a similar manner as the smallest juveniles. At 5 and 17.5 μg Cd/L, however, the last membrane affords considerable protection to the embryo, significantly prolonging its survival time in comparison early juveniles. Generally, the extent to which it can modify the sensitivity of the embryo relative to other life stages may be related to the type and permeability of membrane and whether they remain intact during the toxicity test

In many fish species, larval forms are generally more sensitive than juveniles and adult forms. Newly hatched larvae constitute a particularly critical and sensitive life stage, because at hatching the embryos lose their protective membrane and are fully exposed to potential toxicants (Arufe et al. 2004). A significant characteristic of most larval stages is the fast changing morphology giving rise to the adult forms. Organ systems may become sensitive to the effects of toxicant at certain periods during early development but once developed, they may no longer be vulnerable (Ozoh 1979, Bentivena and Piatkowski 1998). Middaugh and Dean (1977) reported that cadmium was more toxic to the 7-day-old larvae (LC50 = 12 mg Cd/L) of *Fundulus heteroclitus* than the adults (LC50 = 43 mg Cd/L). Similarly, Hilmy et al. (1985) reported that for the larval forms of *Mugil cephalus* the LC50 was 8 mg Cd/L compared with 34 mg Cd/L for juveniles. George et al. (1996) also reported that newly hatched larvae of *Scophthalmus maximus* (yolk sac stage) had a 48-hr LC50 value of 0.18-0.23 mg Cd/L, however, day 4 posthatch larvae showed a 48-hr LC50 of 2 mg Cd/L while the 10-day posthatch larvae showed a 48-hr LC50 of 5 mg Cd/L which indicated decreasing sensitivity with increasing age. Kazlauskienë and Stasiûnaitë (1999) also reported that for rainbow trout, partially and fully hatched larvae were the most sensitive life stage, while eggs, early eye stage and those immediately after fertilization were least sensitive. Williams et al. (1986) reported that the larvae of *Chironomus riparius* showed increased tolerance with increasing age when exposed to cadmium. The most resistant stage (fourth instar) had a 24 h LC50 of 2,400 mg Cd/L, approximately 950 times greater than the corresponding value of 2.1 mg Cd/L recorded for the most sensitive (first instar) stage. The apparent higher sensitivity of larval forms may be related to various factors such as: higher levels of uptake, poorly or underdeveloped organ systems, incompletely formed liver and kidneys, poorly developed immunological systems, and low levels of detoxification proteins. Fish larvae typically do not possess gills, have a large surface-to-volume ratio and possess permeable skin which enables respiration and ionic transport (Tytler and Bell, 1989) as well as the free uptake of metals such as Cd^{2+} (Carpene and George, 1981; Jenkins and Sanders, 1986). As the skin develops it begins to differentiate, becoming multilayered and its permeability to both gases and solutes decreases. Since differentiation occurs gradual during larval development there would appear to be a decreasing sensitivity with increasing age. The skin also secretes a mucus layer which can sequester toxicants such as divalent metal ions (Coombs et al. 1972) further reducing cutaneous absorption. After hatching, marine fish larvae also drink water to maintain their osmotic balance (Brown and Tytler, 1993; Tytler and Blaxter, 1988; Tytler and Ireland, 1994) and actively feed, further increasing the likelihood of uptake from diet and water. However, in some species such as *Scophthalmus maximus,* organogenesis occurs rapidly, usually within 3 to 4 days after hatching. This results in the formation of vital organ systems such as the circulatory system, liver, gills, kidneys and thickening of the skin. However, gills which is one of the major organ for elimination, do not become fully formed until 12-14 days after hatching when the larvae are about 5 mm long (Al-Maghazachi and Gibson, 1984; Segner et al. 1994). In some species such as the Senegalese sole (*Solea senegalensis*) haemopoietic cells in the kidney and were first observed on 6 days after hatching, whereas the thymus was first observed 9 days after hatching (Cunha et al. 2003, Padros et al. 2011). As organs become functional they begin to eliminate or detoxify toxicants, thereby decreasing the sensitivity of the adult forms relative to the early life stages.

http://dx.doi.org/10.5772/55187

4.3. Detoxification mechanisms

Toxicants may induce synthesis of specific proteins specific proteins such as Mix Function Oxygenases and Metallotheinions which may detoxify or sequester toxicants, thus reducing their toxic effects. However, early life stages may lack fully-expressed enzyme systems for efficient detoxification and elimination of toxicants because of slow organ development. In most adult organism detoxification and elimination processes follow one of two pathways depending on whether the toxicant is a metal or organic compound (Figure 1). As previously stated, difference in the development of these mechanism and immature detoxification pathways in early life stages can also be a basis for the apparent increased sensitivity of juveniles exposed to toxicants.

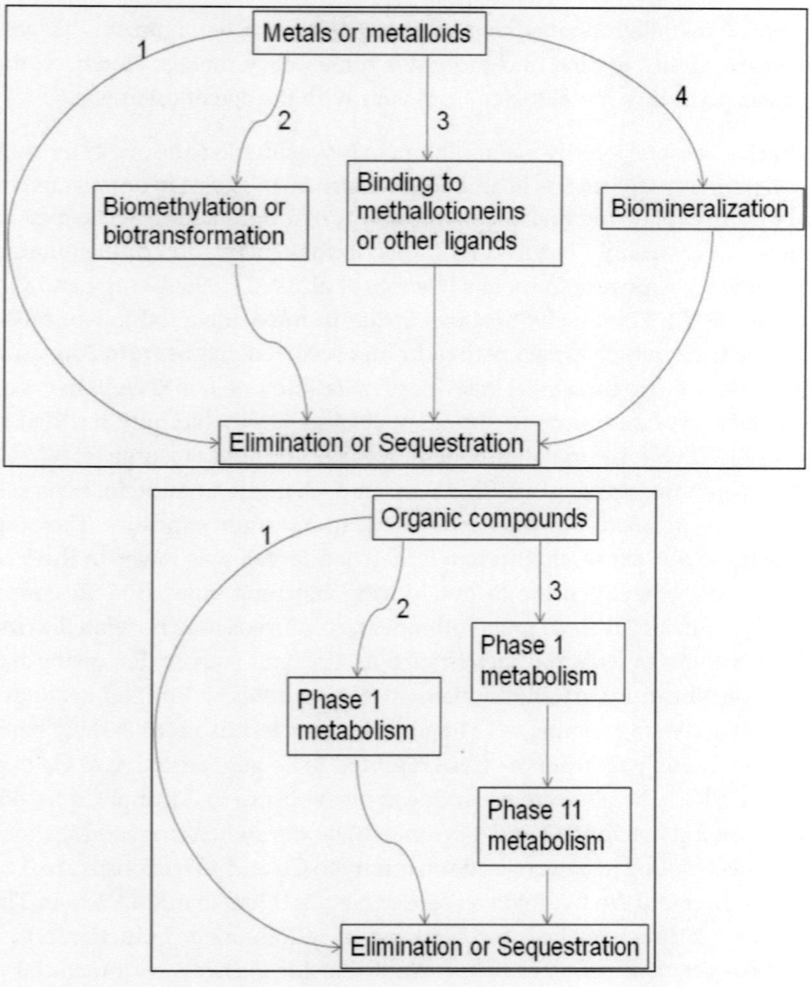

Figure 1. Detoxification pathways for metals and organic compounds

Metallothioneins are non-enzymatic cysteine rich, low molecular weight proteins of about 7 kDa and apparent molecular weight of 13 kDa. The metallothioneins pool is made up of various isoforms each having different physiological roles and different induction pathways and are important in homeostasis of metals such as copper and zinc, and detoxification of heavy metal (Butler and Roesijadi, 2001). Mason and Jenkins (1995) proposed two roles for metallothioneins in the regulation of metals in organisms.

1. They may comprise a non-toxic zinc and copper reservoir available for the synthesis of metalloenzymes, allowing the homeostasis of many cellular processes (Brouwer et al. 1989; Viarengo and Nott 1993; Roesijadi 1996).

2. Metallothioneins can reduce the nonspecific binding of non-essential metals within cells, and so restrict their toxic potential (Roesijadi 1992, 1996; Zaroogian and Jackim 2000).

The induction of metallothioneins confers metal tolerance to organisms (Klaasseen et al. 1999) due to their ability to bind and sequester some heavy metals. However, the ability of metallothioneins to reduce metal toxicity can vary with the age of organism.

The sequestration of metal ions by metallothionein is considered to be one of the most common detoxification pathways for metals in adult organisms. Its presence in organisms can therefore also be used to help explain the variable susceptibility of different life stage to metals. Synthesis of metallothionein is strongly induced by transcriptional activation of metallothionein gene expression following exposure to metals (George et al. 1992, 1996; George and Olsson, 1994; Zafarullah et al. 1989). Laville (1988) showed that in mice, metallothionein mRNA in liver depended on the age at which exposure to cadmium occurred. Exposure to 2mg Cd/kg resulted in a small increase (two- to threefold) in levels of metallothionein mRNA in livers of 7- and 14-day-old mice. However, cadmium treatment of 28- and 56-day-old mice resulted in 12- to 19-fold increases in levels of metallothionein mRNA in liver. George et al. (1996) used metallothionein gene expression (mRNA) to map changes in protein expression during development of *Scophthalmus maximus* in response to cadmium exposure. They reported that metallothionein mRNA expression in newly hatched larvae was lower in the liver at metamorphosis and immediately prior to and during hatching compared to embryos (24 hr postfertilisation). Elevate levels of metallothionein in embryos may be related to its role in the control of homeostasis of essential metals such as zinc and copper. Following hatching (4.5 and 5 days postfertilization) metallothionein mRNA expression dropped to about 50% of the level detected in early-stage embryos (24 and 72 hr after fertilization). Newly hatched larvae feeding on endogenous yolk reserves were reported to be very sensitive to Cd exposure and metallothionein mRNA levels were not induced by exposure to 0.1 ppm Cd for 48 h (George et al. 1996). Following hatching (2 and 4 posthatch) larvae switch from endogenous to exogenous feeding, this resulted in a decreased sensitivity to Cd and 48 h exposure to 0.1 or 0.5 ppm Cd resulted in a threefold - to fivefold increase of metallothionein mRNA levels. These studies therefore indicate a direct relationship between metallothionein induction and decreasing sensitivity. However, Sassi et al. (2012) showed that for gilthead sea bream larvae relative transcript levels of mt were increased at 5 and 10 mg/L of $Cd(2+)$ which they suggested was probably to detoxify excess metals. Zhang et al. 2012 was also able to show that for juvenile grunt (Terapon jarbua) inorganic As(III) and As(V) in the diet and waterborne phases were rapidly biotransformed to the less toxic arsenobetaine (AsB, 89-97%). After exposure to inorganic As, T. jarbua developed detoxified strategies, such as the reduction of As(V) to As(III) followed by methylation to less toxic organic forms, as well as the synthesis of metal-binding proteins such as metallothionein-like proteins.

All organism have at least some ability to metabolize organic compounds. These often involve some enzyme mediate detoxification pathway requiring one or more enzymes such as cytochrome P450 monooxygenase, epoxide hydrolase and other conjugating enzymes (Figure 1) associated with the liver or kidney. In most adult organisms, these pathways are well developed (Shailaja and D'Silva 2003; Tuvikene 1995; Eisler, 1987). In juveniles, induction of these may also occur, once organ systems are fully functional. Oikari et al. (2002) was able to show that in juvenile rainbow trout, exposure to contaminated sediments significantly induced trout liver CYP1A activity. However Sassi et al. (2012) reported that for gilthead sea bream larvae were unable to show transcription of Gpx in following exposure to cadmium. Gpx is responsible for the break down hydrogen peroxide as in adult organisms.

5. Conclusion

The greater sensitivity of early life stages when compared to adults can therefore be explained by a number of physiological, morphological, behavioral and biochemical characteristics. It may appear that in early life stages these responses are either underdeveloped or have not yet developed fully thus contributing to the increased sensitivity of these early life stages when compared to the adults.

Author details

Azad Mohammed

Address all correspondence to: Azad.mohammed@sta.uwi.edu

The University of the West Indies, St Augustine, Trinidad and Tobago

References

[1] Arufe, M. I, Arellano, J, Moreno, M. J, & Sarasquete, C. (2004). Toxicity of commercial herbicide containing terbutryn and triasulfuron to seabream (*Sparus aurata* L.) larvae: a comparison with the Microtox test. Ecotoxicology and Environmental Safety. , 59(2), 209-216.

[2] Al-maghazachi, S. J, & Gibson, R. (1984). The developmental stages of larval turbot, *Scophihalmus maximus* L. Journal of Experimental Marine Biology and Ecology. , 82(1), 35-51.

[3] Beattie, J. H, & Pascoe, D. (1978). Cadmium uptake in rainbow trout, *Salmo gairdneri* eggs andalevins. Journal of Fish Biology. , 13(5), 631-637.

[4] Bentivegna, C. S, & Piatkowski, T. (1998). Effects of tributyltin on medaka (Oryzias latipes) embryos at different stages of development. Aquatic Toxicology., 44(1-2), 117-128.

[5] Bodar, C. W. vd Zee, A., Voogt, P.A., Wynne, H., and Zandee, D.I. (1989). Toxicity of heavy metals to early life stages of Daphnia magna. Ecotoxicology and Environmental Safety. , 17(3), 333-338.

[6] Borlongan, I. G, Coloso, R. M, Mosura, E. F, Sagisi, F. D, & Mosura, A. T. (1998). Molluscicidal activity of tobacco dust against brackishwater pond snails (*Cerithidea cingulata* Gmelin) Crop Protection. , 17(5), 401-404.

[7] Brouwer, M, Winge, D. R, & Gray, W. R. (1989). Structural and functional diversity of copper-metallothioneins from the american lobster *Homarus americanus*. Journal of Inorganic Biochemistry. , 35, 289-303.

[8] Brown, J. A, & Tytler, P. (1993). Hypoosmoregulation of larvae of the turbot, *Scophthalmus maximus:* Drinking and gut function in relation to environmental salinity. Fish Physiology and Biochemistry. , 10(6), 475-484.

[9] Butler, R. A, & Roesijadi, G. (2001). Quantitative reverse transcription polymerase chain reaction of a molluscan metallothionein mRNA. Aquatic Toxicology., 54(1-2), 59-67.

[10] Carpene, E, & George, S. G. (1981). Absorption of cadmium by gills of *Mytilus edulis* (L.). Molecular Physiology. , 1, 23-34.

[11] Coombs, T L, Fletcher, T, & White, A. (1972). Interaction of metal ions with mucus from the plaice, L. Biochemical Journal. , 128(4), 128-129.

[12] Cunha, M, Rodrigues, P, Soares, F, Makridis, P, Skjermo, J, & Dinis, M. T. (2003). Development of the immune system and use of immunostimulants in Senegalese sole (*Solea senegalensis*). In *The Big Fish Bang. Proceedings of the 26th Annual Larval Fish Conference* (Browman, H. I. & Skiftesvik, A. B., eds), Bergen: Institute of Marine Research., 189-192.

[13] Eisler, R. (1987). Polycyclic aromatic hydrocarbon hazards to fish, wildlife, and invertebrates: a synoptic review. U.S. Fish and Wildlife Service Biological Report 85(1.11).

[14] Fisher, S. W, Dabrowski, H, Waller, D. L, Babcokc- Jackson, L, & Zhang, X. (1994). Sensitivity of Zebra Mussels (*Dreissena polymorpha*) life stages to candidate molluscides. Journal of Shellfish Research. , 13, 373-377.

http://dx.doi.org/10.5772/55187

[15] George, S. G, Hodgson, P. A, Tytler, P, & Todd, K. (1996). Inducibility of metallothionein mRNA expression and cadmium tolerance in larvae of a marine teleost, the turbot (*Scophthalmus maximus*). Fundamentals of Applied Toxicology. , 33, 91-99.

[16] George, S, Burgess, D, Leaver, M, & Frenchs, N. (1992). Metallothionein induction in cultured fibroblasts and liver of a marine flatfish, the turbot. *Scophihalmus maximus.* Fish Physiology and Biochemistry. , 10, 43-54.

[17] George, S. G, & Olsson, P. E. (1994). Metallothioneins as indicators of trace metal pollution. In *Biological Monitoring of Coastal Waters and Estuaries* (K. J. M. Kramer. Ed.), CRC Press. Boca Raton FL, 151-178.

[18] Gopalakrishnan, S. (2008). Comparison of heavy metal toxicity in life stages (spermiotoxicity, egg toxicity, embryotoxicity and larval toxicity) of *Hydroides elegans*. Chemosphere. , 71, 515-528.

[19] Green, D. W. J, Williams, K. A, & Pascoe, D. (1986). The Acute and Chronic Toxicity of Cadmium to Different Life History Stages of the Freshwater Crustacean *Asellus aquaticus* (L) Archives of Environmental Contamination and Toxicology., 15(5), , 465-471.

[20] Hardersen, S, & Wratten, S. D. (2000). Sensitivity of aquatic life stages of *Xanthocnemis zealandica* (Odonata: Zygoptera) to azinphos-methyl and carbaryl. New Zealand Journal of Marine and Freshwater Research. , 34(1), 117-123.

[21] Herkovits, J, Cardellini, P, Pavanati, C, & Perez- Coll, C. S. (1997). Susceptibility of early life stages of Xenopus laevis to Cadmium. Environmental Toxicology and Chemistry. , 16(2), 312-316.

[22] Holditch, D. M, & Tolba, M. R. (1981). The effect of temperature and water quality on the *in vitro* development and survival of *A. aqaaticus* (Crustacea; Isopoda) eggs. Hydrobiologia. , 78(3), 227-236.

[23] Hilmy, A. M, Shabana, M. B, & Daabees, A. (1985). Bioaccumulation of cadmium: Toxicity in *Mugil Cephalus.* Comparative Biochemistry and Physiology. , 81(1), 139-143.

[24] Hoang, T. C, & Klaine, S. J. (2007). Influence of organism age on metal toxicity to *Daphnia magna.* Environmental Toxicology and Chemistry. , 26(6): 1198-1204,

[25] Hutchinson, T. H, Solbe, J, & Kloepper-sams, P. (1998). Analysis of the ecetoc aquatic toxicity (eat) database iii- comparative toxicity of chemical substances to different life stages of aquatic organisms. Chemosphere. , 36(1), 129-142.

[26] Jenkins, K. D, & Sanders, B. M. (1986). Relationships between free cadmium ion activity in sea water, cadmium accumulation and subcellular distribution, and growth in Polychaetes. Environmental Health Perspective. , 65, 205-210.

[27] Kennedy, A. J, Millward, R. N, & Steevens, J. A. Lynn, and. Perry, K.D.J.W. (2006). Relative sensitivity of zebra mussel (*Dreissena polymorpha*) life stages to two copper sources. Journal of Great Lakes Research. , 32, 596-606.

[28] Klaassen, C. D, Liu, J, & Choudhuri, S. (1999). Metallothionein:an intracellular protein to protect against cadmium toxicity. Annual Review of Pharmacology and Toxicology. , 39, 267-294.

[29] Kazlauskiene, N, & Stasiunaite, P. (1999). The lethal and sublethal effect of heavy metal mixture on rainbow trout (*Oncorhynchus mykiss*) in its early stages of development. Acta Zoologica Lituanica Hydrobiologia. , 9(2), 47-55.

[30] Laville, J. (1988). Age-Dependent Variation for Inducibility of Metallothionein Genes in Mouse Liver by Cadmium. Developmental Genetics. , 9(1), 13-22.

[31] Lotufo, G. R, & Fleeger, J. W. (1997). Effects of sediment-associated phenanthrene on survival, development and reproduction of two species of meiobenthic copepods. Marine Ecology Progress Series. , 151, 91-102.

[32] Macova, S, Dolezelova, P, Pistekova, V, Svobodova, Z, Bedanova, I, & Voslarova, E. (2008). Comparison of acute toxicity of 2-phenoxyethanol and clove oil to juvenile and embryonic stages of *Danio rerio*. Neuroendocrinology Letters. , 29, 680-684.

[33] Mason, A. Z, & Jenkins, K. D. (1995). Metal detoxification in aquatic organisms. In: Tessier, A., Turner, D.R. (Eds.), Metal Speciation and Bioavailability in Aquatic Systems. John Wiley and Sons Ltd., London. , 479-608.

[34] Middaugh, D. P, & Dean, J. M. (1977). Comparative sensitivity of eggs, larvae, and adults of the estuarine teleosts, *Fundulus heteroclitus* and *Menidia menidia* to cadmium. Bulletin of Environmental Contamination and Toxicology. , 17(6), 645-652.

[35] Mohammed, A, Halfhide, T, & Elias-samlalsingh, N. (2009). Comparative sensitivity of six toxicants of two life stages of the tropical mysid, *Metamysidopsis insularis*. Toxicology and Environmental Chemistry. , 97(7), 1331-1337.

[36] Oikari, A, Fragoso, N, Leppänen, H, Chan, T, & Hodson, P. V. (2002). Bioavailability to juvenile rainbow trout (Oncorynchus mykiss) of retene and other mixed-function oxygenase-active compounds from sediments. Environmental Toxicology and Chemistry. , 21(1), 121-8.

[37] Ozoh, P. T. E. (1979). Malformations and inhibitory tendencies induced to *Brachydanio rerio* (Hamilton-Buchanan) eggs and larvae due to exposures in low concentrations of lead and copper ions. Bulletin of Environmental Contamination and Toxicology. , 21(1), 668-675.

[38] Padrós, F, Villalta, M, Gisbert, E, & Estévez, A. (2011). Morphological and histological study of larval development of the Senegal sole Solea senegalensis: an integrative study. Journal of Fish Biology. , 79(1), 3-32.

[39] Plhalová, L, Mácová, S, Doleželová, P, Maršálek, P, Svobodová, Z, Pišteková, V, Bedánová, I, Voslárová, E, & Modrá, H. (2010). Comparison of Terbutryn Acute Toxicity to *Danio rerio* and *Poecilia reticulata.* Acta Veteriniaria Brno. , 79, 593-598.

[40] Ringwood, A. M. (1990). The Relative Sensitivities of Different Life Stages of *Isognomon californicum* to Cadmium Toxicity. Archives of Environmental Contamination and Toxicology. , 19(3), 338-340.

[41] Roesijadi, G, & Fellingham, G. W. (1987). Influence of Cu, Cd and Zn pre-exposure on Hg toxicity in the mussel *Mytilus edulis*. Canadian Journal of Fisheries and Aquatic Science. , 44(3), 680-684.

[42] Roesijadi, G. (1996). Metallothionein and its role in toxic metal regulation. Comparative Biochemistry and Physiology C. , 113(2), 117-123.

[43] Roesijadi, G. (1992). Metallothioneins in metal regulation and toxicity in aquatic animals. Aquatic Toxicology. , 22(2), 81-114.

[44] Schmieder, P. K, Jensen, K. M, Johnson, R. D, & Tietge, J. E. (2000). Comparative sensitivity of different life-stages of medaka and salmonid fishes to 2,3,7,8-TCDD. Presented at International Symposium on Endocrine-Disrupting Substances Testing in Medaka, Nagoya, Japan, March , 17-20.

[45] Sassi, A, Darias, M. J, Said, K, Messaoudi, I, & Gisbert, E. (2012). Cadmium exposure affects the expression of genes involved in skeletogenesis and stress response in gilthead sea bream larvae. Fish Physiology and Biochemistry (Epub ahead of print) http://link.springer.com/article/10.1007%2Fs10695-012-9727-9?LI=trueAccessed November 17th 2012

[46] Scott, G. R, Sloman, K. A, Rouleau, C, & Wood, C. M. (2003). Cadmium disrupts behavioural and physiological responses to alarm substance in juvenile rainbow trout (*Oncorhynchus mykiss*). The Journal of Experimental Biology., 206(11), 1779-1790.

[47] Segner, H, Storch, V, Reinecke, M, Kloas, W, & Hanke, W. (1994). The development of functional digestive and metabolic organs in turbot. *Scophthalmus maximus.* Marine Biology. , 119(3), 471-486.

[48] Shailaja, M. S, & Silva, D. C. (2003). Evaluation of impact of PAH on a tropical fish, *Oreochromis mossambicus* using multiple biomarkers. Chemosphere., 53, 835-841.

[49] Tuvikene, A. (1995). Responses of fish to Polycyclic aromatic hydrocarbons (PSHs). Annales Zoologici Fennici., 32, 295-309.

[50] Tytler, P, & Bell, M. V. (1989). A study of diffusional permeability of water, sodium and chloride in yolk-sac larvae of cod (*Gadus morhua* L.). Journal of Experimental Biology. , 147, 125-132.

[51] Tytler, P, & Blaxter, J. H. S. (1988). Drinking in yolk-sac halibut *Hippoglossus hippoglossus.* Journal of Fish Biology., 32(3), , 493-494.

[52] Tytler, P, & Ireland, J. (1994). Drinking and water absorption by the larvae of herring *(Clupea harengus)* and the turbot *(Scophthalmus maximus)*. Journal of Fish Biology. , 44(1), 103-116.

[53] Viarengo, A, & Nott, J. A. (1993). Mechanisms of heavy metal cation homeostasis in marine invertebrates. Comparative Biochemistry and Physiology C. , 104(3), 355-372.

[54] Verriopoulos, G, & Morai, M. tou-Apostolopoulou. (1982). Differentiation of the Sensitivity to Copper and Cadmium in Different Life Stages of a Copepod. Marine Pollution Bulletin. , 13(4), 123-125.

[55] Weis, J. S. (2005). Does pollution affect fisheries? Book critique. Environmental Biology of Fishes. , 72(3), 357-359.

[56] Williams, K. A, Green, D. W. J, Pascoe, D, & Gower, D. E. (1986). The acute toxicity of cadmium to different larval stages of *Chironomus riparius* (Diptera: Chironomidae) and its ecological significance for pollution regulation. Oecologia (Berlin). , 70, 362-366.

[57] Zafarullah, M, Olsson, P. E, & Gedamu, L. (1989). Endogenous and heavy metal-ion-induced metallothionein gene expression in salmonid tissues and cell lines. Gene., 83(1), 85-93.

[58] Zaroogian, G, & Jackim, E. (2000). In vivo metallothionein and glutathione status in an acute response to cadmium in *Mercenaria mercenaria* brown cells. Comparative Biochemistry and Physiology C. , 127(3), 251-261.

[59] Zhang, W, Huang, L, & Wang, W. X. (2012). Biotransformation and detoxification of inorganic arsenic in a marine juvenile fish *Terapon jarbua* after waterborne and dietborne exposure. Journal of Hazardous Materials., 221-222:162-9

Chapter 4

Screening of Herbal Medicines for Potential Toxicities

Obidike Ifeoma and Salawu Oluwakanyinsola

Additional information is available at the end of the chapter

http://dx.doi.org/10.5772/54493

1. Introduction

1.1. Herbal medicines in the 21st century

Herbs and herb-derived medicines have played a crucial role in health and disease management for many centuries. Many ancient civilizations show documented evidence for the use of herbs in the treatment of different ailments; as was seen with Mesopotamian, Indian ayurveda, ancient traditional Chinese medicine and Greek unani medicine [1-5]. In Africa, knowledge of traditional medicine as part of wholistic system, was passed through generations by oral communication and indigenous practices [6]. The global demand for herbal medicinal products has increased significantly in recent years. It is estimated that, the world's population will be more than 7.5 billion in the next 10 to 15 years. This increase in population will occur mostly in the southern hemisphere, where approximately 80% of the population still relies on a traditional system of medicine based on herbal drugs for primary healthcare [7].

Use of plants for medicinal purposes is as old as human civilization [8] and continuous efforts [8-17] are being made towards its improvement. About 200,000 natural products of plant origin are known and many more are being identified from higher plants and microorganisms [18-21]. Some plant-based drugs have been used for centuries and for some like cardiac glycosides, there is no alternative conventional medicine. Therefore, medicinal plants and their bioactive molecules are always in demand and are a central point of research. As a result, there is a recent [22] surge in the demand for herbal medicine.

To date, herbs have remained useful not only as remedy for different diseases that affect humans and animals, but also as good starting points for the discovery of bioactive molecules for drug development. The scientific exploitation of herbs used ethnomedicinally for pain relief, wound healing and abolishing fevers has resulted in the identification of a wide range of compounds that have been developed as new therapies for cancer, hypertension, diabetes and as anti-infectives [23]. The ealriest report of the toxicity of herbs originated from Galen, a Greek pharmacist and physician who showed that herbs do not contain only medicinally beneficial constituents, but may also be constituted with harmful substances. [24].

By 2003 in the United States alone, over 1500 herbal products sold were nutraceuticals which are exempt from extensive preclinical efficacy and toxicity testing by the U.S. Food and Drug Administration [25]. This has led to increased concerns about potential harmful effect of these products, which has resulted in efforts to globally harmonize standards of toxicity testing methods that can be used for herbal medicine toxicological characterization including tests for acute high-dose exposure effects, chronic low-dose toxicity tests and specific cellular, organ and system-based toxicity assays. This chapter reviews some of these tests and their applications. Recent biotechnological advancements have rapidly evolved toxicity test methods at molecular and sub cellular levels including next generation sequencing and computer-based modeling and simulation tools which have been used to predict the potential toxicity of novel drug candidates and in some cases, herbal medicine toxicities which may arise from herbs administered alone or concomitantly with other herbs and/or drugs. However, challenges still exist for testing herbal medicines in this exciting field and these will also be discussed.

2. Toxicity of herbs

Despite the growing market demand for herbal medicines, there are still concerns associated with not only their use, but their safety. Less than 10% of herbal products in the world market are truly standardized to known active components and strict quality control measures are not always diligently adhered to [26]. For majority of these products in use, very little is known about their active and/or toxic constituents. In many countries including the U.S, herbal medicines are not subjected to the same regulatory standards as orthodox drugs in terms of efficacy and safety. This raises concern on their safety and implications for their use as medicines. Toxicity testing can reveal some of the risks that may be associated with use of herbs, therefore avoiding potential harmful effects when used as medicine.

In addition, many plants produce toxic secondary metabolites as natural defence from adverse conditions. In some toxicologically and medicinally relevant plant species like *Digitalis purpurea, Hyoscyamus niger, Atropa belladonna, Physostigma venenosum, Podophyllum peltatum* and *Solanum nigrum,* these toxic substances are not distinguished from therapeutically active ingredients. Being stationary autotrophs, plants have evolved different means of adaptation to challenging environments and co-existence with herbivores and pathogenic microorganisms. Thus, they synthesize an array of metabolites characterized as 'phytoanticipins' or as general 'phytoprotectants' that are stored in specialized cellular compartments and released in response to specific environmental stimuli like damage due to herbivores, pathogens or nutrient depletion [27]. Some of the phytochemicals produced by plants against herbivorous insects also end up being harmful to humans, because highly conserved biological similarities are shared between both taxa as seen in most pathways involving protein, nucleic acid,

http://dx.doi.org/10.5772/54493

carbohydrate and lipid metabolism [28]. Human neurochemicals, often with similar biological functions are also reportedly present in insects [28]. These incude signalling molecules, neuropeptides, hormones and neurotransmitters [29-32]; whose functions can be mimicked or antagonized by phytochemicals like alkaloids, flavonoids, terpenoids and saponins. Ecologically, a good number of alkaloids serve as feeding deterrents via agonistic or agonistic activity on neurotransmitter systems [33]. Similarly, some lipid soluble terpenes have shown inhibitory properties against mammalian cholinesterase [34], whilst some interact with the GABAergic system in vertebrates [35]. In addition to these, saponins are potent surfactants that can disrupt lipid-rich cellular membranes of human erythrocytes and microorganisms which explains the potent antimicrobial properties of this group of phytochemicals [36]. Aristolochic acid, a nitrophenanthrene carboxylic acid in *Aristolochia* species and present in some other botanicals has also been identified as a phytochemical toxicant implicated in the development of nephropathies and carcinogenesis [37].

Another implication in the toxicity of certain herbs is the presence of toxic minerals and heavy metals like mercury, arsenic, lead and cadmium [38]. Lead and mercury can cause serious neurological impaiment when a herbal medicinal product contaminated with these metals is ingested. As shown in Table 1, the presence of high levels of arsenic in kelp seaweed may result in toxicosis in some patients [39].

3. Goals of toxicity testing of herbal drugs

The primary aim of toxicological assessment of any herbal medicine is to identify adverse effects and to determine limits of exposure level at which such effects occur. Two important factors which are taken into consideration in evaluating the safety of any herbal drug are the nature and significance of the adverse effect and in addition, the exposure level where the effect is observed. Toxicity testing can reveal some of the risks that may be associated with use of herbs especially in sensitive populations.

An equally important objective of toxicity testing is the detection of toxic plant extracts or compounds derived thereof in the early (pre-clinical) and late (clinical) stages of drug discovery and development from plant sources. This will facilitate the identification of toxicants which can be discarded or modified during the process and create an opportuinity for extensive evaluation of safer, promising alternatives [54]. For certain compounds, modifications such as dosage reduction, chemical group or structural adjustments may improve their tolerability.

3.1. Pre-clinical toxicity testing of herbs

This covers a range of toxicity tests done in non-human experimental models before conducting clinical tests for toxic effects in humans. Generally these tests are classified into non-animal tests and animal studies. Crude extracts or purified compounds obtained by fractionation of the medicinal herb can be evaluated in these tests.

Common name	**Plant source/parts used**	**Intended indications**	**Potential toxicity**
Ginseng	*Panax ginseng* roots	Relieves stress, promotes mental and physical activity	Central nervous system stimulation, hypertension, skin eruptions [40]
St. John's wort	*Hypericum perforatum* aerial parts	Antidepressant, mood stabilizer	Highly potent cytochrome P450 enzyme inducer which affects drug metabolism. Also causes hepatotoxicity and nephrotoxicity in pregnancy and lactation [41]
Kava kava	*Piper methysticum* roots	Sedative, anxiolytic	Hepatotoxic, cytochrome P450 enzyme inhibitor [42]
Ginkgo	*Ginkgo biloba* leaves	Impotence, vertigo, circulatory disorders, improves mental alertness	Gastric irritability, spontaneeous bleeding [43]
Danshen	*Salvia miltiorrhiza* exterior taproot	Angina pectoris, antihyperlipidemic, ischemic stroke	Bleeding, anticoagulant effects [44]
Hawthorn	*Crataegus oxycantha* Flowers, roots, berries	Mild to moderate congestive heart failure	Cardiac arrythmias, lowered blood pressure [45]
Comfrey	*Symphytum officinale* leaves	Anti inflammatory, antidiarrhoel and treatment of thrombophlebitis	Hepatotoxicity, carcinogenicity [46]
Licorice	*Glycyrrhiza glabra* roots	Antiulcer, anti inflammatory, antihypertensive	Hypokalemic myopathy, pseudoaldosteronism, thrombocytopenia [47]
Chaparral, creosote bush	*Larrea tridentata* leaves and twigs	Blood thinner, weight loss, antioxidant, anticancer, anti arthritis	Carcinogenic, nephrotoxic, hepatotoxic [48]
Mistletoe	*Phoradendron spp., Viscum album* leaves and young twigs	Digestive aid, heart tonic, sedative	Hypotension, seizures [49]
Squill	*Urginea maritima* bulbs	Anti-arthritic, bronchial expectorant	Symptoms resembling digitalis toxicity [50]
Kelp (seaweed)	*Liminaria digitata*	Metabolic tonic, thyroid tonic, anti inflammatory	Arsenic poisoning, Hyperthyroidism [39]
Ma-huang	*Ephedra*	Promotes weight loss, mental and physical alertness	Cardiotoxicity, thyrotoxicosis, seizures [51]
Senna	*Senna occidentalis* seeds	Laxative	Skeletal and cardiac muscle degeneration, hepatotoxicity, neurotoxicity [52]
Aloe	*Aloe vera* leaves	Wound healing, laxative	Cytogenetic toxicity [53]

Table 1. Potential toxic effects associated with some common herbal medicines marketed for different indications

http://dx.doi.org/10.5772/54493

3.2. Cell-based cytotoxicity tests

Cytotoxicity assays (CTAs) are performed to predict potential toxicity, using cultured cells which may be normal or transformed cells. These tests normally involve short term exposure of cultured cells to test substances, to detect how basal or specialized cell functions may be affected by the substance, prior to performing safety studies in whole organisms. It can also provide insight towards the carcinogenic and genotoxic dispositions of herb-derived compounds and extracts. The ability of a plant extract to inhibit cellular growth and viability can also be ascertained as an indication of its toxicity. Assessment parameters for cytotoxic effects include inhibition of cell proliferation, cell viability markers (metabolic and membrane), morphologic and intracellular differentiation markers [55]. In conducting CTAs, it is important to critically consider factors such as cell culture systems and methods which affect test outcomes. For example, some cell types maybe incompatible with the solvent used to prepare test solutions. Many plant extracts and compounds are non-polar and prepared as solutions in dimethylsulfoxide (DMSO) prior to CTAs. DMSO has been reported to be cytotoxic at certain concentrations [56] and this effect varies between cell types. Therefore, it is often necessary to pre-determine the maximum tolerable solvent concentration in CTAs especially during validatory stages, and a control using the carrier solvent alone must be used in the CTA.

CTAs are indispensible tools for medium and high throughput screens of different phytochemicals simultaneously, over wide concentration ranges. In addition, they have significant impact in the implementation of the three R's namely; the reduction of number of animals used, refinement of animal test models and replacement of animal in research.

As a herbal product may display cytotoxic effects only against specific cell types, it is important to consider the selection of a wide range of cell types for testing including normal cells of primary origin (usually from rodents), and permanent cell lines; provided they are of high quality and are reproducible over time [57].

CTAs which employ rodent cell lines like the mouse fibroblast cell line BALB/c 3T3 and the Syrian Hamster Embryo cells (SHE, pH 6.7 and pH 7) are robust models for the prediction of genotoxicity and carcinogenity. The tests have been shown to be highly predictive, as inoculation of transformed cells into x-ray irradiated mice induces tumorigenicity. Furthermore, there are no limitations with specific classes of chemicals and formulations that can be tested with these assays as it has been reported to be plausible in the assessment of nanoparticles [58]. Although the applicability of these assays in testing complex mixtures like herbal products is often hindered by non-availability of sufficient evidence in this regard, it is still useful in predicting their toxic effects so long it is makes sufficient contact with the cells [59].

In the BALB/c 3T3 assay, foci scoringis based on the level of malignant transformation, with type III classified as malignantly transformed, according to a previous classification used for cytotoxicity assays involving C3H10T1/2 cells [61]

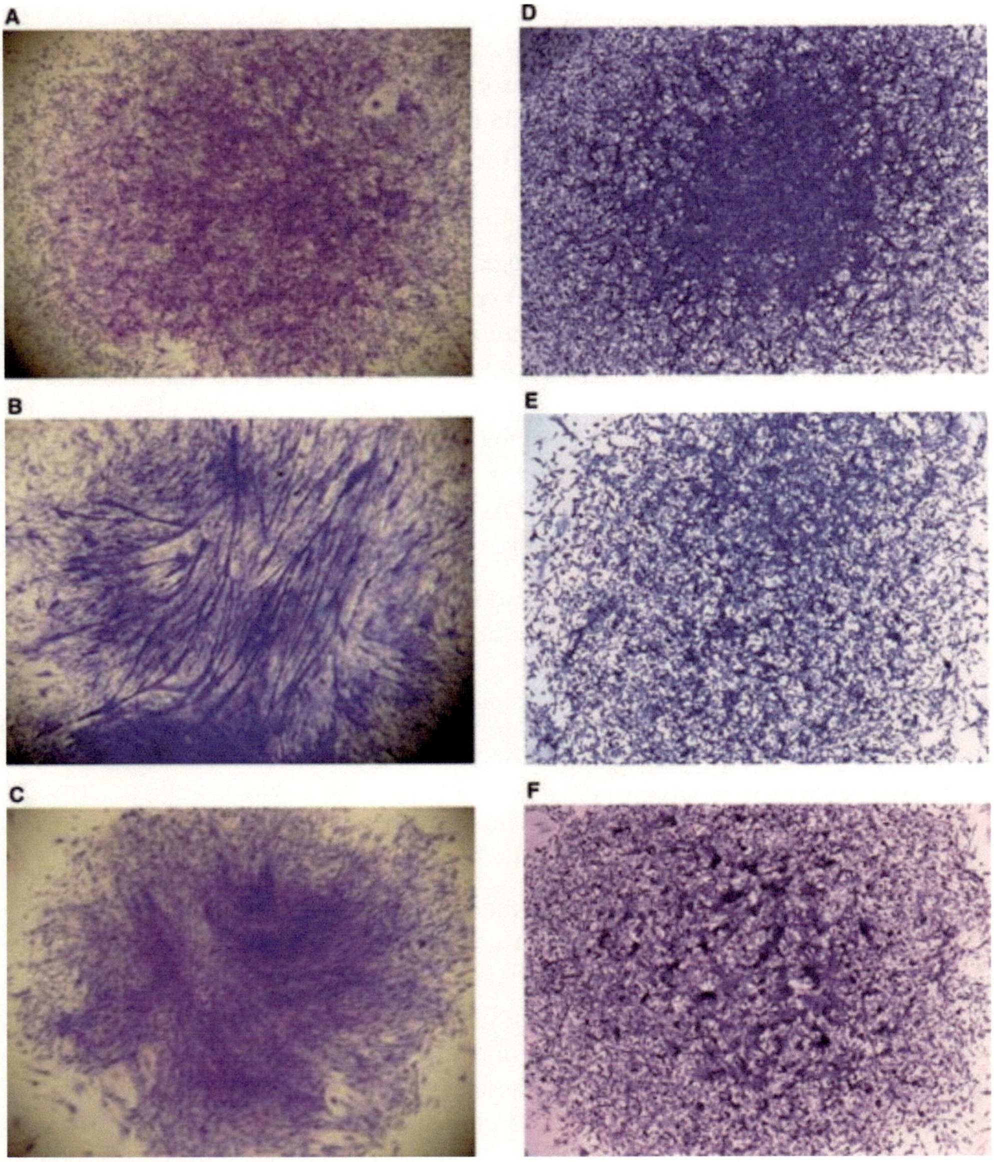

Figure 1. Examples of normal and transformed SHE cells. Plates A, B, C show normal colonies of cells organized in monolayers with no criss-crossing. Plates D, E, F show morphologically transformed colonies comprising stacked cells that are randomly oriented, three-dimensional and criss-crossed throughout; basophilic staining is usually darker. Magnification ×125 [60]

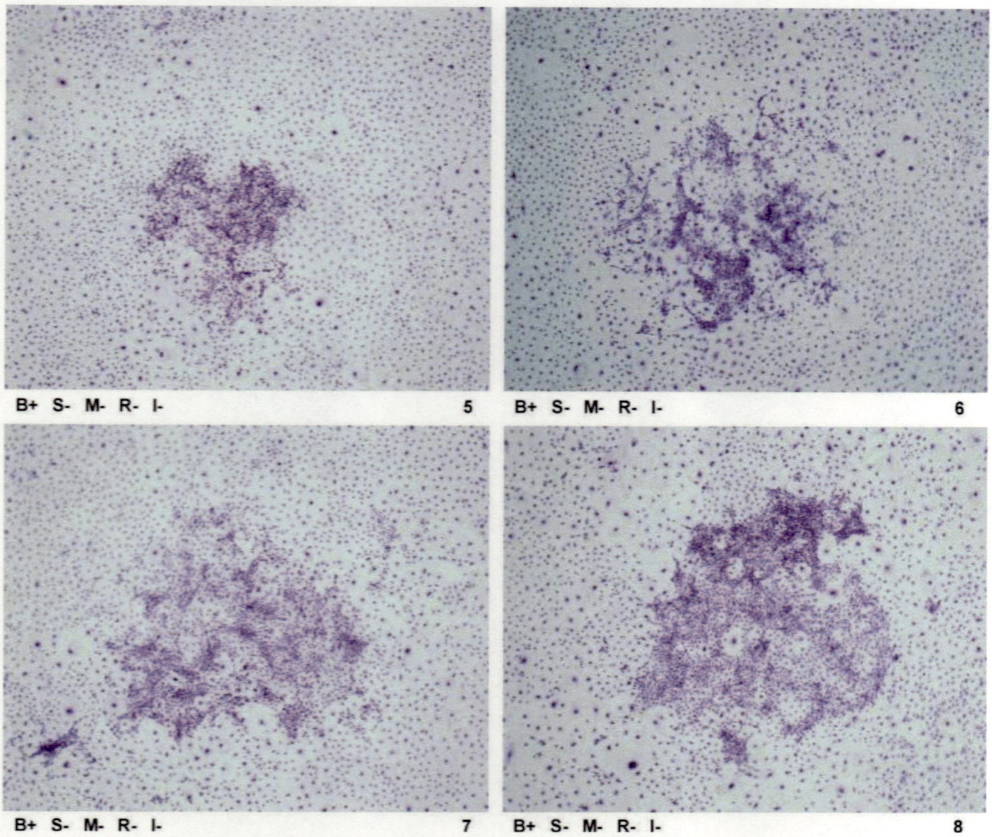

Figure 2. Type I foci: small, non invasive BALB/c 3T3 cells with weak basophilic staining. Under each picture in the catalogue, the characteristics are described as basophilic (B), spindle-shaped (S), multilayer (M), random orientation (R), invasive (I) and were evaluated as absent (–), weak (+/–) present (+), or strong (++). Magnification ×50 [62]

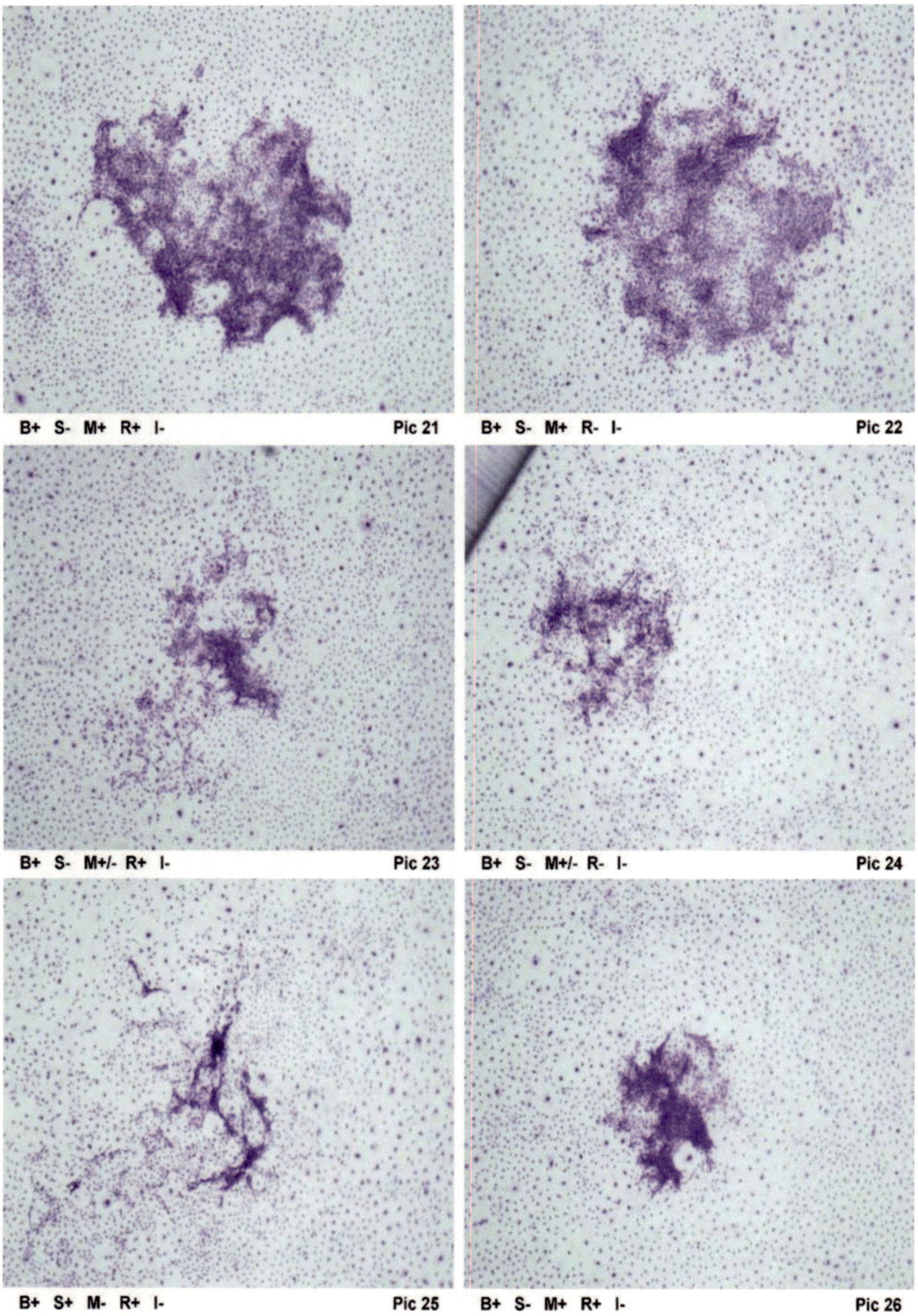

Figure 3. Type II foci: densely packed multi-layered cells, some cells pile up and are criss-crossed. Magnification ×50 [62]

http://dx.doi.org/10.5772/54493

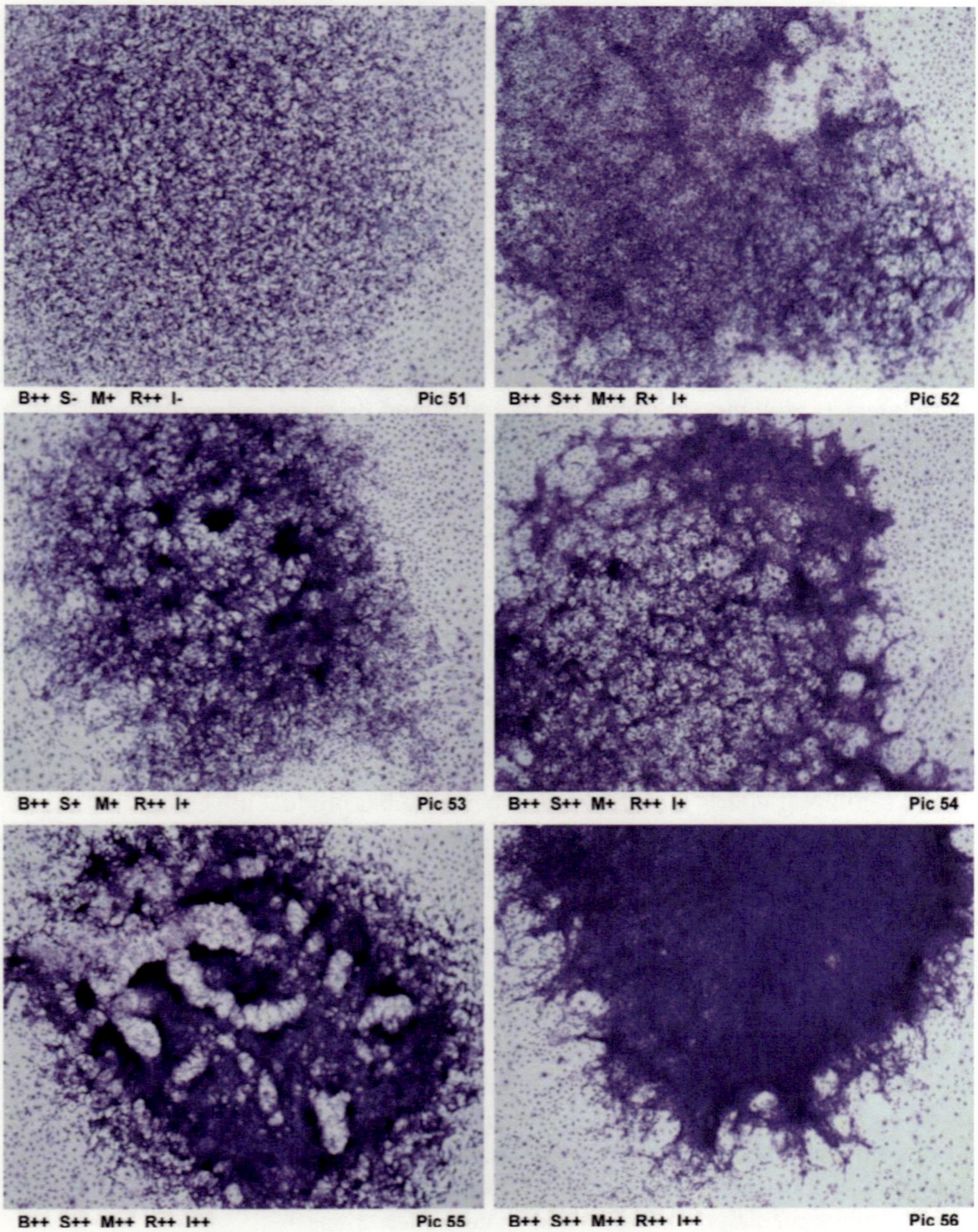

Figure 4. Type III foci: Malignantly transformed colony of morphologically different spindle-shaped cells. Cells are densely multi-layered and criss-crossed. Cells are randomly oriented and grow invasively at foci edge. Magnification ×50 [62]

3.3. Herbal toxicokinetics

Herbal toxicokinetics deals with the prediction of toxicity due to pharmacokinetic disposition of an herb, or purified xenobiotics derived from it, due to genetics or from potential herb-drug interactions [63] Testing usually begins with assays using human liver microsomal Cytochrome P450 isoforms to identify early enough, metabolites which are known to cause toxicological modulation at any level of cellular organization. Modulation of Cytochrome P450 has great significance as this largely affects drug biotransformation to active or inactive forms. For a drug that is dependent on these enzymes for inactivation via conjugation to chemical polar groups prior to elimination, any herb that induces these enzymes would lead to rapid inactivation and clearance of such a drug. Converesly, a herbal medicine that inhibits enzyme activity will lead to high concentrations of a drug whose inactivation relies on the inhibited enzyme. From findings in a recent survey [64], potential adverse drug herb interactions were observed in 40 % of patients receiving conventional therapy and taking a herbal product. Clinically significant drug-herb interactions may occur when an herb interacts with metabolism of a co-administered drug and either reduces its efficacy due to decreased formation of an active metabolite or increases its toxicity due to reduced metabolic elimination. The latter type of interaction potentially predisposes human consumers to adverse reactions or toxic drug effects, especially if the drug has a narrow therapeutic range. This is important because, approximately 73 % of all known drugs are metabolized hepatically by mixed function oxidation reactions, catalyzed by Cytochrome P450 enzymes [65]. Of all its isoforms, CYP3A4, CYP2C9, CYP2C19, CYP1A2 and CYP2D6 are implicated in over 80 % of oxidative drug reactions and are highly subject to inhibition owing to their broad specificity for structurally diverse substrates [66]. Some herbs, notably St. John's Wort (*Hypericum perforatum*), ginkgo (*Ginkgo biloba*), ginseng (*Panax ginseng*), kava (*Piper methysticum*) and garlic (*Allium sativum*) reportedly show significant interaction with some co-administered drugs by modulation of Cytochrome P450 [67]. In order to predict clinically significant effects that can occur when a herbal product inhibits or induces these enzymes, *in vitro* metabolic data can be used to correlate metabolic disposition of a test substance *in vivo* [68].

From the early 1990s onwards, new techniques for generating as much information as possible from one experiment were developed including DNA sequencing, microarrays to study gene expression, protein and metabolite profiling [69]. Further structure-activity relationship of metabolites or pure compounds can be extrapolated from computer-based models and simulation studies. Thereafter, pattern databases of tissue/organ response to drugs which allows for the parallel sequencing of all the relevant genes, measurement of genome transcription, protein expression and quantitation of metabolites produced by direct or indirect actions of the expressed protein. A final screening category for the compound or metabolite utilizes an integrative system biology approach; comprising databases of metabolic pathways, genes, regulatory networks and protein interactions [69].

Despite the high efficiency of these techniques, no single approach is sufficient to predict toxicokinetics *in silico* and harnessing the different assays will be effective in predicting metabolic fate of the test molecule in humans.

3.4. Toxicogenomic screening tools

Herbal toxicogenomics is a collective term that refers to the combination of toxicology with different '–omics' tools that measure the potential toxic outcomes of interactions of the herbal extract or compounds at sub molecular (epigenomics, transcriptomics), molecular (proteomics), cellular, tissue and organ (metabonomics) levels [70]. It is aimed at elucidating molecular mechanisms involved in the expression of toxicity, and to derive molecular patterns (i.e. molecular biomarkers) that predict toxicity or the individual susceptibility to it.

There are three major aspects within this field as outlined below:

DNA microarrays: These are carried out using specially designed microarrays. They usually provide the most information, providing not only clear prediction of cellular response to chemical toxicants, but also mechanisms through which such toxicity is elicited [71]. For an herbal mixture with a diversity of chemical entities, the data obtained cannot usually be extrapolated to that of data libraries of existing chemical compounds.

Proteomics: This high throughput screening tool is applied in protein identification. It is a sequential process of peptide separation and profiling, followed by mass spectrometry and NMR detection. Based on the assumption that a chemically related group of xenobiotics exhibit specific patterns of protein expression, only purified phytochemicals with known chemical structures can have their protein expression profiles correlated to existing databases of those of xenobiotics. The use of proteomics has been considered more advantageous than microarrays which assess gene expression, because they measure proteins which are closer to toxicology endpoints, as not all genes are translated to proteins and expressed proteins are liable to structural changes post-translation [72].

Metabonomics: This is an aspect of toxicity evaluation, performed through the large scale analysis of metabolic profiles of metabolic enzymes and metabolite composition resulting from the action of chemical stressors. This can be a very efficient approach as it can be applied in *in vitro* metabolic profiling, in animal toxicity tests for promising lead selection and in humans during clinical stages of safety testing for the development of biomarkers of safety [73].

3.5. High throughput next generation sequencing

Molecular studies have witnessed rapid developments since DNA was first sequenced in 1997 [74] to the creation of large volumes of DNA sequences at unprecedented speed; also referred to as next generation sequencing (NGS). Apart from its application in personalized medicine, it has also been applied in the creation of large genetic databases of plants, which can serve in the identification of potentially toxic plants, or those that may contain allergens. For example if functional gene transcriptomes present in Aristolochia species are found present in another specie under investigation, it is likely that such a specie may contain aristolochic acid. NGS technology has already been applied in unravelling the genome of Gingko [75] and holds potential for biomarking toxicity in the 21st century.

3.6. Animal tests

The whole animal is usually presumed to be closely correlated to human toxicity as the system incorporates pharmacokinetic (absorption, distribution, metabolism) disposition of the test substance when administered by a route similar to its intended use. It also takes into consideration, other physiological events in an organism that influence toxicity. While cell-based assays measure is predictive of potential toxicity, the whole animal experiment measures the critical toxicity of a test substance, which are the signs of toxicity that manifest as a result of a gradual increase in the dose of the test substance.

Certain drawbacks to animal testing however do exist; the costs of the animals to be used can be prohibitive and subtle differences within species can affect the type of effects that are observed and they are usually more tedious to arrange, in terms of duration of experiments.

4. General tests

Standard guidelines for the conduct of animal toxicity tests have been harmonized by the Organization for Economic Co-operation and Development [76] as part of continuous efforts to internationally harmonize test guidelines.

Before conducting safety study of an herb or its product in animals, some major factors that need to be considered are:

Preparation of test substane: Herbal products can be prepared into different dosage forms like capsules, tablets, ointments, creams and pastes. For correct administration of a pre-defined dose of the product, the product should be quantitatively standardized and administered based on its intended use in humans.

Animal welfare considerations: Guidance on the use of clinical signs as humane end-points for experimental animals used in safety evaluation [77] have been reviewed elsewhere and the reader is advised to look it up. In particular paragraph 62 of the guideline thereof, should always be followed. This paragraph states that "In studies involving repeated dosing, when an animal shows clinical signs that are progressive, leading to further deterioration in condition, an informed decision as to whether or not to humanely kill the animal should be made. The decision should include consideration as to the value of the information to be gained from the continued maintenance of that animal on study relative to its overall condition. If a decision is made to leave the animal on test, the frequency of observations should be increased, as needed. It may also be possible, without adversely affecting the purpose of the test, to temporarily stop dosing if it will relieve the pain or distress, or reduce the test dose."

Animals: Different rodent and non-rodent species are used in animal toxicity tests. In chronic studies, justification is often required for choice of specie or strain of animals used. All animals should be housed in acceptable environmental conditions and adequately catered for in accordance with stipulated guidelines [78].

http://dx.doi.org/10.5772/54493

Regulatory requirements: An independent animal ethics committee usually reviews, approves and supervises animal experiments and ensures that the experiment is well justified and in agreement with provisions for animal welfare. These regulations may differ, dependingon different countries, but basic requirements to be met remain unchanged.

4.1. Acute systemic toxicity

This test measures relative toxicological response of an experimental organism to single or brief exposure to a test substance [79]. Test organisms range from simple systems like brine shrimp to other animals like mice, rats, guinea pigs and rabbits. This test is also used to calculate median lethal dose (LD_{50}) of a substance, using various standardised methods including Lorke's and acute toxic class methods [79, 80]. Exposure routes may be by oral gavage, inhalation/mucosal, dermal; or by injection into the bloodstream, abdomen, or the muscles. Following administration of a test product, animals are observed individually at least once during the first 30 minutes, periodically during the first 24 hours, with special attention given during the first 4 hours, and daily thereafter, for a total of 14 days in the case of delayed toxicities [79]

4.2. Sub-acute/sub-chronic toxicity

This is repeat-dose study performed to expose any deleterious changes in organ, haematological and biochemical indices that may arise in the course of repeated administration of a test substance, usually ranges from weeks to a few months. The terms 'sub-acute' toxicity and 'sub chronic' toxicity can be differentiated on the basis of exposure, the former having a duration period of one month (28-30 days) and the latter ranging from two to three months (60-90 days). The test product or compound is usually administered daily throughout the test period and at the end of the study, data generated will include general parameters such as daily food consumption and water intake measurements and body weight measurements. Other specific endpoints of toxicity assessed will additionally include serum biochemical parameters (Lipid, protein, urea, creatinine, electrolytes, liver transaminases and phosphatase), enzymatic and non-enzymatic liver oxidative stress indicators (thiobarbituric acid reactive substances, reduced glutathione, catalase) and haematological parameters (white blood cells and differentials, red blood cells, haemoglobin, haematocrit, platelets, lymphocytes). Various organs are examined for gross pathological changes and tissue slices obtained from respective organs are prepared for detailed histological examination.

Results of many sub chronic toxicity tests of various plant extracts showed that the major organs usually affected are the liver and kidneys. Hepatotoxic and nephrotoxic effects are mostly to be expected, as the liver acts as the main detoxifying organ for chemical substances, while the kidney is a principal route of excretion for many chemical substances in their active and/or inactive forms [81].

Liver injury associated with the use of herbal medicine ranges from mild elevation of liver enzymes to fulminant liver failure often requiring a new transplant; and carcinogenesis [63]. Established hepatotoxic phytochemicals include podophyllin, eugenol, neoclerodane diterpenes, among others [83-88].

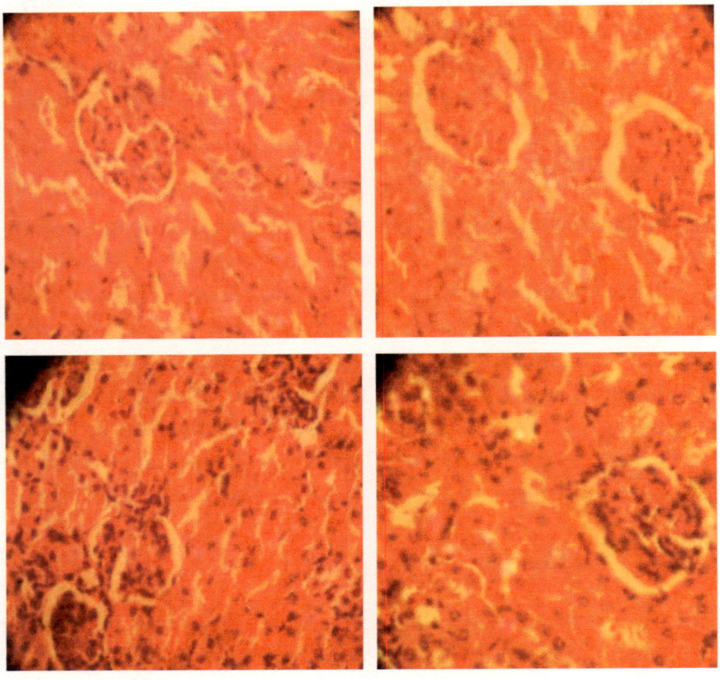

Figure 5. Clockwise from top left: Photomicrographs (×400) of kidney tissue slices from rats treated with (a) aqueous vehicle, (b) 25, (c) 50 and (d) 100 mgkg-1 body weight Hymenocardia acida ethanol leaf extract. Fig. 5a shows normal tubular architecture while Fig. 5b, c and d show alterations ranging from mild cortical oedema to tubular distortions. [82].

5. Chronic toxicity/carcinogenity

Chronic toxicity testing is similar to sub chronic studies except that they are conducted with a larger number of animals to reveal toxicity which may arise during exposure to a substance for a 24 months or for an entire lifespan. Oral, dermal or inhalation are the main routes used here, depending on the intended use in humans. In these long-term studies, mutagenic/carcinogenic propensities of test substances and likely organs where they may accumulate are revealed. End points of toxicity which are studied include dose limits of toxicity, that is, the lowest dose at which no toxicity occurs or no observed adverse effect level (NOAEL), mortality, food consumotion, water intake, hematology and clinical biochemistry measurement, organ gross necropsy ang histopathology. Further informmation on study design and execution can be found in OECD draft guidance document on the design and conduct of chronic toxicity and carcinogenicity studies [89].

5.1. Specialized tests

These are tests suited to reveal specific toxicities, such as reproductive toxicity, developmental toxicity, eye and skin irritancy test (Draize test), neurotoxicity and Genotoxicity.

http://dx.doi.org/10.5772/54493

Ocular/Skin irritancy test:

Named after a US food and Drug Scientist, John Draize, this test was developed in the mid-nineteenth century. Eye and skin irritancy tests involve the topical application of the test substance; usually in rabbit cornea or skin. Irritancy is reversible in nature and distinguished from corrosion which is irreversible. This test has become unpopular due in part to the percieved cruelty to the rabbit its very subjective scoring system, leading to poor reproducibility and high variablility between laboratories [90]. A recently developed short term exposure test using Statens Seruminstitut Rabbit Cornea (SIRC) cells has been demonstrated to be a potential alternative for eye irritancy test in rabbits [91].

Neurotoxicity:

Neurological effects such as convulsions may arise followed acute systemic exposure to some phytomedicines; while cerebrovascular accident, encephalopathy and psychosis can become evident in sub acute, sub chronic and chronic tests for toxicity. It is important to note that the presence of high levels of metals in the herbal medicine can contribute to neurotoxicity [92]. Microbial biosorptive removal using granulated *Cladosporum cladosporioides* and chelation with dithizone have been shown to be effective in removing heavy metal contaminants from herbal extracts [93, 94].

Genotoxicity:

Genotoxicity is a special area in toxicities, as it is often the most difficult to detect. It may be defined as a chemically induced mutation or alteration of the structure and/or segregation of genetic material.Recently, a guidance document on the assessment of genotoxcicity of herbal preparations has been drafted by the European Medicines Agency [95]. The first stage utilizes the Ames test with *S. typhimurium*, although some potent genotoxins like Taxol (*Taxus brevifolia*) and vincristine (*Catharanthus roseaus*) are not reliably identified at this stage and some products rich in flavonoids like quercetin may give false positives. More reliable tests like the mouse micronucleus test and mouse lymphoma assay (MLA) can be used more definitively [95].

Reproductive/developmental toxicity studies:

These studies were developed after it was discovered thousands of offspring of women who used the new drug thalidomide to treat morning sickness were born with serious birth defects [96]. It was later proposed that the drug acts by decreasing transcription efficiency of the genes responsible for angiogenesis in the developing limb bud of the foetus, resulting in truncation of the limb [97]. In designing these tests, a large number of animals are used, which are dosed repeatedly with escalating doses of the herbal test substance before mating, during gestation and after delivery up to the entire lifetime of the new offspring to detect effects of the herb on reproductive performance and/or developing offspring. Toxicity endpoints include spontaneous abortion, premature delivery, and birth defects.

In addition to the use of rodents, research in reproductive and developmental toxicity of traditional Chinese medicine incorporates other animal models like zebrafish and roundworm models and stem cell cultures [98].

5.2. Clinical testing: Clinical/safety trials

After sufficient preliminary investigation showing the safety of an herbal product in pre-clinical studies, further studies can then be initiated in human participants. These type of studies are called clinical trials (CTs) and are carried out in four phases, I – IV [99].

Phase I: These are CTs that are specially designed with a minimum number of human participants that voluntarily consent to partake in assessing the impact of use of the herbal product on vital physiological indices. It is the usually the first stage of testing in healthy humans to determine the safety and maximum tolerable doses of the investigational substance before any further human testing may be carried out. It is however acceptable that for certain herbs with long history of use, this phase may be unecessary [99]

Phase II: Studies carried on a limited number of participants to determine clinical efficacy, also labelled as feasibility studies. In this study, doses that are observed to be relatively safe are used, participants are also monitored for the occurence of adverse effects [99].

Phase III: In this phase, a larger number of participants is used in different centres and the study is designed as a randomized, double-blind, controlled CT. It is a validatory study for clinical efficacy of the herbal product, usually compared with a standard intervention [99].

Phase IV/post-marketing surveilance: Monitoring for rare side effects which may have been unnoticed during Phases I – III but may occur after the product has been introduced to the market [100].

There are critical issues which must be considered to provide justification for the clinical trial of herbal products and guidelines to this effect have been provided by the World Health Organization [99]. These areas of consideration are listed below:

Chemistry-manufacturing-control: Unlike conventional medicines, herbal medicines are frequently monoherbal or polyherbal with wide chemical composition. While it is not required for an active compound to be isolated as it is accepted that the action of the compounds in the product may be synergistic, a means of standardisation has to be used for the product that would be representative of the final product. If the active principle is known, it can serve as the marker for the product. If unknown, a chemical marker of sufficient quantity or a chemical fingerprint of the entire product can be used, within specified limits. Preparation of the herbal medicine intended for administration in a clinical trial also has to be carried out in accordane with WHO guidelines on good manufacturing practices for herbal medicines [101].

Provision of information on the herbal substance and the herbal product is also an important requirement. This includes a description of the source of the plant and its processing, storage conditions and shelf life. Information regarding the product including excepients, dosage form, analytical parameters for active compound or chemical markers, storage conditions over the lenght of the trial and specifications that would be assessed before clinical trial material is released will also need to be furnished.

http://dx.doi.org/10.5772/54493

Non-clinical considerations: This constitutes a supportive background upon which a clinical investigation is based. In general, data on efficacy, toxicity and pharmacokinetics which have been demonstrated or obtained from appropriate literature sources including journal publications and reference pharmacopoiea. A systematic review of earlier trials of the same herb or a related one can be done where possible in order to identify gaps that can be bridged in the proposed trial.

Clinical considerations: At all stages of the trial, ethical standards and quality requirements have to be met. For a phase 1 safety study, the adverse effects related to increasing doses of the test product are observed in human participants recruited within the limits of inclusion based on gender, weight, age and health status. An outline of the basic safety parameters that are monitored are shown in Table 2. The standard intervention is usually the product itself. The study may be randomized, blinded, double blinded or placebo-controlled to minimize bias.

Ethical considerations: All CT protocols require approval by regional ethical board before such trials can be executed. All research that involves human participation, including clinical trials must apply fundamental thical principles and must adhere to standards of good clinical practice [102]. Informed consent of all participants or gaurdians of minor participants must be obtained. It is required that each participant is well informed of any concerns regarding the trial herbal product especially with respect to rarely understood interactions, or known undesirable effects. Risks to participants must be minimized and as such, experienced ethical investigators including clinicians who can promptly identify and treat observed adverse events in participants need to be involved as CT investigators.

Organ/system	Safety parameter
Neurological:	lack of neurologic symptoms
Musculoskeletal:	lack of arthritis or myalgias, normal values of CPK
Skin:	clinical evidence of lack of allergic reactions
Gastrointestinal:	clinical evidence of tolerability
Liver:	normal values of SGOT or SGPT, alkaline phosphatase, total bilirubin,
Kidney:	normal values of BUN or creatinine
Endocrine system and metabolism:	normal values of albumin or total protein, uric acid, glucose, cholesterol, amylase or lipase, sodium/potassium, calcium
Cardiovascular:	normal EKG and blood pressure
Haematopoietic:	normal values of complete blood count
Additionally:	more intensive investigation of any organ system likely to be affected by the product

Table 2. Basic physiological parameters monitored in phase 1 clinical trial [99]

6. Conclusions and perspectives

Summarily, the processes involved in the toxicological evaluation of complex herbal extracts/mixtures and chemically characterized isolated compounds are schematically represented below. It is noteworthy that currently, only chemically characterized phyto compounds are useful candidates for QSAR studies and high throughput toxicogenomic assays, as compound data libraries exists for data comparison.

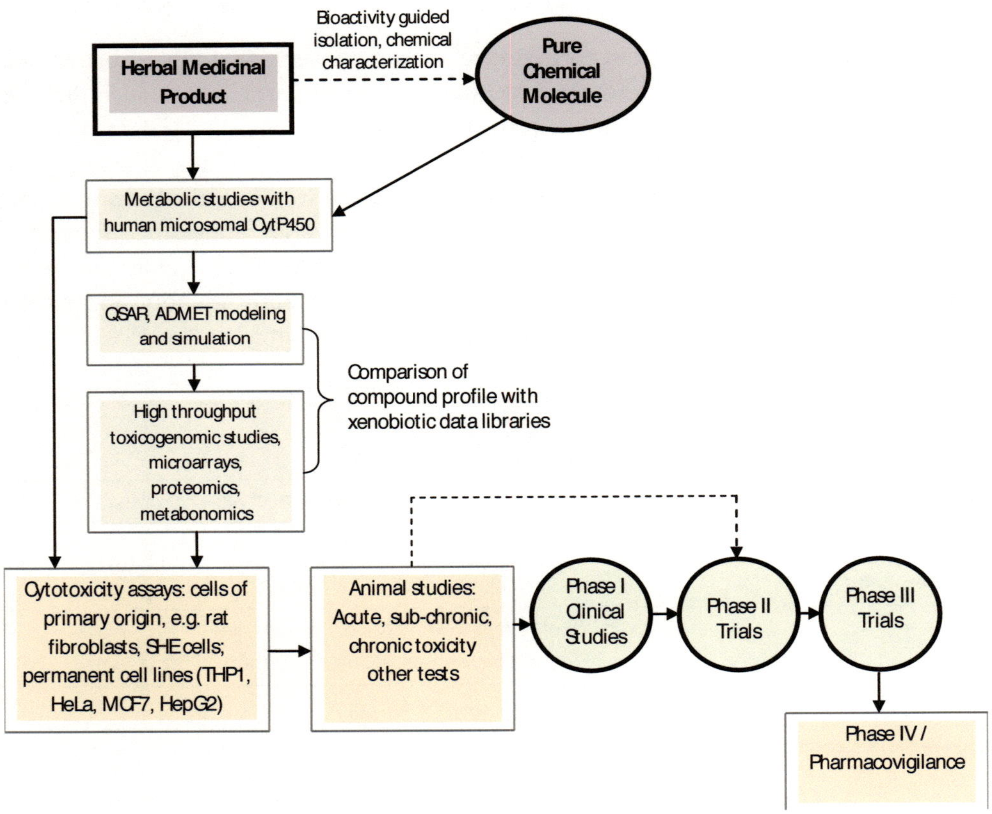

Figure 6. Schematic processes involved in evaluating and establishing the toxicity of medicinal herbs. The broken arrow indicates that for some herbal medicines, phase 1 clinical trials may not always be necessary.

Toxicity testing of herbal medicines in the 21st century tends to begin in a reductionist manner and proceeds through holistic tests to reach clinical conclusions. The challenge however, remains the identification of unique approaches in testing and developing regulations regarding safety of herbal products. Although some drawbacks to animal testing exists; such as the large number of animals used, financial implications and poor validation which affects correlation to humans, animal testing is still relevant as it is still impossible to predict long term carcinogenicity, embryotoxicity and reproductive toxicity using alternative non-animal tests alone.

A major issue in toxicity testing is "Animal welfare". The use of animals in research gave rise to the adoption of the critical 3 R's to consider before conducting animal-based toxicity testing of herbals. This calls for a fundamental paradigm in regulatory toxicology; there is a need to reduce the number of animals, refine the tests methods used in order to minimize pain and suffering of experimental animals, and replace animal tests with validated alternatives employing human cells where possible. Some instances of efforts in this regard are the development of a transcriptomics based *in vitro* screening method to predict embryotoxicity using the embryonic stem cell test. Additionally, the number of rats used for LD_{50} tests can be significantly reduced by the adoption of *in vitro* cell-based assays and chemicals shown to be harmful to cultured cells are excluded from any further LD_{50} tests and animal tests. It is no longer news that, cellular models of toxicity are more rapid and can easily be adapted to high throughput screening.

Next generation sequencing technology and toxicogenomics are strong predictive tools but databases of genetic biomarkers of toxicity of herbal medicines need to be enriched. It will be worthwhile to develop data libraries upon which prediction of the safety herbal extracts can be done to fully exploit these screening tools. As pointed out earlier, this can be achieved by creating genomic signatures of identified phytochemicals which can serve as data library for herbals.

Standardization of an herbal product in terms of parts per million limits of heavy metals will also eliminate product contamination and its associated toxicity. Chemical standardization of medicinal herbs with High Pressure Liquid Chromatography (HPLC) alone or hyphenated with Mass Spectroscopy (HPLC-MS) or Nuclear Mass Resonance Spectroscopy (HPLC-NMR) would also ensure chemical uniformity and detect chemical adulterants in herbal products.

More so, the integration of recent biotechnological innovations like computer-aided modeling and simulation studies, bioinformatics, high throughput screens, toxicokinetic and toxicogenomic tools in a systems toxicology approach with other necessary tests in experimental animals and appropriately designed clinical observation studies will undoubtedly bring about significant advances in predicting and determining herbal medicine safety.

Acknowledgements

The authors gratefully acknowledge Dr. Martins Emeje of the Department of Pharmaceutical Technology and Raw Materials Development, NIPRD, for accepting to review the chapter manuscript.

Author details

Obidike Ifeoma and Salawu Oluwakanyinsola

Department of Pharmacology and Toxicology, National Institute for Pharmaceutical Research and Development, Idu, Abuja, Nigeria

References

[1] Biggs RD. Medicine, surgery and public health in ancient Mesopotamia. Journal of Assyrian Academic Studies 2005; 19(1): 1-19; Aboelsoud NH. Herbal medicine in ancient Egypt. Journal of Medicinal Plant Research 2010; 4(2): 082-086.

[2] Aoelsoud NH. Herbal medicine in ancient Egypt. Journal of Medicinal Plant Research 2010; 4(2): 082-086.

[3] Bhatnagar VK, Hussain SA, Ali M. A brief history of Ayuverda in Hyderabad. Bulletin of the Indian Institute of History of Medicine (Hyderabad) 1994; 24(1): 63-75.

[4] O'Brien KA, Xue CC. The theoretical framework of Chinese medicine. In: Leung PC, Xue CC, Cheng YC, eds. A comprehensive guide to Chinese medicine. River Edge, NJ: World Scientific Publishing Co; 2003.

[5] Shafqat Azmi KA. Development of Unani system of medicine during Asafjahi period. Bulletin of the Indian Institute of History of Medicine (Hyderabad) 1995; 25(1-2): 183-194.

[6] Romero-Daza N. Traditional medicine in Africa. The Annals of the American Academy of Political and Social Science. doi: 10.1177/000271620258300111.

[7] World Health Organization. Traditional medicine. Fact sheet No. 134. www.who.int/mediacentre/factsheets/fs134/cn/. (accessed 12 August 2012).

[8] Mosihuzzaman M. Herbal medicine in healthcare—an overview. Natural Product Communications 2012; 7(6): 807-12.

[9] Osemene KP, Elujoba AA, Ilori MO. An overview of herbal medicine research and development in Nigeria. Research Journal of Medical Sciences 2011; 5(4): 228-232.

[10] Firenzuoli F, Gori L. Herbal medicine today: clinical and research issues. Evidence based Complementary and Alternative Medicine 2007; 4(Suppl 1): 37-40.

[11] Hu J, Zhang J, Zhao W, Zhang Y, Zhang L, shang H. Cochrane systematic reviews of Chinese herbal medicines: an overview. PLoS ONE 2011, 6(12): e28696.

[12] WHO. Herbal medicine research and global health: an ethical analysis. Bulletin of the WHO 2008; 86(8): 577-656.

[13] Verma S, Singh SP. Current and future status of herbal medicines. Veterinary world 2008; 1(11): 347-350.

[14] Vaidya Ashok DB, Devasagayam Thomas PA. Current status of herbal drugs in India: an overview. Journal of Clinical and Biochemical Nutrition 2007; 41(1): PMC2274994.

[15] Yuan R, Lin Y. Traditional Chinese medicine: an approach to scientific proof and clinical validation. Pharmacology and Therapeutics 2000; 86: 191-8.

[16] Schaffner KF. Assessments of efficacy in biomedicine: the turn toward methodological pluralism. In: Callahan D ed. The role of complementary and alternative medicine: accommodating pluralism. Washington DC: Georgetown University Press; 2002. p. 7.

[17] Patwardhan B, Mashelkar RA. Traditional medicine-inspired approaches to drug discovery: can Ayurveda show the way forward? Drug discovery Today 2009; 14(15-16): 804-11.

[18] Kinghorn AD, Pan L, Fletcher JN, Chai H. the relevance of higher plants in lead compound discovery programs. Journal of Natural Products 2011; 74(6): 1539-1555.

[19] Lee KH. Novel antitumor agents from higher plants. Medicinal Research reviews 1999; 19(6); 569-96.

[20] Strobe G, Daisy B, Castillo U, Harper J. Natural products from endophytic microorganisms. Journal of Natural Products 2004; 67(2): 257-68.

[21] Aly AH, Debbab A, Kjer J, Proksch P. Fungal endophytes from higher plants: a prolific source of phytochemicals and other bioactive natural products. Fungal Diversity 2010; 41(1): 1-16.

[22] WHO. The world medicines situation 2011. Traditional medicines: Global situation, issues and challenges. WHO/EMP/MIE/2011.2.3. http://apps.who.int/medicinedocs/documents/s18063en/s18063en.pdf. (accessed 20 August 2012).

[23] Harvey AL. Natural products in drug discovery. Drug discovery Today 2008; 13(19/20): 894-901.

[24] Cheng ZF, Zhen C. The Cheng Zhi-Fan Collectanea of Medical History. Beijing; China: Peking University Medical Press, 2004.

[25] Bent S, Ko R. Commonly used herbal medicines in the United States: a review. The American Journal of Medicine 2004; 116(7): 478-85

[26] Winston D, Maimes S. Adaptogens: Herbs for strength, stamina and stress relief. Rochester, Vermont: Healing Arts Press; 2007.

[27] Kennedy DO, Wightman EL. Herbal extracts and phytochemicals: plant secondary metabolites and the enhancement of human brain function. Advances in Nutrition 2011; 2: 32-50.

[28] Kawashima K, Misawa H, Moriwaki Y, Fujii Y, Fujii T, Horiuchi Y, Yamada T, Imanaka T, Kamekura M. Ubiquitous expression of acetylcholine and its biological functions in life forms without nervous systems. Life Sciences 2007; 80:2206–9.

[29] Nassel DR, Winther AM. Drosophila neuropeptides in regulation of physiology and behaviour. Progress in Neurobiology 2010; 92: 42-104.

[30] Klowden MJ. Physiological systems in insects. London: Academic Press; 2007

[31] Daniels RW, Gelfand MV, Collins CA, Diantonio A. Visualizing glutamatergic cell bodies and synapses in Drosophila larval and adult CNS. Journal of Comp. Neurology 2008; 508: 131-152.

[32] Ismail N, Christine S, Robinson GE, Fahrbach SE. Pilocarpine improves recognition of nestmates in young honey bees. Neuroscience Letters 2008; 439: 178-181.

[33] Wink M. Evolution of secondary metabolites from an ecological and molecular phylogenetic perspective. Phytochemistry 2003; 64: 3-19

[34] Savelev SU, Okello EJ, Perry EK. Butyryl- and acetyl-cholinesterase inhibitory activities in essential oils of Salvia species and their constituents. Phytotherapy Research 2004; 18:315-324.

[35] Rattan RS. Mechanisms of action of insecticidal secondary metabolites of plant origin. Crop Protection 2010; 29: 913-920.

[36] Francis G, Kerem Z, Makkar HPS, Becker K. The biological action of saponins in animal systems: a review. British Journal of Nutrition 2002; 88: 587-605.

[37] Arit VM, Stiborova M, Schmeiser HH. Aristolochic acid as a probable human cancer hazard in herbal remedies: a review. Mutagenesis 2002; 17(4): 265-77.

[38] Dwivedi SK, Dey S. Medicinal herbs: a potential source of toxic metal exposure for man and animals in India. Archives of Environmental Health 2002; 57(3): 229-31.

[39] Amster E, Tiwari A, Schenker MB. Case report: Potential arsenic toxicosis secondary to herbal kelp supplement. Environmental Health Perspectives 2007; 115(4): 606-608.

[40] Chan P, Fu PP. Toxicity of Panax ginseng- An herbal medicine and dietary supplement. Journal of Food and Drug analysis 2007; 15(4): 416-427.

[41] Gregoretti B, Stebel M, Candussio L, Crivellato E, Bartoli F, Decorti G. Toxicity of Hypericum perforatum (St. John's wort) administered during pregnancy and lactation in rats. Toxicology and Applied Pharmacology 2004; 200(3): 201-205.

[42] Gow PJ, Connelly NJ, Hill RL, Crowley P, Angus PW. Fatal fulminant hepatic failure induced by a natural therapy containing kava. The Medical Journal of Australia 2003; 178(9): 442-3.

[43] Sierpina VS, Wollschlaeger B, Blumenthal M. Ginkgo biloba. American Family Physician 2003; 68(5): 923-926.

[44] Wang BQ. Salvia miltiorrhiza: chemical and pharmacological review of a medicinal plant. Journal of Medicinal Plant Research 2010; 4(25): 2813-2820.

[45] Rothfuss MA, Pascht U, Kissling G. Effect of long-term application of Crataegus oxycantha on ischemia and reperfusion induced arrhythmias in rats. Arzneimittelforschung 2001; 51(1): 24-28.

[46] Stickel F, Seitz HK. The efficacy and safety of comfrey. Public Health Nutrition 2000; 3(4A): 501-8.

[47] Celik M, Karakus A, Zeren C, Demir M, Bayarogullari H, Duru M, Al M. Licorice induced hypokalemia, edema and thrombocytopenia. Human and Experimental Toxicology 2012; (Epub ahead of print). www.ncbi.nlm.nih.gov/pubmed/22653692. (accessed 27 July 2012).

[48] Arteaga S, Andrade-Cetto A, Cardenas R. Larrea tridentata (creosote bush), an abundant plant of Mexican and US-American deserts and its metabolite nordihydroguaiaretic acid. Journal of Ethnopharmacology 2005; 98: 231-239.

[49] Spiller HA, willies DB, Gorman SE, Sanftleban J. Retrospective study of mistletoe ingestion. Journal of Toxicology, Clinical Toxicology 1996; 34(4): 405-8.

[50] Tuncok Y, Kozan O, Cavdar C, Guven H, Fowler J. Urginea maritime (squill) toxicity. Clinical Toxicology 1995; 33(1): 83-86.

[51] Woolf AD, Watson WA, Smolinske S, Litovitz T. The severity of toxic reactions to ephedra: comparisons to other botanical products and national trends from 1993-2002. Clinical Toxicology (Philadelphia, Pa.) 2005; 43(5): 345-355.

[52] Barbosa-Ferreira M, Dagli ML, Maiorka PC, Gorniak SL. Sub-acute intoxication by Senna occidentalis seeds in rats. Food and Chemical Toxicology 2005; 43(4): 497-503.

[53] Verma A, Gupta AK, Kumar A, Khan PK. Cytogenetic toxicity of Aloe vera (a medicinal plant). Drug and Chemical Toxiciology 2012; 35(1): 32-25.

[54] Gamaniel KS. Toxicity from medicinal plants and their products. Nigerian Journal of Natural Products and Medicines 2000; 4: 4-8.

[55] O'Brien P, Haskings JR. In vitro cytotoxicity assessment. High Content screening: Methods in Molecular Biology 2006; 356, V, 415-425.

[56] Malinin G. Cytotoxic effect of dimethylsulfoxide on the ultrastructure of cultured Rhesus kidney cells. Cryobiology 1973; 10(1): 22-32.

[57] Elements of a standard test for basal cytotoxicity. In: Using In vitro data to estimate In vivo starting doses for acute toxicity. http://iccvam.niehs.nih.gov/docs/acutetox_docs/guidance0801/gd_s2.pdf

[58] Ponti J, Sabbioni E, Munaro B, Broggi F, Marmorato P, Franchini F, Colognato R, Rossi F. Genotoxicity and morphological transformation induced by cobalt nanoparticles

and cobalt chloride: an in vitro study in Balb/3T3 mouse fibroblasts. Mutagenesis 2009; 24: 439-45.

[59] Breheny D, Zhang H, Massey ED. Application of a two-stage Syrian hamster embryo cell transformation assay to cigarette smoke particulate matter. Mutation Research 2005; 572: 45-57.

[60] Pant K, Aardema MJ. The Syrian Hamster Embryo (SHE) low pH cell transformation assay. Current Protocols in Toxicology, 2008. DOI. 10.1002/0471140856.tx2003s35.

[61] Reznikoff CA, Bertram JS, Brankow DW, Heidelberger C. Qualitative and quantitative studies of chemical transformation of cloned C3H embryo cells sensitive to post-confluence inhibition of cell division. Cancer Research 1973; 33: 3239–3249.

[62] Sasaki K, Bohnenberger S, Hayashi K, Kunkelmann T, Muramatsu D, Poth A, Sakai A, Salovaara S, Tanaka N, Thomas BC, Umeda M. Photo catalogue for the classification of foci in the BALB/c 3t3 cell transformation assay. Mutation Research 2012; 744:42-53.

[63] Maurer HH. Toxicokinetics- variations due to genetics or interactions: Basics and examples. www.gtfch.org/cms/images/stories/media/tb/tb2007/s153-155.pdf. (accessed 20 Aug 2012).

[64] Bush TM, Rayburn KS, Holloway SW, Sanchez-Yamamoto DS, Allen BL, Lam ER, Kantor S, Roth LW. Adverse interactions between herbal and dietary substances and prescription medications: a clinical survey. Alternative Therapies in Health and Medicine 2007; 13: 30-35.

[65] Wienkers LC, Heath TG. Predicting in vivo drug interactions from in vitro drug dicovery data. Nature Reviews Drug Discovery 2005; 4: 825-833.

[66] Williams JA, Hyland R, Jones BC, Smith DA, Hurst S, Goosen TC, Peterkin V, Koup JR, Ball SE. Drug-drug interactions for UDP-glucuronosyltransferase substrates: a pharmacokinetic explanation of typically observed low exposure (AUCi/AUC ratios. Drug Metabolism and Disposition 2004; 32: 1201-1208.

[67] Izzo AA, Ernst E (2009). Interactions between herbal medicines and prescribed drugs: An updated systematic review. Drugs 69(13): 1777-1798.

[68] Guengerich FP (1997). Role of cytochome P450 enzymes in drug-drug interactions. Advances in Pharmacology 43: 7-35.

[69] Bugrim A, Nikolskaya T, Nikolsky Y. Early prediction of drug metabolism and toxicity: systems biology approach and modeling. Drug Discovery Today 2004; 9(3): 127-135.

[70] Youn M, Hoheisel JD, Efferth t. Toxicogenomics for the prediction of toxicity related to herbs from traditional Chinese medicine. Planta Medica 2010; 76(17): 2019-2025.

[71] Waring JF et al. Identifying toxic mechanisms using DNA microarrays. Toxicology 2002; 27: 537-550.

http://dx.doi.org/10.5772/54493

[72] Kennedy S. the role of proteomics in toxicology: identification of biomarkers of toxicity by protein expression analysis. Biomarkers 2002; 7: 269-290.

[73] Beecher C. Metabolomics: the newest 'omics' sciences. Innovations in Pharmaceutical Technology 2002; 2: 57-64.

[74] Schuster SC. Next-generation sequencing transforms today's biology. Nature Methods 2008; 5: 16-18.

[75] Lin X, Zhang J, Li Y, Luo H, Wu Q, Sun C, Song J, Li X, Wei J, Lu A, Qian Z, Khan IA, Chen S. Functional genomics of a living fossil tree, Ginkgo, based on next generation sequencing technology. Physiologia plantarum 2011; 143(3): 207-18.

[76] OECD Guidelines for the testing of chemicals. Available on www.oecd.org/env/testguidelines (accessed 12 August 2012).

[77] OECD (2000), Guidance Document on the recognition, assessment, and use of clinical signs as humane endpoints for experimental animals used in safety evaluation. Series on Testing and Assessment No. 19, ENV/JM/MONO(2000)7, OECD.

[78] National Research Council. Guide for the care and use of laboratory animals. 8th ed. The National Academies Press, Washington DC; 2011. www.nap.edu (accessed 12 August 2012).

[79] OECD (2001), Acute Oral Toxicity - Acute toxic class method, Test Guideline No. 423, OECD Guidelines for the Testing of Chemicals, OECD.

[80] Lorke D. A new approach to practical acute toxicity testing. Archives of Toxicology 1983; 54, 275 – 287.

[81] Abdulrahman FI, Onyeyili PA, Sanni S, Ogugbuaja VO. Toxic effect of aqueous rootbark extract of Vitex doniana on liver and kidney functions. International Journal of Biological Chemistry 2007; 1: 184-195.

[82] Obidike IC, Shehu Idris-Usman M, John-Africa LB, Salawu OA. An Evaluation of acute and sub chronic toxicological effects of Hymenocardia acida leaf extract in adult Wistar rats. Journal of Pharmacology and Toxicology 2011; 6(4): 400-408.

[83] Pak E, Esrason KT, Wu VH. Hepatotoxicity of herbal remedies: an emerging dilemma. Progress in Transplantation 2004; 14(2): 91-6.

[84] Kao WF, Hung ZZ, Tsai WJ et al. Podophyllotoxin intoxication: Toxic effect of Bajiaolian on herbal therapeutics. Human and Experimental Toxicology 1992; 11: 480-7.

[85] Farrell GC, Weltman M. Drug-induced liver disease. In: Ginick G (ed.) Current Hepatology, vol. 16. Chicago: Mosby-year Book Medical Publishers; 1996, 143-208.

[86] Larrey D, Vial T, Pauwels A et al. Hepatitis after germander (Teucrium chamaedrys): another instance of herbal medicine hepatotoxicity. Annals of Internal Medicine 1992; 117: 129-32.

[87] Chitturi S, Farrel GC. Herbal hepatotoxicity: An expanding but poorly defined problem. Journal of Gastroenterology and Hepatology 2000; 15: 1093-1099.

[88] Seeff LB. Herbal hepatotoxicity. Clinics in Liver Disease 2007; 11(3): 5777-96, vii.

[89] OECD. Draft Guidance Document on the Design and Conduct of Chronic Toxicity and Carcinogenicity Studies, Series on Testing and Assessment No. 116, (2009). www.oecd.org/env/testguidelines (accessed 8 August 2012).

[90] Balls M, Botham PA, Bruner LH, Spielmann H. The EC/HO international validation study on alternatives to the Draize eye irritation test. Toxicology in Vitro 1995; 9, 871.929.

[91] Takahashi Y, Koike M, Honda H, Ito Y, Sakaguchi H, Suzuki H, Nishiyama N. Development of the short time exposure (STE) test: an in vitro eye irritation test using SIRC cells. Toxicology in vitro 2008; 22(3): 760-770.

[92] Choi KG. Neurotoxicity of herbal medicine. Journal of the Korean Medical Association 2005; 48(4): 308-313.

[93] Pethkar AV, Gaikaiwari RP, Paknikar KM. Biosorptive removal of contaminating heavy metals from plant extracts of medicinal value. Current Science 2001; 80(9): 1216-9.

[94] Ghosh A, Chakrabarti P, Roy P, Bhadury S,Nag T, Sarkar S. Bioremediation of heavy metals from neem (Azadirachta indica) leaf extract by chelation with dithizone. Asian Journal of Pharmaceutical and Clinical Research 2009; 2(1): 87-92.

[95] www.ema.europa.eu/docs/en_GB/document_library/other/2009/09/WC500003570.pdf. (accessed 20 August 2012).

[96] Botting J. The history of thalidomide. Drug News Perspectives 2002; 15(9): 604-611.

[97] Stephens TD, Bunde CJ, Fillmore BJ. Mechanism of action in thalidomide teratogenesis. Biochemical Pharmacology 2000; 59(12): 1489-99.

[98] Wu C. Overview of developmental and reproductive toxicity research in China: History, funding mechanisms, and frontiers of the research. Birth Defects Research. Part B, Developmental and Reproductive Toxicology 2010; 89(1): 9-17.

[99] World Health Organization. Operational guidance: Information needed to support clinical trials of herbal products. TDR/GEN/Guidance/05.1. 2005; Geneva. http://www.who.int/tdr/publications/documents/operational-guidance-eng.pdf. (accessed 6 August 2012).

[100] World Health Organization. The importance of pharmacovigilance- safety monitoring of medicinal products. A WHO publication; 2002. http://apps.who.int/medicinedocs/en/d/Js4893e/1.html. (accessed 22 August 2012).

[101] WHO guidelines on good manufacturing practice (GMP) for herbal medicines. 2007, Geneva.

[102] Department of Health. Guidelines for Good practice in the conduct of clinical trials with human participants in South Africa. Department of Health: Pretoria, 2006.

Chapter 5

New Trends in Genotoxicity Testing of Herbal Medicinal Plants

Hala M. Abdelmigid

Additional information is available at the end of the chapter

http://dx.doi.org/10.5772/54858

1. Introduction

Although herbal medicinal products (HMP) have been perceived by the public as relatively low risk, there has been more recognition of the potential risks associated with this type of product as the use of HMPs increase. Potential harm can occur via inherent toxicity of herbs, as well as from contamination, plant misidentification, and interactions with other herbal products or pharmaceutical drugs. Regulatory safety assessment for HMPs relies on both the assessment of cases of adverse reactions and the review of published toxicity information. The submission of data on genotoxicity is a precondition for marketing authorization respectively registration of herbal medicinal products (HMPs) with well-established or traditional use in some countries. The assessment of potential genotoxicity of HMPs should describe a stepwise approach, including the possibility to reduce the number of extracts of an herbal drug to be tested by the use of more recent toxicological assessment techniques such as predictive toxicology and "omics". In the regulatory context, safety assessment can have bearing on whether certain products should be restricted, removed from the market, or have augmented safety information placed on labeling.

This chapter discusses the challenges which are faced in the assessment of safety of HMPs and the need for careful judgments on the hazard and risk of HMPs can be made with increased certainty. Hence, it is critical that toxicologists in industry, regulatory agencies and academic institutions develop a consensus, based on rigorous methods, about the reliability and interpretation of endpoints. It will also be important to regulate the integration of conventional methods for toxicity assessments with new "omics" technologies.

Although modern medicine is well developed in most of the world, large sections of the population in developing countries still rely on the traditional practitioners, medicinal plants and herbal medicines for their primary care. Moreover during the past decades, public interest in natural therapies has increased greatly in industrialized countries, with expanding use of medicinal plants and herbal medicines. Many of the plants species used for this purpose have been found to contain therapeutic substances which can be extracted and used in preparation of drugs, but the plant itself can also be used either directly or as an extract for medication, a practice that is particularly popular in developing countries (Ouedraogo *et al.*, 2012). It has been estimated that more than 80% of the world's population utilizes plants as their primary source of medicinal agents, largely due to the high cost of Western pharmaceuticals, but also because the traditional medicines are generally more acceptable from a cultural and spiritual perspective.

The evaluation of these products and ensuring their safety and efficacy through registration and regulation present important challenges. Despite the use of herbal medicines over many centuries, only a relatively small number of plant species has been studied for possible medical applications. Safety and efficacy data are available for an even smaller number of plants, their extracts and active ingredients and preparations containing them (Jordan *et al.*, 2010)

Research in the area of genotoxicity has been prolific, both at the fundamental level and also with respect to comparative analysis of the performance and predictivity of individual tests and combinations of tests for risk assessment. There is an ongoing debate on the need to modify earlier recommended *in vitro* testing batteries (some of which can generate a high number of misleading (false) positives in order to avoid false positives and the triggering of unnecessary testing in animals, whilst at the same time ensuring detection of genotoxic potential that may have human health implications. Optimization of testing batteries to minimize false positives may reduce the likelihood of detecting inherent genotoxic activity (Ouedraogo *et al.*, 2012). Comparative trials have shown conclusively that each *in vitro* test system generates both false negative and false positive results in relation to predicting rodent carcinogenicity. Genotoxicity test batteries (of *in vitro* and *in vivo* tests) detect carcinogens that are thought to act primarily via a mechanism involving direct genetic damage, such as the majority of known human carcinogens. Therefore, these batteries may not detect nongenotoxic carcinogens. Experimental conditions, such as the limited capability of the *in vitro* metabolic activation systems, can also lead to false negative results in *in vitro* tests. The test battery approach is designed to reduce the risk of false negative results for compounds with genotoxic potential, while a positive result in any assay for genotoxicity does not necessarily mean that the test compound poses a genotoxic/ carcinogenic hazard to human. Thus in recommending strategies for genotoxicity testing for risk assessment purposes, a balance needs to be struck that ensures with reasonable certainty that genotoxic substances that are likely to be active *in vivo* are detected. New tests have also been developed and their potential for inclusion in genotoxicity testing strategies, both in basic testing and in follow-up of positive results from basic testing, needs to be considered.

2. History of herbal medicinal products use

Medicinal plants have been widely used by urban and rural populations in treating various diseases, constituting an effective and less expensive therapy (Jordan *et al.*, 2010). Phytotherapy is based on old traditions, widely disseminated through salespeople, healers, faith healers, part of the culture of indigenous people, and rural areas. Of all the 365,000 species of flowering plants, it is estimated that only 8% of them have been systematically studied in terms of constituents. Nevertheless, approximately 7000 substances of pharmaceutical importance have been isolated from plants known for their medicinal properties, and several constituents have been processed into pharmaceuticals (Ouedraogo et al., 2012). Herbal medicines have a long history of use for the prevention and treatment of diseases; their use can be traced to the first written testimonies of humanity, through antiquity and back middle ages till modern time (Williamson, 2003). They have been part of human culture according to the World Health Organization (WHO), nearly 80% of the world populations still rely on medicinal herbs for their primary health care. Herbal medicines are then widely used around the world, and increasingly so in Western nations (Jordan *et al.*, 2010). For instance, 71% of the population in Canada (IPSOS-Reid, 2005) and 80% in Germany (Thomas *et al.*, 2001) used, in their lifetime, traditional medicines under the wording "complementary and alternative medicine". In the United States, about 19% of the adult populations are using herbal medicinal products (HMPs) (Ouedraogo et al., 2012); the herb supplement sales have increased in USA by 23% from 2000 to 2010, reaching a market of more than 5 billion dollars (NBJ, 2011). Europe was estimated to import in 2004 about always 400,000 tons of medicinal plants per annum, with an average market value of US$ 1 billion from Africa and Asia (Wakdikar, 2004). Besides, in developing countries, WHO strongly encourages the use of traditional herbal medicines in primary health care delivery system (Atsamo *et al.*, 2011)

2.1. List of medicinal plants and their uses

The list of medicinal herbs available across the globe is huge. In the following list we have sorted the species that are commonly used due to their wonderful healing effects and therapeutic value.

A plethora of herbs are also utilized for treatment of health disorders. From the table below you shall come to know their medicinal properties and uses. Such herbal medicines are capable of curing health problems completely.

3. International regulation of herbal medicinal products

The legal situation regarding herbal preparations varies from country to country. In some, phytomedicines are well-established, whereas in others they are regarded as food and therapeutic claims are not allowed. Developing countries, however, often have a great number of traditionally used herbal medicines and much folk-knowledge about them, but have hardly any legislative criteria to establish these traditionally used herbal medicines as part of the drug legislation.

For the classification of herbal or traditional medicinal products, factors applied in regulatory systems include: description in a pharmacopoeia monograph, prescription status, claim of a therapeutic effect, scheduled or regulated ingredients or substances, or periods of use. Some countries draw a distinction between "officially approved" products and "officially recognized" products, by which the latter products can be marketed without scientific assessment by the authority (Jordan *et al.*, 2010).

Common Name	Scientific Name	Uses
Acacia	*Acacia greggi*	astringent, demulcent, emollient
Agrimony	*Agrimonia eupatoria*	blood coagulant
Pimenta	*Pimenta dioica*	heals wounds, bruises
Ajwain	*Trachyspermum ammi*	antibacterial, carminative, digestive
Ashok	*Trachyspermum ammi*	relieves menstrual pain, diabetes, uterine disorders
Amla	*Phyllanthus emblica*	Cough, diabetes, laxative, acidity
Ashwagandha	*Withania somnifera*	relieves stress, nerve disorder, restores normal function of body
Brahmi	*Bacopa monnieri*	jaundice, anemia, dropsy
Bael	*Aegle marmelos*	constipation, diarrhea, dysentery
Chirata	*Swertia chirata*	burn, skin diseases, fever
Guggul	*Commiphora wightii*	asthma, hydrocele, diabetes
Guluchi	*Tinospora cordifolia*	jaundice, gout, piles, fever
Kalmegh	*Andrographis paniculata*	gastritis, fever, weakness
Makoi	*Solanum nigrum*	dysentery, diuretic, debility
Pashan Bheda	*Coleus barbatus*	calculus, stones in kidney
Sarpa Gandha	*Ranwolfia serpentina*	insomnia, hypertension
Tulsi	*Ocimum tenuiflorum*	expectorant, cough, cold
Vai Vidanka	*Embelia ribes*	skin disease, helminthiasis
Peppermint	*Mentha piperita*	pain-killer, digestive
Vringraj	*Eclipta alba*	anti-inflammatory, leukemia, stress reliever
Chitrak	*Plumbargo zeylanica*	dyspepsia, inflammation, cough, colic
Harada	*Terminalia chebula*	leprosy, inflammation, vomiting, insomnia
Neem	*Azadirachta indica*	analgesic, astringent, epilepsy

http://dx.doi.org/10.5772/54858

Common Names	Scientific Names	Uses
Lemon Balm	*Melissa officinalis*	digestion, stomach spasms, anti-viral
Angelica	*Angelica sylvestris*	gastritis, cramps, digestion
Chickweed	*Stellaria media*	itching, irritation, rashes
Cleavers	*Galium aparine*	skin diseases, diuretic
Couch grass	*Cynodon dactylon*	rheumatism, cystitis, gout
Dandelion	*Taraxacum officinale*	dissolves kidney and gallstones, diuretics
Elderberry	*Sambucus canadensis*	bronchitis, cold, cough
Garlic	*Allium sativum*	anti-microbial, cardiovascular treatment
Ginger	*Zingiber officinale*	motion sickness, vomiting, flatulence, diarrhea
Lavender	*Lavandula angustifolia*	stress reliever, boosts spirits, stomach disorders
Red Clover	*Trifolium pratense*	rejuvenatory, skin nourishing
Rosemary	*Rosmarinus officinalis*	improves blood supply to brain
Thyme	*Thymus pulegioides*	antifungal, anti-bacterial, expectorant
Yarrow	*Achillea millefolium*	wound cleansing, blood coagulation, digestive

A regulatory framework for HMPs provides consumers greater assurance that the identities of medicinal ingredients have been verified that they have been properly quantified per unit dose, that there has been an assessment of the safety and efficacy of the product prior to granting of market authorization, and that the product is within tolerance limits for contaminants. Requirements for Good Manufacturing Practices (GMP) provide a framework for assuring continuing quality and the ability to deal appropriately and quickly with problems when they do arise. Adverse reaction reporting requirements facilitate the detection of such problems. Four different national regulatory frameworks are summarized below, to illustrate some similarities and differences in the regulation of HMPs. In the United States, HMPs are regulated as dietary supplements, a subset of foods. Under the Dietary Supplement Health and Education Act of 1994 (DSHEA), the dietary supplement manufacturer is responsible for ensuring that a dietary supplement is safe before it is marketed. The United States Food and Drug Administration (FDA) is responsible for taking action against any unsafe dietary supplement product after it reaches the market. Generally, manufacturers do not need to register their products with the FDA, nor obtain FDA approval, before producing or selling dietary supplements unless it is a New Dietary Ingredient, or to verify the acceptability of a structure–function type of claim. The FDA final Rule for current good manufacturing practices (cGMPs) for dietary supplements requires that proper controls are in place for dietary supplements so that they are processed in a consistent manner, and meet quality standards (US Department of Health and Human Services, 2007). The cGMPs apply to all domestic and foreign companies that manufacture, package, label or hold dietary supplements, including those involved with the activities of testing, quality control, packaging and labelling, and distribution in the U.S. The Rule establishes cGMPs for industry-wide uses that are necessary to require that dietary supplements are manufactured consistently as to identity, purity, strength, and composition. Manufacturers, packers, or distributors are required to submit all serious adverse event reports associated with use of the dietary supplement in the United States to the FDA, through the adverse reaction reporting program (Med Watch). FDA's post marketing responsibilities include monitoring safety, e.g. voluntary dietary supplement adverse event reporting, and product information, such as labelling, claims, package inserts, and accompanying literature (US FDA 2009).

In Canada, HMPs are regulated under the Natural Health Products Regulations (NHPR) which came into force on January 1, 2004. These regulations are distinct from the regulations for food and drugs. This is a mandatory pre-market system where each HMP must receive market authorization by obtaining a product license based on evidence that the product is safe under the recommended conditions of use without a prescription, effective for the proposed claims, and of high quality. Each importer, manufacturer, packager and labeller of HMPs requires a site license issued on the basis of evidence of compliance with GMPs created specifically for natural health products (which includes HMPs).

Every license must provide an expedited case report for each serious adverse reaction to their product occurring in Canada and each serious unexpected adverse reaction occurring inside or outside Canada. They must also prepare and maintain an annual summary report with analysis of all adverse reactions, to be provided to the Department of Health upon demand (Government of Canada 2009).

In Australia, HMPs are regulated by the Therapeutic Goods Administration (TGA) as medicines under the Therapeutics Goods Act 1989, using risk-based pre-market assessment procedures based on toxicity of ingredients, dosage form, serious disease claims, side effects/ interactions, and adverse reactions. Listed medicines are considered low risk and are included on the Australian Registry of Therapeutic Goods (ARTG). Herbal medicines that are assessed to be of higher risk are individually evaluated for quality, safety and efficacy for licensing as Registered Medicines. Each Australian manufacturer of HMPs must hold a manufacturing license and comply with the Australian Code of GMP for Medicinal Products. The Code applies to all medicines manufactured in Australia, including complementary medicines such as

http://dx.doi.org/10.5772/54858

HMPs. An adverse reaction reporting system for medicines in Australia is well established. The Australian "Blue Card" scheme covers all medicines and most health professionals. In addition, sponsors of all medicines included in the ARTG are under an obligation to report adverse reactions to the TGA (TGA, 2006).

In the European Union (EU), HMPs are classified as "regular" medicinal products if they claim to treat or prevent illness, or if they are to be administered with a view to restoring, correcting or modifying physiological functions. As such, they are subject to the general regulations for medicines as laid down in the various national medicines laws. A marketing authorization as a HMP is granted based on a "full" dossier in terms of proof of quality, safety and efficacy in almost all Member States but the Committee on Herbal Medicinal Products (HMPC), part of the EMEA, establishes Community herbal monographs to simplify the authorization of HMPs. With respect to GMP compliance, the EU follows the Pharmaceutical Inspection Cooperation Scheme (PIC/S). The competent authority may carry out announced or unannounced inspections of active substance manufacturers in order to verify compliance with the principles of GMPs for active substances placed on the Community market. The Marketing Authorization Holder (MAH) must ensure that they have an appropriate system of pharmacovigilance and risk management in place in order to assure responsibility and liability for its products on the market and to ensure that appropriate action can be taken, when necessary. Specifically, the MAH must have an approved system of reporting adverse reactions. In the United Kingdom, the Medicines and Healthcare products Regulatory Agency (MHRA) provides transitional provisions where an HMP legally on the UK market as an unlicensed herbal remedy in accordance with the Medicines Act 1968 can continue to be marketed as an unlicensed herbal remedy until April 30, 2011. At that time all manufactured HMPs will be required to have either a Traditional Herbal Registration or a Marketing Authorization based on the European Directive. The Traditional Herbal Registration is a simplified UK registration scheme that began in 2005 with specific standards of safety and quality, agreed indications based on traditional usage, and systematic patient information allowing the safe use of the product (MHRA, 2009).

4. The assessment of HMPs

Although HMPs are widely considered to be of lower risk compared with synthetic drugs, they are not completely free from the possibility of toxicity or other adverse effects (De Smet, 2004). High profile issues such as adverse reactions associated with *Ephedra* and *Aristolochia* have shown that HMPs can produce toxicity in humans. While inherent toxicity of certain herbs is well known, adverse effects from the use of HMPs may also result from contamination of products with toxic metals, adulteration with pharmacologically active synthetic compounds, misidentification or substitution of herbal ingredients, or improperly processed or prepared products (Van Breemen *et al.*, 2008; Chan, 2009). Interactions may also occur between drugs, foods and other HMPs taken concomitantly (Goldman *et al.*, 2008).

Recently, there has been increased discussion on the safety assessment of herbs. Protocols and guidance documents on safety and toxicity testing of HMPs have been issued by the International Life Sciences Institute, the Institute of Medicine, the Union of Pure and Applied Chemistry (Mosihuzzaman and Choudhary, 2008), the European Medicines Agency (EMEA) (e.g. EMEA, 2007, 2009), and most recently by the European Food Safety Authority (EFSA, 2009). These guidance documents discuss the assessment of the safety of herbs for use in both foods and medicines. The types of testing described in these guidance documents represent the ideal type of information that could be obtained in order to adequately characterize the toxicity of a specific herb or a finished herbal product ready for the marketplace.

International regulatory systems for HMPs can be quite variable in terms of safety and toxicity testing requirements. In countries where HMPs are less strictly regulated than synthetic drugs, and where limited toxicity testing is required, or where HMPs are regulated as intermediate products classified separately from foods and drugs, where less stringent requirements exist for certain sub-types of products (e.g. traditionally used herbs where their long-term use is considered evidence for safety), pre-market assessment may be based on limited information. Even in countries where HMPs are assessed in detail before market authorization is given, pharmacovigilance is a critical activity to promote the safe use of HMPs throughout their life cycle. As the use of HMPs grows around the world, the identification of safety signals becomes of increased importance. The identification and investigation of safety signals associated with HMPs are subject to the same challenges as signals arising from pharmaceutical drugs. There are, however, challenges unique to HMPs. There are often deficiencies in both the quantity of information (e.g. under-reporting of adverse reactions, general lack of toxicological information on herbs) and the quality of information (e.g. poor quality of adverse reaction case reports or lack of information on the quality of HMPs associated with case reports submitted to regulatory authorities or published in the scientific literature). These factors present challenges when signals of safety concerns arise.

In the regulatory context, safety assessment can have bearing on whether certain products should be restricted, removed from the market, or have augmented safety information placed on labelling. In instances where little toxicity information exists on a specific herbal product or its ingredients, regulatory decisions on risk mitigation activities are likely to take a cautious approach, until further information is obtained which can potentially clarify the toxicity of the product, and reduce uncertainty in the risk assessment of HMPs. From the post-market perspective, an integrative approach is necessary to investigate safety signals for any product type. Clinical assessment of adverse reaction reports, either submitted to the regulatory authority, or published in the scientific literature, needs to be considered along with available toxicological and pharmacological information in order to fully characterize potential safety concerns. While challenges exist for the assessment of HMP safety, efforts are being made to add quality information to the herbal safety knowledge base so that judgments on the hazard and risk of HMPs can be made with increased certainty.

An adverse reaction (AR) is defined as a noxious and unintended response to a marketed health product, which occurs at doses normally used or tested for the diagnosis, treatment or pre-

http://dx.doi.org/10.5772/54858

vention a disease or the modification of an organic function (Health Canada, 2009a). In the literature, there are few clinical studies with most herbs despite the fact that many have been employed for centuries as traditional medicines; therefore, surveillance for HMP-related ARs consists mainly of voluntary reporting from consumers and Health Care Practitioners (HCP) and published reports which are usually single reports or small case series. Due to the lack of clinical trials for most HMPs, post-market pharmacovigilance is a critical source of safety information; however, the assessment of ARs associated with HMPs offers unique challenges in the quantity and quality of available information (Gardiner *et al.*, 2008.).

5. Genotoxicity assessment

Genotoxicity can be due to many physico-chemical agents that result in a wide variety of possible damages to the genetic material, ranging from various DNA adducts to single- and double-strand breakages, DNA–DNA and DNA–protein cross-links or even chromosomal breakage (Cavalcanti *et al.*, 2010; Wang *et al.*, 2012). The major challenge in genotoxicity testing resides in developing methods that can reliably and sensibly detect either such a vast array of damages or a general cellular response to genotoxic insult. It is recognized that no single test can detect every genotoxin, therefore the concept of tests battery has been implemented in many regulatory guidelines.

In the last decades, numerous damage signalization and repair mechanisms, complex and extremely efficient, have been unravelled, both in prokaryote, eukaryote and mammalian systems (Bootsma *et al.*, 2001). Although DNA alterations, both in the sequence of nucleotides and in the arrangement of DNA strands, can also arise from mistakes in the repair process, agents interfering with damage signalization repair mechanisms are generally not considered in safety testing. They should however be detected as they could impair indirect genotoxicity by facilitating the activity of genotoxic agents such as direct genotoxins, reactive oxygen species, and radiations (Johnson and Loo, 2000; Kelly *et al.*, 2001; Ouedraogo *et al.*, 2012).

5.1. Aims and rationale of genotoxicity assessment

5.1.1. Potential health effects of genotoxic substances (both cancer and other diseases)

Genetic alterations in somatic and germ cells are associated with serious health effects, which in principle may occur even at low exposure levels. Mutations in somatic cells may cause cancer if mutations occur in proto-oncogenes, tumor suppressor genes and/or DNA damage response genes, and they are responsible for a variety of genetic diseases (Erickson, 2010). Accumulation of DNA damage in somatic cells has also been proposed to play a role in degenerative conditions such as accelerated aging, immune dysfunction, cardiovascular and neurodegenerative diseases (Hoeijmakers, 2009; Slatter and Gennery, 2010; Frank, 2010). Mutations in germ cells can lead to spontaneous abortions, infertility or heritable damage to the offspring and possibly to the subsequent generations.

5.1.2. Scope of genotoxicity assessment

In view of the adverse consequences of genetic damage to human health, the assessment of mutagenic potential is a basic component of chemical risk assessment. To this aim, both the results of studies on mutation induction ("mutagenicity") and tests conducted to investigate other effects on genetic material are taken into consideration. Both the terms "mutagenicity" and "genotoxicity" are used in this opinion. Definitions of these terms given below are taken from the REACH "Guidance on information requirements and chemical safety assessment" (ECHA, 2008b).

"**Mutagenicity**" refers to the induction of permanent transmissible changes in the amount or structure of the genetic material of cells or organisms. These changes may involve a single gene or gene segment, a block of genes or chromosomes. The term clastogenicity is used for agents giving rise to structural chromosome aberrations. A clastogen can cause breaks in chromosomes that result in the loss or rearrangements of chromosome segments. Aneugenicity (aneuploidy induction) refers to the effects of agents that give rise to a change (gain or loss) in chromosome number in cells. An aneugen can cause loss or gain of chromosomes resulting in cells that have not an exact multiple of the haploid number.

"**Genotoxicity**" is a broader term and refers to processes which alter the structure, information content or segregation of DNA and are not necessarily associated with mutagenicity. Thus, tests for genotoxicity include tests which provide an indication of induced damage to DNA (but not direct evidence of mutation) via effects such as unscheduled DNA synthesis (UDS), sister chromatid exchange (SCE), DNA strand-breaks, DNA adduct formation or mitotic recombination, as well as tests for mutagenicity." The tests mentioned in the definition of "Genotoxicity" above that do not detect mutagenicity but rather primary DNA damage are commonly termed "indicator" tests. DNA adduct formation, for example, occurs when a substance binds covalently to DNA, initiating DNA repair, which can either return the DNA to its original state or, in the case of mis-repair, result in a mutation.

For an adequate evaluation of the genotoxic potential of a chemical substance, different end-points (i.e. induction of gene mutations, structural and numerical chromosomal alterations) have to be assessed, as each of these events has been implicated in carcinogenesis and heritable diseases. An adequate coverage of all the above-mentioned end-points can only be obtained by the use of multiple test systems (i.e. a test battery), as no individual test can simultaneously provide information on all end-points. All the above mentioned endpoints should be examined in hazard identification irrespective of the expected level of human exposure. A battery of *in vitro* tests is generally required to identify genotoxic substances. *In vivo* tests may be used to complement *in vitro* assays in specific cases, e.g. when the available information points to the involvement of complex metabolic activation pathways, which are expected not to be replicated by *in vitro* exogenous metabolic activation systems, or in case of high or "moderate and sustained" human exposure (Eastmond *et al.*, 2009). Further *in vivo* testing may be required to assess whether the genotoxic effect observed *in vitro* is also expressed *in vivo*. The choice of *in vivo* follow-up tests should be guided by effects observed in the *in vitro* studies (genetic end-point) as well as by knowledge of bioavailability, reactivity, metabolism and target organ specificity of the substance. Clear evidence of genotoxicity in somatic cells *in vivo* has to be

http://dx.doi.org/10.5772/54858

considered an adverse effect *per se*, even if the results of cancer bioassays are negative, since genotoxicity is also implicated in other somatic diseases than cancer. Another important issue that should be kept in mind is that one of the original purposes of performing genotoxicity tests is to identify substances that are germ cell mutagens. A substance that is a somatic cell mutagen should also be considered a potential germ cell mutagen, unless it can be demonstrated that the substance or a genotoxic metabolite cannot reach the germ cells. In addition, a germ cell mutagen is expected to be also a somatic cell mutagen.

5.2. Review of key issues in genotoxicity assessment

The methods most frequently used for the assessment of genotoxic activity of herbal medicinal products in *vitro* and *in vivo* are described below. This list is not meant to be comprehensive of all existing methods, but more a consideration of the strengths, limitations and opportunity for further developments of the most widely used genotoxicity assays. Positive results of an *in vitro/in vivo* test indicate that the tested substance is genotoxic under the conditions of the assay performed; negative results indicate that the test substance is not genotoxic under the conditions of the assay performed.

5.2.1. Conventional methods

The Organization for Economic Co-operation and Development (OECD, 2012) and the European Centre for the Validation of Alternative Methods (ECVAM, 2012) have largely investigated the validation of mutagenicity tests and should be referred to more for details.

5.2.1.1. Detection of phytochemical compounds bearing structural alerts for genotoxicity activity

Structural alerts or "toxicophores" are defined as molecules or molecular functionalities that are associated with toxicity. Their presence in compounds or a molecular structure alerts the investigator to their potential toxicity (Ouedraogo *et al.*, 2012). A few well-characterized compounds include (i) 1–2 unsaturated pyrrolizidine alkaloids esters from many Boraginaceae, Asteraceae and Fabaceae (Prakash *et al.*, 1999b; Fang *et al.*, 2011) that exhibit a large variety of genotoxicities, including DNA binding, DNA cross-linking, DNA–protein cross-linking, sister chromatid exchange, and chromosomal aberrations (Roeder, 2000; Fu *et al*, 2004); (ii) aristolochic acids (AA), nitro-polyaromatic compounds responsible for terminal nephropathies observed after intoxication by many *Aristolochia* species (Fang *et al.*, 2011); a series of studies confirmed that they are genotoxic in both bacterial and mammalian cells, yielding highly persistent and molecules non-repaired DNA adducts; (iii) allylalkoxybenzenes (e.g. eugenol, methyleugenol,estragole) and safrole (4-allyl-1,2 methylenedioxybenzene), potentially genotoxic components from some essential oils (Smith *et al.*, 2010). The notion of threshold for genotoxic insult is still a matter of heavy debates; consequently such compounds should be proscribed from herbal medicines or at least severely limited (Ouedraogo *et al.*, 2012).

5.2.1.2. Analytical methods

Analytical methods with suitable detection limits have been developed for the characterization and quantification of many known molecules or molecular functionalities associated with genotoxicity; they are now being implemented in official pharmacopeias. Such methods are based on spectrophotometry (the Ehrlich reagent for pyrrolizidine alkaloids), thin layer Chromatography (TLC), and gas chromatography/mass spectroscopy (GC/MS) and liquid chromatography/mass spectroscopy (LC/MS and LC/MS/MS) (Fu *et al.*, 2007; Napoli *et al.*, 2010).

5.2.1.3. In silico methods

These predictive methods generally refer to a computational experiment, mathematical calculation, scientific analysis of substances data through a computer-based analysis (Valerio-Jr, 2009; Ouedraogo *et al.*, 2012). Computer models used for genotoxicity prediction fall into three principal categories (Votano et al., 2004): (i) rule-based expert systems such as DEREK that estimates the presence of a DNA-reactive moiety in a given molecule; (ii) quantitative structure–activity relationship models (QSAR) such as TOPKAT that use "electro-topological" descriptors (atom-type, bond-type and group-type E-state) rather than chemical structure to predict mutagenic reactivity with DNA (Votano *et al.*, 2004; Snyder and Smith, 2005); and (iii) three-dimensional computational DNA-docking model to identify molecules capable of noncovalent DNA interaction (Snyder and Smith, 2005).

In silico prediction systems are cheaper, rapid, higher reproducibility, have low compound synthesis requirements, can undergo constant optimization, and have potential or replace the use of animals (Valerio-Jr, 2009). Their limitations are the lack of available toxicity data, inappropriate (simplistic) modeling of some endpoints and poor domain applicability of models (Cronin, 2002). The application of *in silico* methods to complex mixtures such as herbal extracts is by evidence limited to the detection of known phytochemical compounds bearing known or new structural alerts for genotoxicity reduce activity; they could however help to elucidate which compounds are responsible for a proven effect.

5.2.2. Most commonly used In vitro methods

By evidence, the absence of known phytochemical compounds bearing structural alerts for genotoxic activity in an herbal medicine does not mean the absence of potential genotoxicity. It is highly possible that many genotoxic natural molecules have not been identified yet and, therefore, complementary testing methods have been developed. The most commonly used methods for assessing the genotoxic potential of substances are listed below:

5.2.2.1. Investigations on non-mammalian cells

All these tests can be performed both in the absence and in the presence of an exogenous metabolizing system, often a rat liver S9 (microsomal) suspension. These studies which indicate gene (point) mutation includes: bacterial reverse mutation test and SOS-chromotest in *Salmonella typhimurium* and *Escherichia coli.*

http://dx.doi.org/10.5772/54858

Prokaryotic organisms: the Ames test

The *Ames test*, a bacterial reverse mutation assay, is performed with histidine dependent auxotrophic mutants of *Salmonella typhimurium* (strainsTA97, TA98, TA100, TA102, TA1535, TA1537, etc.) or tryptophan dependent auxotrophic mutants of *Escherichia coli* (WP2 isogenic strains uvr) (Maron and Ames, 1983). In the presence of a mutagenic agent, a selective pressure, from a medium depleted in the essential amino acid, results in reverse mutations and the growth of colonies that are simply counted. Several different strains of *Salmonella* must be used, because each strain individually assays for a particular type of mutagen (i.e., one strain for base pair substitutions and a separate strain for frameshift mutations) (Ogura *et al.*, 2008).

Prokaryotic organisms: SOS-chromotest

Tests based on the response of *Escherichia coli* and *Salmonella typhimurium* to genotoxic agents involves the triggering of a complex system of genes known as the "SOS response". The SOS-chromotest procedure is based on the *Escherichia coli* PQ37 strain in which the β-galactosidase (β -Gal) gene, lacZ, is placed under the control of sfiA, one of the SOS genes, through an operon fusion which (Nieminen *et al.*, 2002). The Vitotox assay involves genetically modified *Salmonella typhimurium* that harbor a luciferase gene under control of the *recN* or *pr1* promoter. In the presence of a DNA damaging compound, the SOS response leads to β -Gal or luciferase expression, respectively, which is then an indirect measure of the genotoxic activity of a test compound. The bacterial toxicity needs to be assessed, e.g. by measurement of alkaline phosphatase (Nieminen *et al.*, 2002). The Vitotox test has a high predictivity for bacterial mutagenicity and the number of false-positive scores due to cytotoxicity is relatively low (Westerink *et al.*, 2010).

Eukaryotic organisms: *Saccharomyces cerevisiae*

The most widely used *Saccharomyces cerevisiae* assay, (Nohynek *et al.*, 2004), relies on the diploid D7 strain. When compounds mutate the DNA of this yeast strain, easily scorable phenotypes (color of colonies, growth on particular media) are produced at three separate genomic sites. Additionally, each one of these phenotypic changes specifies separate type of mutation and repair mechanism. The RadarScreen assay is based on a *RAD54* promoter-linked by β -Gal reporter assay in yeast; *RAD54* is involved in DNA recombination events and repair mechanisms, especially those involving double-stranded DNA breaks during both mitosis and meiosis. Upon DNA damage and β -Gal expression, the substrate d-luciferino- β -galactopyranoside liberates luciferin that is luminometrically measured (Westerink *et al.*, 2010). The RadarScreen assay has a high predictivity for clastogenicity; the number of false-positive scores due to cytotoxicity is relatively low (Westerink *et al.*, 2010).

Eukaryotic organisms: *Aspergillus nidulans*

Because of its parasexual cycle, the filamentous fungus *Aspergillus nidulans* constitutes an excellent system for studying mitotic crossing over, since its cells spend a substantial part of their cell cycle in the G2 phase during the germination period; two copies of each chromosome during that period of the cell cycle significantly favors a mitotic recombination event, visually detected by simple plating tests (Souza-Junior *et al.*, 2004).

5.2.2.2. *Investigations on mammalian cells*

There are circumstances where the performance of the above tests does not provide appropriate or sufficient information for the assessment of genotoxicity. The first circumstance is the case of compounds that are excessively toxic to microorganisms (e.g. antibiotics, antifungal compounds). It is also the case of compounds thought or known to interfere with the mammalian cell replication system (e.g. topoisomerase inhibitors, nucleoside analogues or inhibitors of DNA metabolism) that most likely will not be detected. Guidelines consequently recommend performing additional *in vitro* mammalian cell tests. Different cell lines are used, some of which are metabolically competent to allow detection of genotoxins needing metabolic activation. Alternatively, for non-metabolizing cell lines, microsomal or S9activation as in the *Ames test* can be applied.

***In vitro* mammalian cell gene mutation test**

The *in vitro* mammalian cell gene mutation test can detect gene mutations, including base pair substitutions and frame-shift mutations. Suitable cell lines include L5178Y mouse lymphoma cells, the CHO, CHO-AS52 and V79 lines of Chinese hamster cells, and *TK6* human lymphoblastoid cells. In these cell lines the most commonly-used genetic endpoints measure mutation at thymidine kinase (*tk*) and hypoxanthine-guanine phosphoribosyl transferase (*hprt*) loci, and a transgene of xanthine-guanine phosphoribosyl transferase (*xprt*). The *tk, hprt,* and *xprt* mutation tests detect different spectra of genetic events. The autosomal location of *tk* and *xprt* may allow the detection of genetic events (e.g. large deletions) not detected at the hemizygous *hprt* locus on X-chromosomes. Preference is often given to the L5178Y mouse lymphoma assay (MLA *tk* +/-). This test can detect not only gene mutations, but also other genetic events leading to the inactivation or loss of heterozygosity (LOH) of the thymidine-kinase gene, such as large deletions or mitotic recombination. While the standard protocol allows discrimination between gross DNA alterations and point mutations on the basis of colony size, the use of additional analytical methods can give information about the specific event that has occurred (Wang *et al.*, 2009).

***In vitro* mammalian chromosomal aberration test**

The *in vitro* chromosomal aberration (CA) test detects structural aberrations and may give an indication for numerical chromosome aberrations (polyploidy) in cultured mammalian cells caused by the test substance. However, this test is optimized for the detection of structural aberrations. The *in vitro* chromosomal aberration test may employ cultures of established cell lines or primary cell cultures. Cells in metaphase are analyzed for the presence of chromosomal aberrations. Additional mechanistic information can be provided using FISH or chromosome painting. The test has been widely used for many decades but it is resource intensive, time consuming and it requires good expertise for scoring. Only a limited number of metaphases are analyzed for each assay.

***In vitro* mammalian cell micronucleus test**

The purpose of the *in vitro* mammalian cell micronucleus test (MNvit) is to identify substances that cause structural and numerical chromosomal damage in cells that have undergone cell division during or after the exposure to the test substance. The assay detects micronuclei in the cytoplasm of interphase cells and typically employs human or rodent cells lines or primary cell cultures.

The *in vitro* mammalian cell micronucleus test (OECD, 2010a) can be conducted in the presence or in the absence of cytochalasin B (cytoB), which is used to block cell division and generate binucleate cells. The advantage of using cytoB is that it allows clear identification that treated and control cells have divided *in vitro* and provides a simple assessment of cell proliferation. The *in vitro* micronucleus test can be combined with kinetochore staining or fluorescence *in situ* hybridisation (FISH) to provide additional mechanistic information, e.g. on non-disjunction, which is not detected in the standard *in vitro* micronucleus assay. The MNvit is rapid and easy to conduct and it is the only *in vitro* test that can efficiently detect both clastogens and aneugens. The MNvit was formally validated based on the retrospective evaluation of available data (Corvi *et al.*, 2008).

Micronuclei are acentric chromosomal fragments or whole chromosomes left behind during mitotic cellular division, appearing in the cytoplasm of interphase cells as small additional nuclei. The detection of micronuclei, manual or, as more recently described, automated (Westerink *et al.*, 2011), provides a readily measurable index of chromosome breakage and loss.

Unscheduled DNA synthesis (UDS) assay

The unscheduled DNA synthesis (UDS) assay measures chemical induced DNA excision repair by detecting labeled thymidine (3H-TdR) incorporation. The induction of DNA repair mechanisms is presumed to have been preceded by DNA damage, indicating the DNA damaging ability of a chemical (Bakkali *et al.*, 2008). A core limitation of the UDS assay is its inability to indicate if a xenobiotic is mutagenic; indeed, it provides no information regarding the fidelity of DNA repair and it does not Identify DNA lesions handled by mechanisms other than excision repair (Lambert *et al.*, 2005).

Sister chromatid exchanges (SCE) assay

Various cytomolecular protocols have been used to perform the sister chromatid exchanges (SCE) assay (Bakkali *et al.*, 2008; Hseu *et al.*, 2008). This method relies on the differential staining of sister chromatids during replication to visualize reciprocal genetic exchanges between them. Such an exchange arises when, during DNA replication, two sister chromatids break and rejoin with one another (Wilson and Thompson, 2007); this natural mechanism is increased by exposure to genotoxic agents capable of inducing DNA damage (Djelic *et al.*, 2006).

***In vitro* comet assay (single-cell gel electrophoresis assay)**

In this well-established, highly sensitive, rapid, and simple genotoxicity test, isolated cells embedded in agarose are lysed, washed to remove membranes and proteins, briefly electrophoresed, stained and examined under epifluorescence microscopy; strand breaks, coming from either strand breakage or excision repair, result in DNA extending towards the anode in a structure resembling a "comet" (Speit *et al.*, 2009; Berthelot-Ricou *et al.*, 2011). Depending on experimental conditions, the migrating DNA (comet tail or derived parameters) reflects the amount of single- or double-strand breaks, alkalilabile sites, including incomplete excision repair sites, but also of DNA–DNA and DNA–protein cross-links (Santos *et al.*, 2009;Verschaeve *et al.*, 2010). A broad spectrum of DNA damage can then be detected either by visual classification of comet morphologies ("visual scoring") or from morphological parameters obtained by image analysis and integration of intensity profiles using in-house or commercially available systems. There are only few limitations of the comet assay with regard to its application and interpretation. Short-lived primary DNA lesions such as single strand breaks, which may undergo rapid DNA repair, could be missed when using inadequate sampling times. Another limitation is that indirect mechanisms related to cytotoxicity (e.g. DNA fragmentation in apoptosis) can lead to positive effects (Speit *et al.*, 2005).

5.2.2.3. Plant in vitro cultures in the evaluation of genotoxicity

Adventitious roots (e.g. *Allium cepa*) or primary roots (e.g. *Vicia faba, Crepis capillaris, and Pisum sativum*) are the most frequently used for assessing chromosome or DNA damage in higher plant bioassays (Maluszynska and Juchimiuk, 2005). It follows that to conduct such tests, plant breeding is necessary. Nevertheless, the development of tissue *in vitro* culture and transformation techniques make other tissues attractive as sources of mitotic cells. An example is a culture of transformed roots, so called hairy roots, obtained after the transformation with *Agrobacterium rhizogenes*. Transformed root lines, which are characterized by lateral branching, easily provide many root tip cells. It allows them to be used in cytogenetic analysis in basic plant genome research. Additionally, "genetic identity" is a feature of transformed roots which is very important in case the plant is not self-fertile. Unfortunately, a number of altered karyotypes have been found in hairy roots of the majority of species, both during transformation and in long-term *in vitro* culture. However, *C. capillaris* hairy roots are a rare example of karyotype and morphology stability after transformation and during long–term culture. Their fast growth, genetic stability and simple conditions of *in vitro* culture, together with simple karyotypes, make them convenient for evaluating chromosome damage. An additional advantage of *C. capillaris* hairy roots is its higher sensitivity to mutagens compared to primary roots. A comparison of the sensitivity of cells of root meristems of seedlings and hairy roots was based on a response to two mutagens: MH (maleic acid hydrazide) and X-ray. Chromosomal aberrations and SCEs tests were used to analyse chromosome changes, whereas TUNEL assay was applied for in situ detection of DNA fragmentation. The responses of the transformed roots to analyzed mutagens were significantly stronger than the responses of the primary roots, both on the DNA and chromosome level. The cytogenetic effect of MH was similar in seedlings treated with 2 mM MH and in hairy roots treated with a four times lower concentration of mutagen. Furthermore, the same dose of MH caused the death of hairy roots, while it did not affect seedling growth. There were also differences in the frequency of chromosomal aberrations in hairy roots and seedling roots to the same doses of X-rays. Monitoring of DNA breakage in the TUNEL test after MH treatment showed a higher frequency of labelled nuclei in hairy roots than in seedlings, even though the mutagen concentration used to treat hairy roots was four times lower. Irradiation with the

http://dx.doi.org/10.5772/54858

same dose caused DNA fragmentation in nuclei with a two times higher frequency in hairy roots than in seedlings (Maluszynska and Juchimiuk, 2005). This suggests that all the described features of *C. capillaris* hairy roots, especially their relatively high sensitivity, make them a promising new system for plant bioassaying.

Advantages and limitations of *in vitro* genotoxicity assays

It is recognized that *in vitro* genotoxicity assays are extremely useful. Their set-ups are small and use minimal amounts of test substances, allowing low costs, high numbers of replicates, miniaturization and automation; they have generally been validated to detect an impressive number of genotoxic agents and mechanisms. However, these simple cellular models are often thought to be a too reductionist approach. The main limitations of in vitro models include the artificial and non-physiological conditions in which the cells are maintained which do not reflect the body temperature, the blood electrolyte concentrations, the extracellular matrix or the extent of cell–cell interactions within tissues. Most cell systems represent only one cell type, often cancerous in origin, with uncertain DNA damage signalization and repair status and possibly further degenerated during maintenance culture. Moreover, culture media are not always homeostatic during experiments (Hartung, 2011).

5.2.3. *In vivo methods for genotoxicity assessment*

5.2.3.1. *In vivo mammalian investigations*

In order to overcome some limitations of the investigations, *in vivo* methods have been also developed, not to replace them, but to complete their information on a whole organism. Despite the mainstream willingness to substitute animal experimentation with in vitro models, animal studies *in vitro* remain core component of toxicity assessment of drugs and plant-based medicinal products. Number of test animals, gender, suitable controls, and dose and time parameters is important components of these experiments and are generally specified in the relevant guidelines (Hartung, 2011). At various periods after the treatment, the blood samples are collected by venipuncture (usually from the tail), the animals are sacrificed and organs (liver, kidney, femurs, tibias...) are removed for the analysis.

***In vivo* micronucleus assay**

Blood sample and bone marrow are collected by venipuncture and removed from the femur, respectively; they are then smeared, stained and scored as described for the in vitro assay. As a measure of toxicity of test compounds on bone marrow, the polychromatic erythrocytes: normochromatic erythrocytes ratio is scored; the incidences of micronuclei are also calculated to highlight clastogenic properties (Nohynek *et al.*, 2004). The frequency of micronucleated reticulocytes can also be determined.

***In vivo* unscheduled DNA synthesis (UDS) assay**

The *in vivo* UDS is generally evaluated in the hepatocytes of treated animals following the same detection systems as its corresponding *in vitro* model.

Mouse spot test

The "mouse spot test", a rapid screening test to detect gene mutations and recombination in mice somatic cells (Lambert *et al.*, 2005), is based on the observation that genotoxic compounds can induce color spots on the coat of mice exposed *in utero*. The color spots arise when mouse melanoblasts, heterozygous for several recessive coat color mutations, lose a dominant allele through a gene mutation, chromosomal aberration or reciprocal recombination, allowing the recessive gene to be expressed.

Transgenic rodent (TGR) mutation assay

Transgenic animals carry multiple copies of chromosomally integrated plasmid and phage shuttle vectors that harbor reporter genes to detect, quantify and sequence mutations *in vivo*. The frequency of mutations occurring in the animal is scored by recovering shuttle vector and analyzing the phenotype of the reporter gene in a bacterial host; the molecular analysis of the gene can provide further mechanistic information (Lambert *et al.*, 2005). Some deletions and insertion mutations may however not be detected in phage-based TGR. The test does not involve a large number of animals and a major advantage is that mutations can be evaluated in any tissue; the protocol is reproducible but requires well-trained experts, is not yet automated and the assay cost is superior to most of the other genotoxicity assays (Lambert *et al.*, 2005).

***In vivo* comet assay**

After treatment and sacrifice animals, blood lymphocytes and/or cells, dissociated from organs by mincing a small piece into very fine fragments, are treated as per the same protocols as *in vitro* studies (Cavalcanti *et al.*, 2010; Ouedraogo *et al.*, 2012). The *in vivo* comet assay detects low levels of DNA damage, requiring small numbers of cells per sample.

Somatic mutation and recombination test (SMART)

In view of minimizing the number of higher organisms used in toxicological research, a somatic mutations and recombination test (SMART) in the wings of *Drosophila melanogaster* ("wing-spot test") has been developed. This test, based on the loss of heterozygosity for two recessive markers (Carmona *et al.*, 2011b), is a tool to evaluate gene mutations, chromosome aberrations and rearrangements related to mitotic recombination. Recently, the comet assay has been adapted to be used *in vivo* in *Drosophila melanogaster* (Carmona *et al.*, 2011b; Ouedraogo *et al.*, 2012).

5.2.3.2. In vivo Investigations on plant cells

Plant mutagenicity bioassays have been in existence for many years. Now, plant bioassays are well-established systems and are used for screening and monitoring environmental chemicals with mutagenic and carcinogenic potential (Maluszynska and Juchimiuk, 2005). The International Program on Chemical Safety (IPCS) collaborative study on higher plant genetic systems for screening and monitoring environmental pollutants was initiated in 1984. It is a cooperative venture of the United Nations Environment Program, the International Labour Organization and the World Health Organization. Its goal was to develop methodologies for improving the assessment of risks from chemical exposure. Under the sponsorship of the IPCS, 17 laboratories from diverse regions of the world participated in evaluating the utility of four plant bioassays for detecting genetic hazards of environmental chemicals. Using plant bioassays for testing and monitoring environmental chemicals or pollutions has many advantages. They are easy to handle, inexpensive and in many cases more sensitive than other available systems (Maluszynska and Juchimiuk, 2005). There are some limitations as well, such as the longer life cycle of most plants than bacteria, yeast or *Drosophila* and some biochemical differences between plants and mammals. The differences between plant and animal cells have led to the lack of general recognition of plant genotoxicity assays. Limited data from plant bioassays are applicable only when we wish to extrapolate them directly to human. There are many reports on the excellent correlation of the plant system with the mammalian system. Higher plant bioassays are based on the detection of chromosomal aberrations, sister chromatid exchanges, and recently, on the analysis of DNA strand breaks. In some systems, point mutations are analyzed, e.g. chlorophyll mutations in leaves, waxy mutations or embryo mutations of *Arabidopsis*.

Cytogenetic tests

Cytogenetic tests analyze the frequency and type of chromosome aberrations in mitotic cells and the frequency of micronuclei in interphase cells. Genotoxic agents cause DNA damage, which is either repaired or otherwise leads to alterations of the DNA. Chromosome aberrations are the consequence of DNA double strand break which was unrepaired or repaired improperly. Broken chromosome ends without telomeres become "sticky" and may fuse with other broken chromosome ends. The result of these chromosomal rearrangements are acentric fragments, dicentric bridges observed in mitotic cells of the first cell cycle after mutagenic treatment or micronuclei in the interphase cell in the next cell cycle.

***Allium* test**

The classical test for studying the effects of chemicals on plant chromosomes is the *Allium* test, which was developed by Levan in 1938 (Maluszynska and Juchimiuk, 2005). It uses the root tips from bulbs. *Allium* has eight pairs of relatively large chromosomes; this allows for the easy detection of chromosome aberrations. The plant material is available all year round. The micronucleus test was developed parallel to chromosome aberration assays. Micronuclei are extranuclear bodies of chromatin material formed as a consequence of chromosome breakage or aneuploidy. The frequency of cells with micronuclei is a good indicator of the cytogenetic effects of tested chemicals. Similarly, chromosome available all year round. The micronucleus test was developed parallel to chromosome aberration assay. Micronuclei are extranuclear bodies of chromatin material formed as a consequence of chromosome breakage or aneuploidy. The frequency of cells with micronuclei is a good indicator of the cytogenetic effects of tested chemicals. Similarly, chromosome aberration and micronuclei tests are conducted with other plant species such as *Vicia faba, Crepis capillaris, and Hordeum vulgare* (Maluszynska and Juchimiuk, 2005).

***Tradescantia* test**

One of the most suitable plants for detecting different types of xenobiotics is *Tradescantia*. This plant is especially useful for evaluating a hazardous condition in the environment. There are two main tests: the stamen hair mutation (Trad-SH) test and the micronucleus assay (Trad-MCN). The first is based on the heterozygosity for flower colour in *Tradescantia* clones. Clone 4430 is a hybrid of *T. hirsutiflora* and *subacaulis* reproduced only asexually, through cloning. The visual marker for mutation induction is a phenotypic change in the pigmentation of the stamen cells from the dominant blue colour to recessive pink. The *Trad-MCN* test is based on the frequency of micronuclei in tetrad cells induced in male meiotic cells by the tested mutagen. These tests may be used under laboratory, or in situ exposure conditions, for monitoring air or water, or for testing radioactive or chemical agents.

Sister chromatid Exchanges

The sister chromatid exchange (SCE) test is a well-known, highly sensitive cytogenetic tool for detecting DNA damage. The test is based on DNA segregation, which occurs in chromosomes according to a semiconservative model of DNA replication. SCE involves symmetrical exchange at one locus between sister chromatids that does not alter chromosome length and genetic information. Sister chromatids are visualized through the methods of incorporating bromodeoxyuridine (BrdU) into chromosomal DNA and different staining of chromatids containing DNA with BrdU and chromatids without BrdU. The frequency of SCEs per chromosome set increases after treatment with genotoxic agents. SCE method can be applied in both plant and mammalian cells. Plant species used for SCE test should have a low number of chromosomes, relatively large, such as *Vicia faba* and *Allium cepa*. *Crepis capillaris* is especially convenient for analyzing the frequency of SCE. This species has only three pairs of morphologically differentiated chromosomes.

Detection of DNA breaks

The development of molecular biology and the application of molecular techniques in cytogenetic studies have made progress in the methods of detection and the estimation of genotoxicity of different agents.

The comet assay

The Comet assay was established for investigating the process of apoptosis in animal cells and then it was adapted to plant cells (Maluszynska and Juchimiuk, 2005). This test allows not only the detection of single and double stranded DNA breaks in the nucleus, but also the measuring of the level of DNA migration through an agarose gel in an electric field. This is also a useful tool to investigate the capacity of DNA repair of damage induced by different types of mutagens and various damage levels in different cell types The Comet assay was used to detect DNA damage in nuclei of several plant species isolated from leaves or root tissue after mutagenic treatment.

TUNEL test

Another test used to identify apoptosis that has found application in genotoxicity studies is the TUNEL (TdT-mediated dUTP nick end labeling) test (Maluszynska and Juchimiuk, 2005). The polymerization of labelled nucleotides to DNA strand breaks in situ is catalyzed by terminal deoxynucleotidyl transferase. The advantages of the TUNEL test include detec-

http://dx.doi.org/10.5772/54858

tion of DNA breaks at a single nucleus, short time of assay and easy screening of labelled nuclei. This test is recommended for the preliminary evaluation of genotoxicity of any new tested agent.

FISH – new perspectives for plant bioassays

Changes in chromosomal morphology are usually detected with classical cytogenetic techniques. However, the traditional methods of chromosome staining can fail in the analysis of small changes in chromosome structure. Fluorescent in situ hybridization (FISH) gives new possibilities to study chromosomal aberrations in plant mutagenesis. It allows the detection and a more detailed localization of chromosomal rearrangements, both in mitotic and interphase nuclei. Additionally, it helps to understand the mechanisms of the formation of chromosomal aberrations. Until now, DNA probes required for each chromosome have made possible detailed identification of chromosome aberrations using FISH, mainly in human genotoxic studies ((Maluszynska and Juchimiuk, 2005). Even DNA probes for particular plant chromosomes are limited; there are few examples when FISH employing chromosome region-specific DNA probes (e.g. centromere, telomere, rDNA) is helpful in chromosome aberration analysis. Furthermore, detailed analysis of chromosomal rearrangements in interphase nuclei using FISH is especially important in tissues in which mutagenic treatment caused a decrease in the frequency of cell divisions.

Transgenic plants as a bioindicators

A new approach to biomonitoring, which involves transgenic plants, is based on the integration into the plant genome of a marker gene of known sequences that will serve as target for mutagenic influences. The transgene can be introduced in an active or inactive state and mutation permits the evaluation of the mutagenicity of the tested agents. Two different transgenic systems were designed to study mutagenic influence via point mutations and homologous recombination events (HR). To analyze point mutations, plants carry one copy of transgene (GUS) per haploid genome inactivated by point mutation. The plants used to screen HR events possess one copy per haploid genome of an overlapping, nonfunctional, truncated version of the GUS marker gene as recombination substrate. GUS is activated via strand-break-induced HR between two repeats. The frequency of point mutation and homologous recombination can be measured by GUS gene-reactivation assay. To date, mainly transgenic *Arabidopsis* and tobacco plants have been used for the biomonitoring of environmental factors (Maluszynska and Juchimiuk, 2005).

5.3. "Omics" technologies

The term "omic" is derived from the Latin suffix "ome" meaning mass or many. "Omics" studies involve a high number of measurements per endpoint to acquire comprehensive, integrated understanding of biology and to simultaneously identify the different factors (e.g., genes, RNA, proteins and metabolites) rather than each of those individually (Ouedraogo *et al.*, 2012). "Toxicogenomics" aim to study the interaction between the structure and activity of the genome and the adverse biological effects of exogenous agents. This discipline is based on the concept that the toxic effects of xenobiotics on biological systems are generally reelected at cellular level by their impact on the expression of genes (transcriptomics) and proteins (proteomics) and on the production of small metabolite (metabonomics) (Ouedraogo *et al.*, 2012).

5.3.1. Transcriptomics

Transcriptomics analyze the expression level by measuring the transcriptome, the genome-wide mRNA expression. Transcriptomics uses high density and/or high-throughput methods of assessing mRNA expression of genes.

5.3.1.1. Microarrays and qrt-PCR

Microarrays ("DNA microarrays", "DNA arrays", "DNA chips", "biochips", "gene chips"), the most common approach used for gene expression profiling, are generated by immobilizing a high number of oligonucleotides on an extremely small surface (up to 200,000 spots/cm^2). Based on the target sequences, significant changes of mRNA can be estimated for thousands of genes (Ouedraogo *et al.*, 2012). Specialized sub-sets of gene expression changes and quantitative real-time reverse transcriptase-polymerase chain reactions (qrt-PCR)-based approaches that focus on specific genes have also been developed. The latter is a highly recommended confirmatory tool for quantifying gene expression with improvements in sensitivity and specificity.

5.3.1.2. Open systems

Other technologies such as serial analysis of gene expression (SAGE), massively parallel signature sequencing (MPSS) and total gene expression analysis (TOGA) are also successfully used to detect changes in transcriptomes (Ouedraogo *et al.*, 2012). In contrast to microarray technology (which can only measure transcript abundances with pre-selected, known probe and sequence), these approaches are "open systems" and thus suited for gene discovery; they offer linear gene expression quantification over a wide dynamic range.

5.3.1.3. Specific genes targeting

Published microarrays genomics studies have been quite inconclusive for genotoxicity prediction; they nevertheless pointed to some genes, *GADD45a*, p53R2, *Ephx*, *Btg2* and *Cbr3 Perp* (Ouedraogo *et al.*, 2012) of which a robust induction of expression was noted for a series of genotoxins with apparently high sensitivity and specificity. There is a considerable interest in genes involved in tissue development, cell death, cell-to-cell signaling, cycle and cellular growth, proliferation, DNA damage signaling and DNA repair (Jordan *et al.*, 2010).

5.3.1.4. Limitations of transcriptomics

Changes in genes expression levels may predict major changes in the proteins profiles in cells, tissues or organisms but there are cases where a functional protein is not produced despite

http://dx.doi.org/10.5772/54858

gene expression; and so, changes in the transcriptome do not necessarily reflect a change in the profile of "end-products" (Ouedraogo *et al.*, 2012).

5.3.1.5. Proteomics

Proteomics is the study of a broad spectrum of proteins within a cell or tissue, including proteins expression, structural status, functional states and their interactions with other cellular components. Key technologies rely on two-dimensional gel electrophoresis coupled to mass spectrometry on antibody microarrays and on LC–MS–MS of proteins fragments, a technique known as *"shotgun proteomics"* and its specific platform variations, called ICAT (isotope coding affinity tags) and MuDPIT (multi-dimensional protein identification technology). Affinity chromatography, fluorescence resonance energy transfer and surface plasmon resonance are also used to identify protein–protein or protein–DNA interactions. X-ray tomography is used to determine the location of proteins or protein complexes in labeled cells. Techniques are available but a large database of proteomics "fingerprint' is still needed for compounds of known toxicity; once available for a series of known carcinogens, it will be possible to identify changes in biochemical pathways and to assess the toxicity of unknown compounds. The products of the genes identified so far in transcriptomics studies are probably promising candidates as proteomic markers.

5.3.2. Metabonomics

Toxicometabonomics concern the analysis, either in organs, blood or urine, of metabolites and metabolic pathways modifications that follow a toxic insult. This implies the quantitative and qualitative study of a wide range of low molecular weight (LMW) molecules produced as the net result of cellular by nuclear magnetic resonance (NMR) spectroscopy, Fourier transform infrared and near-infrared spectroscopy or mass spectrometry (MS). The latter technique generally requires pre-separation of the metabolic components by gas chromatography (GC), liquid chromatography (LC) or capillary electrophoresis (CE) (Ouedraogo *et al.*, 2012). So far metabonomics have been scarcely applied to genotoxicity studies; major applications concern the urinary profiling of damaged bases excreted upon DNA excision repair and the search for activated metabolites of precarcinogens.

5.4. Next Generation Sequencing (NGS)

The advent of the human genome project helped to foster the development of faster and cheaper DNA sequencing. Sanger sequencing (Sanger *et al.*, 1977) also now known as *'first generation sequencing'*, has dominated the past few decades. The need to conduct large-scale sequencing projects more economically has led to the rapid development of a variety of *next-generation sequencing* (NGS) technologies. The development of NGS platforms represents a great advance in technology. In comparison to Sanger sequencing, the NGS platforms are able to produce orders of magnitude more sequence data through massively parallel processes, which result in substantial quantities of data at a low cost per base. With the challenge issued by the US Food and Drug Administration's (FDA), biomarkers are set to have an ever more important role in the drug development process (Wollard *et al.*, 2011). NGS could have a central role in the discovery of new genomic biomarkers, owing to the many different types of experiment that can be performed on a single machine. From a single sample, it could be possible to generate complementary data sets from *genome DNA sequencing, miRNA,* and both *transcriptome sequencing* and *quantification* to *epigenetic changes* of DNA methylation, *histone post-translational modifications* and even *protein translation* (ribosome profiling). The challenge will be around developing data analysis tools that could simultaneously analyze across these vast data sets, looking for biomarker signatures. NGS can be used in the very early stages of target identification to provide detailed genomics data in the same way as traditional tools, such as *microarrays. RNA-Seq* can be used to perform differential gene expression studies of diseased versus normal tissue. Data from NGS of whole human exomes are being successfully applied to identify mutations in genes underlying rare Mendelian disorders, which could also inform target identification. In addition, using NGS has enabled the resolution of genetic linkage studies, a finding that has potential in identifying new drug targets from complex trait genetics studies (Wollard et al., 2011).

NGS has also proved to be a useful tool in the characterization of therapeutically relevant mutations in mice (D'Ascenzo *et al.*, 2009), which can often contribute important information to target validation. Through exome or targeted region capture sequencing, underlying mutations can be rapidly isolated without the requirement for lengthy genetic mapping studies. NGS promises to facilitate this area of research by uncovering all of the common and rare genetic variation in human populations. With a comprehensive genetic map of all human variation produced by NGS, researchers will be able to perform more detailed experiments to detect genetic variation underlying the response to medicines.

5.5. Computational methods to predict genotoxicity

Decades of mutagenesis and clastogenesis studies have yielded enough structure-activity-relationship (SAR) information to make feasible the construction of computational models for prediction of endpoints based on molecular structure and reactivity. It is expected that the right balance of *in vivo, in vitro* and computational toxicology predictions applied as early as possible in the discovery process will help to reduce the need for actual genotoxicity testing. The current trend is to make simpler predictions, closer to the mechanism of action, and to follow them up with *in vitro* or *in vivo* assays.

Computer–assisted prediction models, so-called predictive tools, will likely play an essential role in the proposed repertoire of "alternative methods". Acceptable prediction models already exist for those toxicological endpoints which are based on well-understood mechanism, such as mutagenicity and skin sensitization, whereas mechanistically more complex endpoints such as acute, chronic or organ toxicities currently cannot be satisfactorily predicted (Merlot, 2010). A potential strategy to assess such complex toxicities will lie in their dissection into models for the different steps or pathways leading to the final endpoint. Integration of these models should result in a higher predictivity. Despite these limitations, computer-assisted prediction tools already today play a complementary role for the assessment of chemicals for

http://dx.doi.org/10.5772/54858

which no data is available or for which toxicological testing is impractical due to the lack of availability of sufficient compounds for testing.

However, the broad application of such predictions has been hampered by their lack of accuracy (Simon-Hettich *et al.*, 2006). It is generally deemed that this lack of accuracy is due to the complexity of the predicted endpoints, rather than to the poor performance of data analysis methods. The focus, therefore, is on modeling more simple endpoints, such as off-target activity, to increase accuracy and to combine the results with experiments from other fields (e.g. -omics) to try to make a link with potential modes of action. Of the several approaches to predicting the effects of small molecules from the structure, most algorithms can be put into two classes: *expert systems* and *statistical modeling*.

Expert systems, such as *Oncologic* (Woo *et al.*, 1995) or *Derek* for Windows (http://www.lhasalimited.org), are a repository of expert knowledge. The computer is there to store and then use on demand a piece of knowledge that has been formalized and input by human experts. The power of the system is linked to the amount of expert time invested in feeding it and to the availability of reliable and high-quality datasets. Its expansion, therefore, is limited by the time it takes for humans to collect and digest lots of information. Although the information contained in these systems is considered reliable enough, it suffers from a lack of sensitivity (Valerio-Jr *et al.*, 2007). The direct consequence is that many side effects are likely to be missed. Medicinal chemists have to use this tool cautiously because the outcome of the program requires a deep understanding of the system to interpret results (Mustin *et al.*, 2008).

On the other hand, *statistical modeling* software – such as *Topkat* (http://accelrys.com/products/discovery-studio/toxicology), *PASS* (Anzali *et al.*, 2001), *TPSSVM* (Kawai *et al.*, 2008) and *Multicase* (http://www.multicase.com/)–aims to analyze existing data and automatically build models, with a reduced need for human intervention. Just as for *expert systems*, the first step consists of assembling a relevant training set of compounds with experimental biological data. The system will then perform a statistical analysis that shall be reviewed by a scientist. These systems require a lot of attention for the selection of modeling techniques and structural descriptors. They have several advantages over *expert systems*, however: a model can be optimized on internal data more quickly and objectively than through an expert analysis. It can also be combined with a quantitative structure–activity relationship *(QSAR)* when only a single chemical series is involved. Although statistical analysis highlights trends in diverse structures (i.e. all molecules containing a given fragment are flagged as potentially toxic), the QSAR handles the more subtle structural changes that, in a set of similar compounds, flag some compounds as toxic and others as less harmful. The combination of statistical analysis and QSAR, therefore, facilitates lead optimization and the removal of toxicophores (Merlot, 2010).

6. Applications to herbal medicines

As genotoxicity testing aims to yield information types of damage, including gene mutations, structural chromosome aberrations (clastogenicity) and numerical chromosome aberrations (aneugenicity), standard test batteries have been developed (Kirkland *et al.*, 2005) which include the assessment, and without metabolic activation, these tests have been developed for single chemicals and applying them to herbs has been quite a challenge. The current EU guidelines for herbal products (EMEA, 2007) define the Ames test as the primary endpoint that, if negative, accepts the drug as probably "non genotoxic". This is not entirely satisfying however and there are still heavy debates on the topic (EMEA, 2008); indeed (i) the Ames test does not detect every genotoxic insult; and (ii) some common compounds, including flavonoids, yield very positive Ames tests but are not carcinogens. Given the number of herbal products on the market and relatively low budgets available for research, there are still relatively few herbs for which safety assessment according to the current guidelines has been done. Nonetheless, some herbal products and their secondary metabolites were assessed for genotoxicity by various techniques. The Ames test has been widely used to assess the mutagenicity of herbal products, including for example extracts from *Calendula officinalis L., Echinodorus macrophyllus* (Kunth) *Micheli, Mouriri pusa* Gardner, *Phyllantus orbicularis* Kunth, *Punica granatum L., Parthenium hysterophorus L.*and a green tea *catechins* preparation (Santos *et al.*, 2009; Nohynek *et al.*, 2004). Among these extracts, *Punica granatum* whole extract and the enriched fractions of flavonoids and tannins from *Mouriri pusa* were found to give a positive genotoxic test. The genotoxicity of Copaiba oil (*Copaifera langsdorffii* Desf.) was demonstrated by *in vitro* micronucleus and comet assays. Metabonomics techniques have already been used toxicity studies of Guan Mutong (*Aristolochia manshuriensis* Kom.) (Ouedraogo *et al.*, 2012) and its toxic component aristolochic acid I was suggested to possess genotoxic potency also by QSA modeling. In the in vitro comet assay, artesunate, a semisynthetic derivative from artemisinin (*Artemisia annua* L.) induced DNA breakage in a dose-dependent manner.

There is certainly a need for the development of validated methods to rapidly pinpoint indicators of genotoxicity that yield warning signals and indicate which drugs need further assessment through a complete test battery.

Author details

Hala M. Abdelmigid[1,2*]

Address all correspondence to: halaabdelmigid@yahoo.com

1 Botany department, Faculty of Science, El Mansoura University, KSA

2 Biotechnology Dept. Faculty of Science, Taif University, KSA

References

[1] Anzali, S, et al. (2001). Discriminating between drugs and non-drugs by prediction of activity spectra for substances (PASS). J. Med. Chem. , 44, 2432-2437.

[2] Atsamo, A. D, Nguelefack, T. B, Datté, J. Y, & Kamanyi, A. (2011). Acute and subchronic oral toxicity assessment of the aqueous extracts from the stem *Erythrina senegalensis* DC (Fabaceae) in rodents. Journal of Ethnopharmacology , 134, 697-702.

[3] Bakkali, F, Averbeck, S, Averbeck, D, & Idaomar, M. (2008). Biological effects of essential oils-areview. Food and Chemical Toxicology, 46, 446-475.

[4] Berthelot-ricou, A, & Perrin, J. Di Giorgio, C., De Meo, M., Botta, A., Courbiere, B., (2011). Comet assay on mouse oocytes: an improved technique to evaluate genotoxic risk on female germ cells. Fertility and Sterility. , 95, 1452-1457.

[5] Bootsma, D, Kraemer, K. H, Cleaver, J. E, & Hoeijmakers, J. H. (2001). Nucleotide excision repair syndromes: xeroderma pigmentosum, cockayne syndrome and trichothiodystrophy. In: Scriver, C.R., Beaudet, A.L., Sly, W.S., Valle, D. (Eds.), The Metabolic and Molecular Bases of Inherited Disease. McGraw-Hill, New York, , 677-703.

[6] Cavalcanti, B. C, Ferreiraa, J. R. O, Moura, D. J, Rosa, R. M, Furtado, G. V, Burbano, R. R, Silveira, E. R, Lima, M. A. S, Camara, C. A. G, Saf, J, Henriques, J. A. P, Rao, V. S. N, Costa-lotufo, L. V, Moraes, M. O, & Pessoa, C. (2010). Structure-mutagenicity relationship of kaurenoic acid from Xylopia sericeae (Annonaceae). Mutation Research , 701, 153-163.

[7] Chan, T. Y. K. (2009). Aconite poisoning. Clin. Toxicol. 47 (4), 279-285.

[8] Corvi, R, Albertini, S, Hartung, T, Hoffmann, S, Maurici, D, Pfuhler, S, Van Benthem, J, & Vanparys, P. (2008). ECVAM retrospective validation of the *in vitro* micronucleus test (MNT). Mutagenesis , 271, 271-283.

[9] Cronin, M. T. D. (2002). The current status and future applicability of quantitative structure-activity relationships (QSARs) in predicting toxicity. Alternatives to Laboratory Animals: ATLA , 30, 81-84.

[10] Ascenzo, D, et al. (2009). Mutation discovery in the mouse using genetically guided array capture and resequencing. Mamm. Genome , 20, 424-436.

[11] De Smet, P. A. (2007). Clinical risk management of herb-drug interactions. British Journal of Clinical Pharmacology, 63, 258-267.

[12] Djelic, N, Spremo-potparevic, B, Bajic, V, & Djelic, D. (2006). Sister chromatid exchange and micronuclei in human peripheral blood lymphocytes treated with thyroxine *in vitro*. Mutation Research , 604, 1-7.

[13] Eastmond, D. A, Hartwig, A, Anderson, D, Anwar, W, Cimino, M. C, Dobrev, I, Douglas, G. R, Nohmi, T, Phillips, D. H, & Vickers, C. (2009). Mutagenicity testing for chemical risk assessment: update of the WHO/IPCS Harmonized Scheme. Mutagenesis , 24, 341-349.

[14] Echa, . Guidance for the Implementation of REACH. Guidance on information requirements and chemical safety assessment. Chapter R.7.a: Endpoint specific guidance. Section R.7.7 Mutagenicity and carcinogenicity, European Chemicals Agency,

Helsinki.Availableat:http://guidance.echa.europa.eu/docs/guidance_document/information_requirements_r7a_en.pdf, 377.

[15] ECVAMhttp://ecvam.jrc.it/consulted January (2012).

[16] EFSA(2009). Scientific Opinion of the Scientific Committee on Existing approaches incorporating replacement, reduction and refinement of animal testing: applicability in food and feed risk assessment. The EFSA Journal 1052, 1077.

[17] EMEA(2007). Guideline on the assessment of genotoxic constituent's substances/preparations.

[18] EMEA(2008). Overview of comments received on draft in herbal 'guideline the assessment of genotoxic constituents in herbal substances/preparations' (Emea / hmpc/ 107079/2007).

[19] Erickson, R. P. (2010). Somatic gene mutation and human disease other than cancer: an update. Mutat. Res. , 705, 96-106.

[20] Fang, Z, Zhang, Z, Wang, Y. -Y, Cao, X. -L, Huo, Y. -F, & Yang, H. L., (2011). Bioactivation of herbal constituents: simple alerts in the complex system. Expert Opinion on Drug Metabolism&Toxicology, 7, 1-19.

[21] Frank, S. A. (2010). Evolution in health and medicine Sackler colloquium: Somatic evolutionary genomics: mutations during development cause highly variable genetic mosaicism with risk of cancer and neurodegeneration. Proc. Natl. Acad. Sci. USA. 107 Suppl , 1, 1725-1730.

[22] Fu, P. P, Xia, Q, Lin, G, & Chou, M. W. (2004). Pyrrolizidine alkaloids-genotoxicity, metabolism enzymes, metabolic activation, and mechanisms. Drug Metabolism Reviews , 36, 1-55.

[23] Fu, P. P, Xia, Q, Chou, M. W, & Lin, G. (2007). Detection, hepatotoxicity, and tumorigenicity of pyrrolizidine alkaloids in Chinese herbal plants and herbal dietary supplements. Journal of Food&DrugAnalysis, 15, 400-415.

[24] Gardiner, P, Sarma, D. N, Dog, T. L, Barrett, M. L, et al. (2008). The state of dietary supplement adverse event reporting in the United States. Pharmacoepidemiol. Drug Saf. , 17, 962-970.

[25] Goldman, R. D, Rogovik, A. L, Lai, D, & Vohra, S. (2008). Potential interactions of drug-natural health products and natural health products-natural health products among children. J. Pediatr e4., 152, 521-526.

[26] Government of Canada(2009). Natural Health Products Regulations. Available: http.justice.gc.ca/en/showtdm/cr/SOR-2003

[27] Hartung, T. (2011). From alternative methods to a new toxicology. European Journal of Pharmaceutics and Biopharmaceutics, , 77, 338-349.

[28] Health Canada(2009a). Release of the Guidance Document for Industry Reporting Adverse Reactions to Marketed Health Products. July 09, 2009. http://www.hc-sc.gc.ca/

dhp-mps/pubs/medeff/_guide/guidancedirectrice_reportinnotification/index-eng.php (accessed September 28, 2009).

[29] Hoeijmakers, J. H. (2009). DNA damage, aging, and cancer. New Engl. J. Med. , 361, 1475-1485.

[30] Hseu, Y, Chen, C, Chen, S. -C, Chen, Y. -L, Lee, J. -Y, Lu, M. -L, Wu, F. -J, Lai, F. -Y, & Yang, J. -S. H.-L., (2008). Humic acid induced genotoxicity in Wu, human peripheral blood lymphocytes using comet and sister chromatid exchange assay. Journal of Hazardous Materials , 153, 784-791.

[31] IPSOS-Reid(2005). Baseline Natural Health Products Survey among Consumers.

[32] Johnson, M. K, & Loo, G. (2000). Effects of epigallocatechin gallate and quercetin on oxidative damage to cellular DNA. Mutation Research , 459, 211-218.

[33] Jordan, S. A, Cunningham, D. G, & Marles, R. J. (2010). Assessment of herbal medicinal products: challenges, and opportunities to increase the knowledge base for safety assessment. Toxicology and Applied Pharmacology , 243, 198-216.

[34] Kawai, K, et al. (2008). Predictive activity profiling of drugs by topologicalfragment-spectra-based support vector machines. J.Chem.Inf.Model., 48, 1152-1160.

[35] Kelly, M. R, Xu, J, Alexander, K. E, & Loo, G. (2001). Disparate effects of similar phenolic phytochemicals as inhibitors of oxidative damage to cellular DNA. Mutation Research , 485, 309-318.

[36] Kirkland, D, Aardema, M, Henderson, L, & Muller, L. (2005). Evaluation of the ability of a battery of three in vitro genotoxicity tests to discriminate rodent carcinogens and non-carcinogens I. Sensitivity, specificity and relative predictivity. Mutation Research , 584, 1-256.

[37] Lambert, I. B, Singer, T. M, Boucher, S. E, & Douglas, G. R. (2005). Detailed review of transgenic rodent mutation assays. Mutation Research, 590, 1-280. Levan, A. 1938. The effect of colchicine on root mitoses in *Allium*. Hereditas 1938; , 24, 471-86.

[38] Maluszynska, J, & Juchimiuk, J. (2005). Plant genotoxicity: A molecular Cytogenetic approach in plant bioassays Arh Hig Rada Toksikol 2005;, 56, 177-184.

[39] Marshall, P. A. (2007). Using *Saccharomyces cerevisiae* to test the mutagenicity of household compounds: an open ended hypothesis-driven teaching lab. Cellbioed , 6, 307-315.

[40] Maron, D. M, & Ames, B. N. (1983). Revised methods for the *Salmonella* mutagenicity test. Mutation Research, 113, 173-215.

[41] MHRA(2009). Herbal medicines regulation and safety. United Kingdom Medicines and Healthcare products Regulatory Agency. Available at: http://www.mhra.gov.uk/Howwe regulate/Medicines/Herbalmedicines/index

[42] Mosihuzzaman, M, & Choudhary, M. I. (2008). Protocols on safety, efficacy, standardization, and documentation of herbal medicine (IUPAC technical report). Pure Appl. Chem. , 80, 2195-2230.

[43] Muster, W, et al. (2008). Computational toxicology in drug development. Drug Discov. Today , 13, 303-310.

[44] Napoli, E. M, Curcuruto, G, & Ruberto, G. (2010). Screening the essential oil composition of wild Sicilian fennel. Biochemical Systematics and Ecology , 38, 213-223.

[45] NBJ(2011). NBJ Supplement Business Report.

[46] Nieminen, S. M, Maki-paakkanen, J, Hirvonen, M. R, Roponen, M, & Von Wright, A. (2002). Genotoxicity of gliotoxin, a secondary metabolite of *Aspergillus fumigatus*, in a battery of short-term test systems. Mutation Research , 520, 161-170.

[47] Nohynek, G. J, Kirkland, D, Marzin, D, Toutaina, H, Leclerc-ribaud, C, & Jinnai, H. (2004). An assessment of the genotoxicity and human health risk of topical use of kojic acid [5-hydroxy-2-(hydroxymethyl)-4H-pyran-4-one]. Food and Chemical Toxicology , 42, 93-105.

[48] Oecd, . OECD Guideline for the Testing of Chemicals: *In Vitro* Mammalian Cell Micronucleus Test (TG 487). Available at: http://www.oecd-ilibrary.org/environment/test-mammalian-cell-micronucleustest_en, 9789264091016.

[49] OECDhttp://www.oecd-ilibrary.org/environment/oecd-guidelines-for-thetesting-of-chemicals-section-health-effects 20745788 consulted (January2012). , 4.

[50] (Ogura, R., Ikeda, N., Yuki, K., Morita, O., Saigo, K., et al., 2008. Genotoxicity studies on green tea catechin. Food and Chemical Toxicology 46, 2190-2200). 46, 2190-2200.

[51] Ouedraogo, M, Baudoux, T, Stévigny, C, Nortier, J, et al. (2012). Review of current and "omics" methods for assessing the toxicity (genotoxicity, teratogenicity and nephrotoxicity) of herbal medicines and mushrooms. Journal of Ethnopharmacology , 140(2012), 492-512.

[52] Prakash, A. S, Pereira, T. N, Reilly, P. E. B, & Seawright, A. A. (1999b). Pyrrolizidine alkaloids in human diet. Mutation Research , 443, 53-67.

[53] Roeder, E. (2000). Medicinal plants in China containing pyrrolizidine alkaloids. Die Pharmazie , 55, 711-726.

[54] Sanger, F, et al. (1977). DNA sequencing with chain-terminating inhibitors. Proc.Natl. Acad. Sci. U. S. A , 74, 5463-5467.

[55] Santos, D. B, Schiar, V. P, Ribeiro, M. C, Schwab, R. S, et al. (2009). Genotoxicity of organo selenium compounds in human leukocytes *in vitro*. Mutation Research , 676, 21-26.

[56] Simon-hettich, B, et al. (2006). Use of computer-assisted prediction of toxic effects of chemical substances. Toxicology , 224, 156-162.

[57] Slatter, M. A, & Gennery, A. R. (2010). Primary immunodeficiencies associated with DNA-repair disorders. Expert Rev. Mol. Med. 12:e9.

[58] Smith, B, Cadby, P, Leblanc, J, & Setzer, C. R.W., (2010). Application of the margin of exposure (MoE) approach to substances in food that are genotoxic and carcinogenic example: methyleugenol, CASRN: 93-15-2. Food and Chemical Toxicology Snyder, R.D., Smith, M.D., 2005. Computational prediction of genotoxicity: room for improvement. DDT10., 48, 89-97.

[59] Souza-jonior, S. A. Gonc¸ alves, E.A.L., Catanzaro-Guimaraes, S.A., Castro-Prado, M.A.A., (2004). Loss of heterozygosity by mitotic recombination in diploid strain of *Aspergillus nidulans* in response to castor oil plant detergent. Brazilian Journal of Biology , 64, 885-890.

[60] Speit, G, Vasquez, M, & Hartmann, A. (2009). The comet assay as an indicator test for germ cell genotoxicity. Mutation Research , 681, 3-12.

[61] TGA(2006). The regulation of complementary medicines in Australia-an overview. Australian Government Department of Health and Ageing, Therapeutic Goods Administration. Available:http://www.tga.gov.au/cm/cmreg-aust.htm

[62] Thomas, K. J, Nichol, J. P, & Coleman, P. (2001). Use and expenditure on complementary medicine in England: a population based survey. Complement TherMedicine, 9, 2-11.

[63] US Department of Health and Human Services, 2007. Food and Drug Administration. Current good manufacturing practice in manufacturing, packaging, labelling, or holding operations for dietary supplements; final rule. Fed. Regist. 72, 34752-34958.

[64] Fda, U. S. (2009). Dietary supplements. Available: http://www.fda.gov/Food/DietarySupplements/default.htm (accessed October 1, 2009).

[65] Valerio-jr, L. G. (2009). *In silico* toxicology for the pharmaceutical sciences. Toxicology and Applied Pharmacology: , 241, 356-370.

[66] Valerio-jr, L. G, et al. (2007). Prediction of rodent carcinogenic potential of naturally occurring chemicals in the human diet using high-throughput QSAR predictive modeling. Toxicol. Appl. Pharmacol. , 222, 1-16.

[67] Van Breemen, R. B, Fong, H. H. S, & Farnsworth, N. R. (2008). Ensuring the safety of botanical dietary supplements. Am. J. Clin. Nutr. 87.

[68] Verschaeve, L, Juutilainen, J, Lagroye, I, Miyakoshi, J, et al. (2010). *In vitro* and *in vivo* genotoxicity of radiofrequency fields. Mutation Research , 705, 252-268.

[69] Votano, J. R, Parham, M, Hall, L. H, Kier, L. B, et al. (2004). Three new consensus QSAR models for the prediction of Ames genotoxicity. Mutagenesis , 19, 365-377.

[70] Wakdikar, S. (2004). Biotechnology issues for developing countries- global health care challenge: Indian experiences and new prescriptions. Electronic Journal of Biotechnology , 7, 214-220.

[71] Wang, J, Sawyer, J. R, Chen, L, Chen, T, Honma, M, Mei, N, & Moore, M. M. (2009). The mouse lymphoma assay detects recombination, deletion, and aneuploidy. Toxicol. Sci., 109, 96-105.

[72] Westerink, W. M, Stevenson, J. C, Horbach, G. J, & Schoonen, W. G. (2010). The development of RAD51C, Cystatin A, and Nrf2 luciferase-reporter in metabolically competent HepG2 cells for the assessment of mechanism-based genotoxicity assays and of oxidative stress in the early research phase of drug development. Mutation Research 696, 21-40., 53.

[73] Williamson, E. (2003). Drug interactions between herbal and prescription medicines. Drug Safety, 26, 1075-1092.

[74] Wilson 3rdD.M., Thompson, L.H., (2007). Molecular mechanisms of sister-chromatid exchange. Mutation Research , 616, 11-23.

[75] Woollard, P, Mehta, N, Vamathevan, J, & Van Horn, S. Bonde, B; Dow, D. (2011). The application of next-generation sequencing technologies to drug discovery and development. Drug Disco. Today , 16, 512-519.

[76] Woo, Y. T, et al. (1995). Development of structure-activity relationship rules for predicting carcinogenic potential of chemicals. Toxicol. Lett. , 79, 219-228.

Section 2

Drug Testing and Development

Chapter 6

Animal Models in Drug Development

Ray Greek

Additional information is available at the end of the chapter

http://dx.doi.org/10.5772/53893

1. Introduction

The use of specific chemicals to treat specific diseases and disorders dates to 1910 when Paul Ehrlich and Sahachiro Hata discovered that salvarsan, also known as arsphenamine and compound 606, killed the microorganism that caused syphilis. Their research relied on animal models of syphilis as, even currently, syphilis cannot be grown in culture medium. Arsphenamine was the first synthetic drug to actually target and kill a disease-causing organism and is credited with starting the pharmaceutical age. Ehrlich is also credited with coining the term *magic bullet* in reference to a drug that would kill a microorganism without damaging or otherwise affecting the host of the microorganism: the patient. As I will explain, despite being an inspirational concept that led to advances in science and medicine, the notion of a magic bullet proved incomplete. Salvarsan and Ehrlich's concept of a magic bullet are important to current concepts in drug testing because: 1) salvarsan was initially called compound 606 as it was the 606th compound tested on animals in an attempt to find a treatment for syphilis; and 2) the concept of a magic bullet was based on the scientific process known as reductionism. In this chapter, I will explore the reductionist approach of using animal models in drug development, especially in toxicity testing.

2. Reductionism and complexity

The use of animals as models for human anatomy and pathophysiology dates back millennia but the modern version began with Claude Bernard in the 19th century. Bernard was a firm believer in the reductionist approach to medical science and that approach has indeed served biomedical science well for decades. A review of reductionism will allow us to contrast this approach to understanding the material universe with systems biology, which is needed in order to fully understand complex living systems. [1-13]

Ernst Mayr defines reductionism as: "The belief that the higher levels of integration of a complex system can be fully explained through a knowledge of the smallest components." [[14] p290] For example, physics attempts to describe the universe in terms of a few elementary particles, and the relationships among them. Reductionism has been very successful in describing many aspects of the material universe, including allowing successful predictions to be made. Reductionism is associated with Newton, Descartes, and determinism and the reliance on animal models in medical science arose during the time of Newtonian physics vis-à-vis reductionism and determinism. Newton said: "Therefore to the same natural effects we must, as far as possible, assign the same causes" and went on to explain that this rule applies "to respiration in a man and in a beast, the descent of stones in Europe and America, the light of our culinary fire and of the sun, the reflection of light in the earth and in the planets."[[15] p3-5] Both Newton and Claude Bernard subscribed to the position that similar causes yield similar effects. Indeed, this concept was one of the breakthroughs that led to the systematic method of inquiry known as the *resoluto-compositive method* or method of analysis and synthesis. This concept of causal determinism rests on two claims. First, all events have causes, and second, for qualitatively identical systems, the same cause is followed by the same effect. Causal determinism is a presupposition of much scientific activity. The idea that results in the laboratory can be extended to form expectations about qualitatively similar systems outside the laboratory is embodied in this idea, as is the claim that experiments should be replicable. [16] This was how science viewed the universe, including animate bodies, when the animal model was embraced by science in the 19th century.

Claude Bernard was a strict causal determinist, meaning that if X caused Y in a monkey it was also cause Y in a human. Bernard stated: "Physiologists... deal with just one thing, the properties of living matter and the mechanism of life, in whatever form it shows itself. For them genus, species and class no longer exist. There are only living beings; and if they choose one of them for study, that is usually for convenience in experimentation."[[17] p 111] Further complicating matters, Bernard and many of his colleagues rejected the notion of evolution put forth by Darwin. [17-19] Bernard thought that organs and other tissues were interchangeable among animals and that all differences could be accounted for based on scaling; the chief difference between humans and animals being a soul.[19] This thinking persists even in recent times as exemplified by the baboon heart transplant in to the recipient Baby Fae, performed by the creationist surgeon Leonard Bailey of Loma Linda University in 1984. [[20] p162-3]

However, recent advances in other disciplines of science, namely chaos and complexity along with evolutionary biology, have called into question the use of reductionism as the sole factor in studying complex systems. Moreover, the developments in evolutionary biology and genetics are cause for further concern regarding the use of one complex evolved system, say a mouse, to predict responses to perturbations such as disease and drugs for another differently evolved complex system, say a human. For example, we now understand that the same gene can be used in different ways among species and that knocking out a gene in one species is not predictive for the function of that gene in another species.[21-27] This has implications for drug development.

http://dx.doi.org/10.5772/53893

Reductionism was used to study simply systems as opposed to complex systems. Animals, including humans, are complex systems and as such exhibit the characteristics listed below [from [28]].

1. Complex systems are robust, meaning they have the capacity to resist change. [8, 9, 29-35] This can be illustrated by the fact that knocking out a gene in one strain of mouse may produce no noticeable effects.
2. Redundancy tends be a part of complex systems and may explain some aspects of robustness. For example, many members of the kingdom Animalia exhibit gene redundancy. [8, 9, 29-35]
3. Different parts of a complex system are linked to and affect one another in a synergistic manner. In other words, there is positive and negative feedback in a complex system. [36] This is why overloading one part of a complex system with say vitamins, may not result in a healthier individual. The feedback system results in the rest of the system acting to simply excrete the unneeded vitamins.
4. Complex systems are also modular. But failure in one module does not necessarily spread to the system as a whole as redundancy and robustness also exist. [37-40]
5. The modules do communicate though. For example, genes tend to be part of networks, genes interact with proteins, proteins interact with other proteins and so on.
6. Complex systems communicate with their environment—are dynamic. [37-40]
7. Complex systems are very dependent upon initial conditions. [39] For example, very small changes in genetic makeup can result in dramatic differences in response to perturbations of the living system.
8. The causes and effects of the events that a complex system experiences are not proportional to each other. Perturbations to the system have effects that are nonlinear, in other words large perturbations may result in no change while small perturbations may cause havoc. [37-40]
9. The whole is greater than the sum of the parts. [1, 8, 9, 30, 39]
10. Complex systems have emergent properties. An emergent property cannot be predicted by full knowledge of the component parts. For example, the formation of a flock of birds and hurricanes are examples of emergent phenomenon as is perhaps consciousness. [39]

Reductionism is essentially *divide and conquer*. By dividing a system into its parts and ascertaining the functions of all the parts of the system, one can deduce the function of the entire system. The gears of a Swiss watch, for example, are capable of description on their own, without reference to the system from which they are removed. Conversely, the individual components of a complex system must be described based on the *interaction* of the parts. Describing individual components in isolation, regardless of how detailed such a description is, cannot fully describe the complex system as a whole. The whole is greater than the sum of the parts. A complex system must be described based on the *organization* of the individual components. [41, 42]

Miska states:

The basic analytical method that is behind most biomedical research can be traced back over 300 years to Descartes's essay Discourse on Method, which argued that an animal is a clock-like machine in which the parts and their relationships to one another are precise and unchangeable, and in which causes and effects can be understood by taking the pieces apart. This so-called 'reductionist' approach to understanding biology and medicine has been very productive, but is now up against problems that require different frameworks, institutionally and intellectually. [43]

Nicolis & Prigogine defined complexity as the ability of a system "to switch between different modes of behavior as the environmental conditions are varied."[44] In other words, complex systems are able to adapt to their environments just as life on this planet has adapted resulting in different species. But these adaptions mean that two complex systems that were originally identical would now be less similar and behave differently in certain circumstances. An example of this would be the susceptibility to disease between monozygotic twins. [45-56] Van Regenmortel states:

Reductionists tend to disregard the fact that all biological systems possess so-called emergent properties that arise through the multiple interconnections and relations existing between individual components of the system. These emergent, relational properties do not exist in the constituent parts and they cannot be deduced or predicted from the properties of the individual, isolated components [[57]p258]. Examples of emergent properties are the viscosity of water (individual water molecules have no viscosity), the colour of a chemical, a melody arising from notes, the saltiness of sodium chloride, the specificity of an antibody and the immunogenicity of an antigen. [58]

Living complex systems are the result of various evolutionary processes and as such are arguably the *most complex* of all complex systems. Species differ because of the presence of different genes, mutation in the same genes, a difference in the number of the same allele (copy number variants), the same genes may be regulated or expressed differently, alternative splicing, the presence of modifier or background genes, differences in gene networks and protein networks, and convergent evolution where two species share a trait but the trait evolved independently in each. Individuals of the same species may differ for many of the above reasons but also because of dissimilarities in environmental exposures. [50] Importantly, each of the above means that different species as well as individuals of the same species manifest differences in the initial conditions of their complex system. The above also translates into differences in other characteristics of a complex system such as robustness and redundancy.

The progress in these two areas of science, complexity science and evolutionary biology, results in strong theoretical concerns regarding the use of animals as predictive models in drug development. We should expect animals and humans to share responses to perturbations at the level of organization where complex systems can be described as simple systems but not for perturbations occurring at the level of organization where the system as a whole is studied or where parts of the systems that are themselves complex are studied. I will next examine the empirical evidence and place it in the context of these theoretical concerns.

3. Prediction in science

The third relevant advance in science since animal models were mandated for use in drug development is the formal evaluation of animal models in terms of their predictive value for humans. Animal models are used for ascertaining the properties of absorption, distribution, metabolism, elimination and toxicity (ADMET). As all of these properties influence toxicity, an examination of the ability of animal models to predict these properties is important, as is the straightforward examination of animal models for toxicity itself. The answer to the question of the predictive ability of animal models was hinted at by the fact that Ehrlich and Hata ultimately tested the 606th compound of a series in their attempt to find a treatment for syphilis. Previous compounds had successfully treated syphilis in animal models but had failed for various reasons in humans. Even salvarsan resulted in side effects in humans that were unforeseen in animal models.

The ability to predict facts about the material universe is a hallmark of science. Hypotheses are generated that make predictions about the phenomena under study and the success or failure of these predictions can falsify or strengthen the hypothesis. This use of the term *predict* differs from determining whether a modality, practice, or test is *predictive* for its purpose. For example, a CT scan of the chest is a predictive test for diagnosing a pneumothorax, because the CT scan, as opposed to a chest x-ray, is successful in locating the pneumothorax essentially 100% of the time. In order to evaluate a modality like CT scans, a blood test for cancer, or even the use of dogs for catching drug smugglers in airports, the calculations in table 1 are employed.

When evaluating the predictive value of methods, practices, or tests for use in biomedical science, positive predictive value (PPV) and negative predictive value (NPV) > 0.9 are sought. If a single test alone cannot yield such high values then a combination of tests can be evaluated in hopes that the combination will meet the criteria. Such evaluations have been made for toxicity testing using animal models as well as other animal model-based tests in drug development. Profound *inter*-species differences, as well as inter-individual human differences, have been revealed for absorption [[59] p 8-10] [[60] pp 5, 9, 45, 50, 66-7, 90, 102-3,] [61-64], distribution [65, 66], metabolism [67-77], elimination [78, 79], and toxicity [64, 80-91], which results in predictive values for these animal models that are far below those required in biomedical science. For example, Litchfield conducted a classic study in 1962 comparing toxicity among three species: humans, rats, and dogs. The positive predictive values for the animal models were between 0.49 and 0.55. [92] Similarly, Suter compared toxicities for ergoloid mesylates, bromocriptine, ketotifen, cyclosporine, FK 33-824, and clozapine in animals and humans. The sensitivity for toxicity for the animal tests was 0.52 and the predictive value positive was 0.31. [93] Fourches et al. evaluated animal human data for 1061 compounds known to cause hepatotoxicity in humans and found that the concordance or sensitivity among species was around 39-44%.[94] The positive and negative predictive values could not be calculated from the article but would be well below 0.39. Smith and Caldwell studied twenty-three chemicals and discovered that only four were metabolized the same in humans and rats. [70] Sietsema [95], compared the oral bioavailability of 400 drugs in humans with three other species (see Figure 1) and concluded the data was consistent with a "scatter-gram." Similar results have been obtained from other studies.[84, 96-101]

		Gold Standard	
		GS+	**GS-**
Test	**T+**	**TP**	**FP**
	T-	**FN**	**TN**

T+ = Test positive
T- = Test negative
T = True
F = False
P = Positive
N = Negative
GS+ = Gold standard positive
GS- = Gold standard negative

Sensitivity = TP/(TP+FN)

Specificity = TN/(FP+TN)

Positive Predictive Value = TP/(TP+FP)

Negative Predictive Value = TN/(FN+TN)

Table 1. Binomial classification method for calculating sensitivity, specificity, positive predictive value, and negative predictive value when comparing a modality, practice, or test with a gold standard.

http://dx.doi.org/10.5772/53893

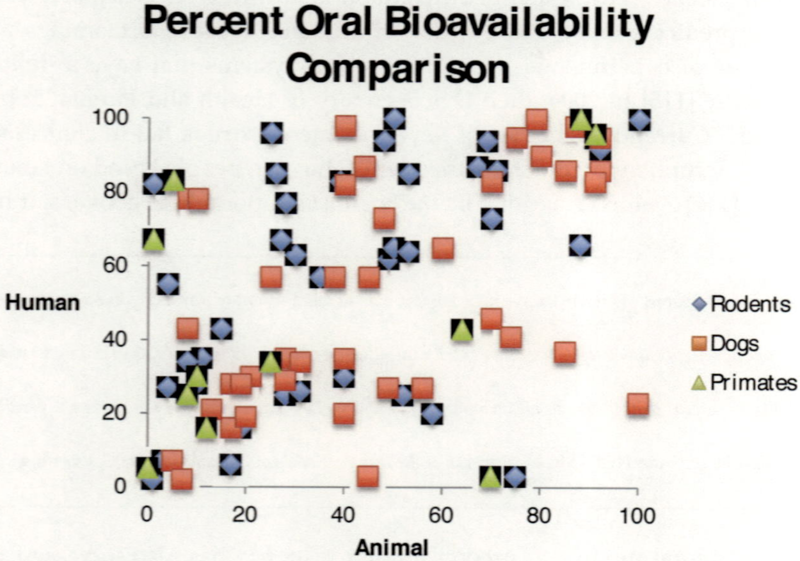

Figure 1. Variation in bioavailability among species. (Based on data from [95].)

The fact that animal models lack predictive ability is well known.[102-110] This shortcoming includes the inability of animal models to be predictive modalities for carcinogenicity.[111, 112] Salsburg stated: "Thus the lifetime feeding study in mice and rats appears to have less than a 50% probability of finding known human carcinogens. On the basis of probability theory, we would have been better off to toss a coin..."[111]

The general attitude in the drug development-related sciences reflects the empirical evidence. Cook et al:

Over many years now there has been a poor correlation between preclinical therapeutic findings and the eventual efficacy of these [anti-cancer] compounds in clinical trials [109, 110].... The development of antineoplastics is a large investment by the private and public sectors, however, the limited availability of predictive preclinical systems obscures our ability to select the therapeutics that might succeed or fail during clinical investigation. [108]

Reuters quoted Francis Collins, Director of the NIH, as stating that: "about half of drugs that work in animals may turn out to be toxic for people. And some drugs may in fact work in people even if they fail in animals, meaning potentially important medicines could be rejected."[113] Alan Oliff, former executive director for cancer research at Merck Research Laboratories in West Point, Pennsylvania asserted in 1997: "The fundamental problem in drug discovery for cancer is that the [animal] model systems are not predictive at all."[114] Björquist and Sartipy stated: "Furthermore, the compound attrition rate is negatively affected by the inability to predict toxicity and efficacy in humans. These shortcomings are in turn caused by the use of experimental pre-clinical model systems that have a limited human clinical relevance..."[115] In 2006, then U.S. Secretary of Health and Human Services Mike Leavitt declared: "Currently, nine out of ten experimental drugs fail in clinical studies because we cannot accurately predict how they will behave in people based on laboratory and animal studies."[116] Zielinska, writing in *The Scientist* supported the above, stating:

Mouse models that use transplants of human cancer have not had a great track record of predicting human responses to treatment in the clinic. It's been estimated that cancer drugs that enter clinical testing have a 95 percent rate of failing to make it to market, in comparison to the 89 percent failure rate for all therapies... Indeed, "we had loads of models that were not predictive, that were [in fact] seriously misleading," says NCI's Marks, also head of the Mouse Models of Human Cancers Consortium... [117]

The inability of animal models to predict human response has also increased the cost of drug development as the cost for the 90-95% of drugs that fail must be recouped from the ones that go to market.[91, 118-121] Lost revenue has also resulted from the drugs that would have been marketable had animal models not derailed them in development. This lack of predictive ability for animal models is largely to blame for the cost of new medications and for the fact that the drug development pipeline is drying up.[115, 122, 123] Because animal models fail to predict drugs destined to fail, these drugs go to clinical trials and marketing which consumes roughly 95% of the cost for drug development.[124, 125] Catherine Shaffer, Contributing Editor of *Drug Discovery & Development*, wrote in 2012: "Drug development is an extremely costly endeavor. Estimates of the total expense of advancing a new drug from the chemistry stage to the market are as high as $2 billion. Much of that cost is attributable to drug failures late in development, after huge investments have been made. Drugs are equally likely to fail at that stage for safety reasons, as for a lack of efficacy, which is often well-established by the time large trials are launched."[120] Roy estimates the real cost is even higher: "The true amount that companies spend per drug approved is almost certainly even larger today. Matthew Herper of Forbes recently totaled R&D spending from the 12 leading pharmaceutical companies from 1997 to 2011, and found that they had spent $802 billion to gain approval for just 139 drugs: a staggering $5.8 billion per drug."[125] Kenneth Kaitin, director of Tuft's Center for the Study of Drug commenting on Pharma's drying pipeline in the March 7, 2011 *New York Times*, stated: "This is panic time, this is truly panic time for the industry." Even when a drug does reach the market, there is a great amount of uncertainty regarding safety. For example, over 1000 drugs that reached the market were discovered to result in hepatotoxicity. [126]

Kirschner addressed this issue, asking: "could we develop a better way of predicting whether a drug will work or have intolerable side effects?" He then explains the problem in terms similar to what I have presented above:

In part, this problem stems from the fact that we rarely have a situation in which one gene can be linked to one disease and targeted by one drug. The nature of our biological system is that we have relatively few genes — say 20,000 basic core genes — that are used over and over again in different contexts. So when we investigate targets, we need to better appreciate how these function in different contexts. Moreover, there are many overlapping and redundant pathways, so we need to better understand genes not as individual elements with individual functions but within the context of the circuits in which they operate. This approach requires not just a wiring diagram, but a quantitative wiring diagram... [127]

4. This leads us to current efforts at improving drug development

4.1. Twenty-first century science

Today we have options for drug development and toxicity testing that did not exist until the 21st century, for example microdosing and pharmacogenomics. Two points need be emphasized before I address these two advances, however. First, animal models fail to meet the ends for which they are used; they are not predictive modalities for human response. Therefore using animal models is akin to relying on bloodletting as a treatment for cancer when oncologists have no cures for the cancer in question. Just as bloodletting is not effective as a treatment for cancer, regardless of whether or not other options are available, so employing animal models as they are currently utilized is nonsensical.

Second, technology is available, or is being developed, that will at least predict human response for certain properties important in drug development. However, regardless of how much time is needed in order for these technologies to be developed, animal models are simply ineffective and hence should be abandoned. Lack of effective technology does not justify the utilization of methods proven to be ineffective. Regardless of the technologies available, drug development must be human-based both when reductionism is used and when complexity is relevant. Basing drug development decisions on drug targets identified from animal models has not been effective. Human tissues can be studied instead and this will allow targets to be established in a more reliable manner. Humans must also be studied when responses to drugs are occurring at higher levels of organization; where the system is complex.

In 2006, the FDA approved microdosing for Phase 0 clinical trials.[128, 129] Microdosing is the process whereby very small doses of a drug are administered to human volunteers after which positron emission tomography (PET) and accelerator mass spectrometry (AMS) are used to assess pharmacokinetic (PK) data.[130-132] While animal models are used to inform the dose for the first administration of the drug, the usual range for drugs is 100ng to 100μg. If all drugs were initially administered at a dose of 1ng and subsequently increased, this would obviate the use of unreliable animal models and ensure that the first-in-human dose was lower than the most toxic substance currently known.[133, 134] This would be a reliably safe method for conducing first-in-human trials. Although in practice microdosing is currently only used to evaluate PK (as opposed to pharmacodynamics, which is abbreviated as PD), it could be used for evaluating the other properties of interest. For example, by increasing the dose incrementally, the drug could be evaluated for toxicity. This solves the problem of unanticipated catastrophic reactions such as occurred in the TGN1412 trial [135] and allows toxicity to be determined very early in the drug development process. Long term carcinogenicity studies could not be conducted in this fashion however animal models are not predictive for carcinogenicity and human data from long terms use is the *de facto* method now used. Nothing would be lost by eliminating long-term carcinogenicity studies in animals until predictive technologies are developed. According to the Centers for Disease Control and Prevention (CDC): "Most of what we know about chemicals and cancer in humans comes from scientists' observation of workers. The most significant exposures to cancer-causing chemicals have occurred in workplaces where large amounts of toxic chemicals have been used regularly."[136]

The concept of microdosing, used in combination with pharmacogenomics (see below) would allow go-no go decisions to be made early and reliably in drug development as well as matching drug to patient. The transition to full-scale clinical trials would also be seamless. As the dose was increased, an evaluation of efficacy could be made. By starting the dose at 1ng and increasing, the entire clinical trial could be conducted much more reliably and efficiently, drugs destined to fail could be eliminated earlier thus saving money, and the drugs could be matched to genotype before being marketed thus further saving money and decreasing side effects. This leads us to the concepts of pharmacogenomics and personalized medicine.

Personalized medicine seeks to individualize medicine both in terms of treatment and diagnosis while pharmacogenomics matches drugs to patients. Rashmi R Shah, previous Senior Clinical Assessor, Medicines and Healthcare products Regulatory Agency, London stated in 2005: "During the clinical use of a drug at present, a prescribing physician has no means of predicting the response of an individual patient to a given drug. Invariably, some patients fail to respond beneficially as expected whereas others experience adverse drug reactions (ADRs)."[137] Shah echoed comments by Allen Roses, then-worldwide vice-president of genetics at GlaxoSmithKline (GSK), who stated that fewer than half of the patients prescribed some of the most expensive drugs derived any benefit from them: "The vast majority of drugs - more than 90% - only work in 30 or 50% of the people."[138] That individual humans respond very differently to disease and drugs [139, 140], including vaccines [141, 142], has long been appreciated. During the Korean War, Alving observed that black soldiers had an increased probability, compared with white soldiers, of developing anemia when from antimalarials. This was discovered to be secondary to a commonly occurring enzyme deficiency in the black soldiers.[143] Variation in disease susceptibility and response to drugs has been noted to exist between sexes [144-150] and ethnic groups [151-159] as well as between monozygotic twins.[45-52, 56]

Many advances have been made in linking drugs to genes, in part because of spin-offs from the Human Genome Project. Differences between humans including single nucleotide polymorphisms, copy number variants, differences the regulation and expression of the same genes, differences in gene networks, and the influence of background genes can result in a drug being efficacious for one patient but not another. Diseases vary intra-species as well. Michael Snyder, chair of genetics at Stanford University School of Medicine, recently stated: "However, the bulk of the differences among individuals are not found in the genes themselves, but in regions we know relatively little about. Now we see that these differences profoundly impact protein binding and gene expression."[160, 161] Hunter et al studied a mouse model of cancer and discovered differences in metastatic efficiency secondary to background genes. Hunter et al:

Because all tumors were initiated by the same oncogenic event, differences in the metastasis microarray signature and metastatic potential are probably due to genetic background effects rather than different combinations of oncogenic mutations. Consistent with our observations in metastasis, several laboratories have shown similar strain differences with regard to oncogenesis, aging and fertility in transgenic mouse models.[162-164] Data on both primary tumors and metastases reinforce the notion that tumorigenesis and metastasis are complex phenotypes involving both inherent genetic components and cellular responses to extrinsic stimuli. [165]

Thein likewise stated: "As the defective genes for more and more genetic disorders become unravelled, it is clear that patients with apparently identical genotypes can have many different clinical conditions even in simple monogenic disorders." Thein assessed β–thalassemia and noted that the clinical manifestations are very diverse, ranging from life threatening to asymptomatic. Thein: "The remarkable phenotypic diversity of the β–thalassemias is prototypical of how a wide spectrum of disease severity can be generated in single gene disorders.... relating phenotype to genotype is complicated by the complex interaction of the environment and other genetic factors at the secondary and tertiary levels..."[166]

Agarwal and Moorchung reinforce the above stating: "It is now increasingly apparent that modifier genes have a considerable role to play in phenotypic variations of single-gene disorders." This is due to factors such as: "Oligogenic disorders occur because of a second gene modifying the action of a dominant gene. It is now certain that cancer occurs due to the action of the environment acting in combination with several genes."[167] Friedman and Perrimon explain that there are "hundreds of potential regulators of known signaling pathways." [168] *PLoS Biology,* in an editorial said the following about mouse models of autoimmune diseases: "These results fall in line with mounting evidence that background genes are not silent partners in gene-targeted disease models, but can themselves facilitate expression of the disease. This finding underscores the notion that genes are not solitary, static entities; their expression often depends on context. With genetically complex diseases, having the requisite combination of susceptibility genes does not always lead to disease."[169]

Liu et al explain why the same genes can result in very outcomes:

A general view is that critical genes involved in biological pathways are highly conserved among species. To understand human autoimmune diseases, a great deal of effort has been devoted to the study of murine models that mirror many pathologic properties observed in the human disease. We have found that lymphocytes from humans with different autoimmune disease all carry a common conserved gene expression profile. Therefore, we wanted to determine if lymphocytes from common murine models of autoimmune disease carried a gene expression profile similar to the human profile and if both mouse models carried a shared gene expression profile. We identified numerous differentially expressed genes (DEGs) in the autoimmune strains compared to non-autoimmune strains. However, we found very little overlap in the gene expression profile between human autoimmune disease and murine models of autoimmune disease and between different murine autoimmune models. Our research further confirms that murine models of autoimmunity do not perfectly match human autoimmune diseases. [26]

Weiss et al continues this theme:

In contrast to these single gene effects, many drug treatment response phenotypes are complex, produced by multiple coding and regulatory variants in multiple genes that often interact in a signalling pathway. In these cases, each variant could contribute to the variance in the phenotype and there is no clear model of genetic inheritance. Genetic factors that influence whether a drug treatment response is complex include mode of inheritance (recessive versus dominant or additive); pleiotropy; incomplete penetrance; and epistasis, due to gene–environment interactions and environmental phenocopies. All of these factors contribute to the complexity of the response phenotypes. [170]

Gabor Miklos states:

There is enormous phenotypic variation in the extent of human cancer phenotypes, even among family members inheriting the same mutation in the adenomatous polyposis coli (APC) gene believed to be causal for colon cancer. In the experimental mouse knockout of the catalytic gamma subunit of the phosphatidyl-3-OH kinase, there can be a high incidence of colorectal carcinomas or no cancers at all, depending on the mouse strain in which the knockout is created, or into which the knockout is crossed... [27]

Because of advances alluded to above, society is seeing the death of the blockbuster and the arrival of the "niche buster." [171] Herscu et al write: "The era of the 'blockbuster drug mod-

http://dx.doi.org/10.5772/53893

el' is ending, and the development of personalized pharmaceutical system is on the rise." [172] This is also due to the fact that diseases are being categorized into more types and individuals even within the same type react differently to drugs. Herscu et al write:

Diabetes mellitus, for example, was simply divided into juvenile or adult onset types for many years. Now we have pre-diabetes; Type I, broken into immune-related and other causes; Type 2, broken into secretory defect and insulin-resistant types; and more than 11 types that have been linked to specific genetic defects. However, even diabetic patients in a precisely defined category with shared genetic markers differ because they exist at different points along the continuum of the disease depending on their diet, exercise, comorbid conditions and other factors. These phenotypic dissimilarities are the source of inter-patient variability, which confounds both clinical trials and treatment results. [172]

Iressa was one of the first medications administered to patients based on genotype. Iressa did not perform well in clinical trials and was to be abandoned but clinicians were adamant that it helped some people with cancer. By genotyping the patients that responded well to Iressa, researchers were able to confirm that, in certain genotypes, Iressa was efficacious. Numerous drug responses have been matched to specific mutations. [77, 173-176] The Personalized Medicine Coalition notes that personalized medicine will allow patients and physicians to:

- select optimal therapy and reduce "trial-and-error" medicine;
- reduce adverse drug reactions;
- improve the selection of drug targets;
- increase patient compliance with therapy;
- reduce the time, cost, and failure rate of clinical trials;
- revive drugs that failed clinical trials or were withdrawn from the market;
- avoid withdrawal of marketed drugs;
- shift the emphasis in medicine from reaction to prevention; and
- reduce the overall cost of healthcare.[177]

5. Conclusion

We are currently living in what will become known as the Age of Personalized Medicine. While much has yet to be discovered, society is already benefitting from personalized medicine applied to specific drugs and diseases. Contrast this with using a different species in an attempt to predict human response to drugs and disease. While animals can be used in basic science pursuits, empirical evidence from drug development, placed in the context of the scientific theories of Complexity and Evolution, demands that animal testing be replaced with human-based drug development. Implementing human-based testing early in the development process is how drugs should be developed now and it will be how drugs are developed in the future.

Author details

Ray Greek*

Address all correspondence to: AFMA@AFMA-curedisease.org

Americans For Medical Advancement, Goleta, CA, USA

References

[1] Ahn AC, Tewari M, Poon CS, Phillips RS. The limits of reductionism in medicine: could systems biology offer an alternative? PLoS Med. 2006 May;3(6):e208. Digital Object Identifier: 05-PLME-ES-0675R1 [pii] 10.1371/journal.pmed.0030208. http://www.ncbi.nlm.nih.gov/entrez/query.fcgi?cmd=Retrieve&db=PubMed&dopt=Citation&list_uids=16681415

[2] Bornholdt S. Systems biology. Less is more in modeling large genetic networks. Science. 2005 Oct 21;310(5747):449-51. Digital Object Identifier: 310/5747/449 [pii] 10.1126/science.1119959. http://www.ncbi.nlm.nih.gov/entrez/query.fcgi?cmd=Retrieve&db=PubMed&dopt=Citation&list_uids=16239464

[3] Butcher EC. Can cell systems biology rescue drug discovery? Nat Rev Drug Discov. 2005 Jun;4(6):461-7. Digital Object Identifier: nrd1754 [pii] 10.1038/nrd1754. http://www.ncbi.nlm.nih.gov/entrez/query.fcgi?cmd=Retrieve&db=PubMed&dopt=Citation&list_uids=15915152

[4] Department of Systems Biology. Harvard Medical School. Systems Biology. Boston: Harcard; 2010 [cited 2011 August 22]; Available from: https://sysbio.med.harvard.edu/.

[5] Editorial. End of the interlude? Nat Biotechnol. 2004 Oct;22(10):1191. Digital Object Identifier: nbt1004-1191 [pii] 10.1038/nbt1004-1191. http://www.ncbi.nlm.nih.gov/entrez/query.fcgi?cmd=Retrieve&db=PubMed&dopt=Citation&list_uids=15470438

[6] Editorial. In pursuit of systems. Nature. 2005 May 5;435(7038):1. Digital Object Identifier: 435001a [pii] 10.1038/435001a. http://www.ncbi.nlm.nih.gov/entrez/query.fcgi?cmd=Retrieve&db=PubMed&dopt=Citation&list_uids=15874978

[7] Hood L. Leroy Hood expounds the principles, practice and future of systems biology. Drug Discov Today. 2003 May 15;8(10):436-8. Digital Object Identifier: S1359644603027107 [pii]. http://www.ncbi.nlm.nih.gov/entrez/query.fcgi?cmd=Retrieve&db=PubMed&dopt=Citation&list_uids=12801791

[8] Kitano H. Computational systems biology. Nature. 2002 Nov 14;420(6912):206-10. Digital Object Identifier: 10.1038/nature01254 nature01254 [pii]. http://www.ncbi.nlm.nih.gov/entrez/query.fcgi?cmd=Retrieve&db=PubMed&dopt=Citation&list_uids=12432404

[9] Kitano H. Systems biology: a brief overview. Science. 2002 Mar 1;295(5560):1662-4. Digital Object Identifier: 10.1126/science.1069492 295/5560/1662 [pii]. http://www.ncbi.nlm.nih.gov/entrez/query.fcgi?cmd=Retrieve&db=PubMed&dopt=Citation&list_uids=11872829

[10] Oltvai ZN, Barabasi AL. Systems biology. Life's complexity pyramid. Science. 2002 Oct 25;298(5594):763-4. Digital Object Identifier: 10.1126/science.1078563 298/5594/763 [pii]. http://www.ncbi.nlm.nih.gov/entrez/query.fcgi?cmd=Retrieve&db=PubMed&dopt=Citation&list_uids=12399572

[11] Schaffner KF. Theories, Models, and Equations in Systems Biology. In: Boogerd F, Bruggeman FJ, Hofmeyr J-HS, Westerhoff HV, editors. Systems Biology: Philosophical Foundations. Netherlands: Elsevier; 2007. p. 145-62.

[12] Strange K. The end of "naive reductionism": rise of systems biology or renaissance of physiology? Am J Physiol Cell Physiol. 2005 May;288(5):C968-74. Digital Object Identifier: 288/5/C968 [pii] 10.1152/ajpcell.00598.2004. http://www.ncbi.nlm.nih.gov/entrez/query.fcgi?cmd=Retrieve&db=PubMed&dopt=Citation&list_uids=15840560

[13] Vidal M. A unifying view of 21st century systems biology. FEBS Lett. 2009 Dec 17;583(24):3891-4. Digital Object Identifier: 10.1016/j.febslet.2009.11.024. http://www.ncbi.nlm.nih.gov/pubmed/19913537

[14] Mayr E. What evolution Is: Basic Books; 2002.

[15] Thayer HS. Newton's Philosophy of Nature: Selections from His Writings: Dover Publications; 2005.

[16] Shanks N, Greek R. Animal Models in Light of Evolution. Boca Raton: Brown Walker; 2009.

[17] Bernard C. An Introduction to the Study of Experimental Medicine. 1865. New York: Dover; 1957.

[18] Elliot P. Vivisection and the Emergence of Experimental Medicine in Nineteenth Century France. In: Rupke N, editor. Vivisection in Historical Perspective. New York: Croom Helm; 1987. p. 48-77.

[19] LaFollette H, Shanks N. Animal Experimentation: The Legacy of Claude Bernard. International Studies in the Philosophy of Science. 1994;8(3):195-210. Digital Object Identifier:

[20] Milner R. Darwin's Universe: Evolution from A to Z: University of California Press; 2009.

[21] Darlison MG, Pahal I, Thode C. Consequences of the evolution of the GABA(A) receptor gene family. Cell Mol Neurobiol. 2005 Jun;25(3-4):607-24. Digital Object Identifier: 10.1007/s10571-005-4004-4. http://www.ncbi.nlm.nih.gov/entrez/query.fcgi?cmd=Retrieve&db=PubMed&dopt=Citation&list_uids=16075381

[22] Enna SJ, Williams M. Defining the role of pharmacology in the emerging world of translational research. Advances in pharmacology. [Historical Article]. 2009;57:1-30. Digital Object Identifier: 10.1016/S1054-3589(08)57001-3. http://www.ncbi.nlm.nih.gov/pubmed/20230758

[23] Geerts H. Of mice and men: bridging the translational disconnect in CNS drug discovery. CNS Drugs. 2009 Nov 1;23(11):915-26. Digital Object Identifier: 10.2165/11310890-000000000-00000. http://www.ncbi.nlm.nih.gov/pubmed/19845413

[24] Jankovic J, Noebels JL. Genetic mouse models of essential tremor: are they essential? J Clin Invest. 2005 Mar;115(3):584-6. Digital Object Identifier: 10.1172/JCI24544. http://www.ncbi.nlm.nih.gov/entrez/query.fcgi?cmd=Retrieve&db=PubMed&dopt=Citation&list_uids=15765140

[25] Kieburtz K, Olanow CW. Translational experimental therapeutics: The translation of laboratory-based discovery into disease-related therapy. Mt Sinai J Med. 2007 Apr;74(1):7-14. Digital Object Identifier: 10.1002/msj.20006. http://www.ncbi.nlm.nih.gov/entrez/query.fcgi?cmd=Retrieve&db=PubMed&dopt=Citation&list_uids=17516559

[26] Liu Z, Maas K, Aune TM. Comparison of differentially expressed genes in T lymphocytes between human autoimmune disease and murine models of autoimmune disease. Clin Immunol. 2004 Sep;112(3):225-30. Digital Object Identifier: 10.1016/j.clim.2004.03.017 S1521661604001081 [pii]. http://www.ncbi.nlm.nih.gov/entrez/query.fcgi?cmd=Retrieve&db=PubMed&dopt=Citation&list_uids=15308114

[27] Miklos GLG. The human cancer genome project--one more misstep in the war on cancer. Nat Biotechnol. 2005 May;23(5):535-7. Digital Object Identifier: nbt0505-535 [pii] 10.1038/nbt0505-535. http://www.ncbi.nlm.nih.gov/entrez/query.fcgi?cmd=Retrieve&db=PubMed&dopt=Citation&list_uids=15877064

[28] Greek R, Menache A, Rice MJ. Animal models in an age of personalized medicine. Personalized Medicine. 2012 2012/01/01;9(1):47-64. Digital Object Identifier: 10.2217/pme.11.89. http://dx.doi.org/10.2217/pme.11.89

[29] Csete ME, Doyle JC. Reverse engineering of biological complexity. Science. 2002 Mar 1;295(5560):1664-9. Digital Object Identifier: 10.1126/science.1069981 295/5560/1664

[pii]. http://www.ncbi.nlm.nih.gov/entrez/query.fcgi?cmd=Retrieve&db=PubMed&dopt=Citation&list_uids=11872830

[30] Kitano H. A robustness-based approach to systems-oriented drug design. Nat Rev Drug Discov. 2007 Mar;6(3):202-10. Digital Object Identifier: nrd2195 [pii] 10.1038/nrd2195. http://www.ncbi.nlm.nih.gov/entrez/query.fcgi?cmd=Retrieve&db=PubMed&dopt=Citation&list_uids=17318209

[31] Morange M. The misunderstood gene. Cambridge: Harvard University Press; 2001.

[32] Morange M. A successful form for reductionism. The Biochemist. 2001;23:37-9. Digital Object Identifier:

[33] Pearson H. Surviving a knockout blow. Nature. 2002 Jan 3;415(6867):8-9. Digital Object Identifier: 10.1038/415008a 415008a [pii]. http://www.ncbi.nlm.nih.gov/entrez/query.fcgi?cmd=Retrieve&db=PubMed&dopt=Citation&list_uids=11780081

[34] Horrobin DF. Modern biomedical research: an internally self-consistent universe with little contact with medical reality? Nat Rev Drug Discov. 2003 Feb;2(2):151-4. Digital Object Identifier: 10.1038/nrd1012 nrd1012 [pii]. http://www.ncbi.nlm.nih.gov/entrez/query.fcgi?cmd=Retrieve&db=PubMed&dopt=Citation&list_uids=12563306

[35] Monte J, Liu M, Sheya A, Kitami T. Definitions, Measures, and Models of Robustness in Gene Regulatory Network. Report of research work for CSSS05. 2005 [cited 2007 March 30]; Report of research work for CSSS05, 2005]. Available from: http://www.santafe.edu/education/csss/csss05/papers/monte_et_al._cssssf05.pdf.

[36] Jura J, Wegrzyn P, Koj A. Regulatory mechanisms of gene expression: complexity with elements of deterministic chaos. Acta Biochim Pol. 2006;53(1):1-10. Digital Object Identifier: 20061177 [pii]. http://www.ncbi.nlm.nih.gov/entrez/query.fcgi?cmd=Retrieve&db=PubMed&dopt=Citation&list_uids=16505901

[37] Alm E, Arkin AP. Biological networks. Curr Opin Struct Biol. 2003 Apr;13(2):193-202. Digital Object Identifier: S0959440X03000319 [pii]. http://www.ncbi.nlm.nih.gov/entrez/query.fcgi?cmd=Retrieve&db=PubMed&dopt=Citation&list_uids=12727512

[38] Ottino JM. Engineering complex systems. Nature. 2004 Jan 29;427(6973):399. Digital Object Identifier: 10.1038/427399a 427399a [pii]. http://www.ncbi.nlm.nih.gov/entrez/query.fcgi?cmd=Retrieve&db=PubMed&dopt=Citation&list_uids=14749808

[39] Sole R, Goodwin B. Signs of Life: How Complexity Pervades Biology: Basic Books; 2002.

[40] Kauffman SA. The Origins of Order: Self-Organization and Selection in Evolution Oxford University Press; 1993.

[41] Van Regenmortel M. Reductionism and complexity in molecular biology. Scientists now have the tools to unravel biological complexity and overcome the limitations of reductionism. EMBO Rep. 2004 Nov;5(11):1016-20. Digital Object Identifier: 7400284

[pii] 10.1038/sj.embor.7400284. http://www.ncbi.nlm.nih.gov/entrez/query.fcgi?cmd=Retrieve&db=PubMed&dopt=Citation&list_uids=15520799

[42] Van Regenmortel MHV. Basic Research in HIV vaccinology is hampered by reductionist thinking. Frontiers in Immunology. [Review]. 2012 2012-July-9;3. Digital Object Identifier: 10.3389/fimmu.2012.00194. http://www.frontiersin.org/Journal/Abstract.aspx?s=1247&name=immunotherapies_and_vaccines&ART_DOI=10.3389/fimmu.2012.00194

[43] Miska D. Biotech's twentieth birthday blues. Nat Rev Drug Discov. 2003 Mar;2(3):231-3. Digital Object Identifier: 10.1038/nrd1036 nrd1036 [pii]. http://www.ncbi.nlm.nih.gov/entrez/query.fcgi?cmd=Retrieve&db=PubMed&dopt=Citation&list_uids=12612649

[44] Nicolis G, Prigogine I. Exploring complexity: An introduction. New York: W.H. Freeman and Co; 1989.

[45] Bell JT, Spector TD. A twin approach to unraveling epigenetics. Trends Genet. 2011 Mar;27(3):116-25. Digital Object Identifier: 10.1016/j.tig.2010.12.005.

[46] Bruder CE, Piotrowski A, Gijsbers AA, Andersson R, Erickson S, de Stahl TD, et al. Phenotypically concordant and discordant monozygotic twins display different DNA copy-number-variation profiles. Am J Hum Genet. 2008 Mar;82(3):763-71. Digital Object Identifier: S0002-9297(08)00102-X [pii] 10.1016/j.ajhg.2007.12.011. http://www.ncbi.nlm.nih.gov/entrez/query.fcgi?cmd=Retrieve&db=PubMed&dopt=Citation&list_uids=18304490

[47] Dempster EL, Pidsley R, Schalkwyk LC, Owens S, Georgiades A, Kane F, et al. Disease-associated epigenetic changes in monozygotic twins discordant for schizophrenia and bipolar disorder. Human molecular genetics. 2011 Sep 22;20(24):4786-96. Digital Object Identifier: 10.1093/hmg/ddr416. http://www.ncbi.nlm.nih.gov/pubmed/21908516

[48] Fraga MF, Ballestar E, Paz MF, Ropero S, Setien F, Ballestar ML, et al. Epigenetic differences arise during the lifetime of monozygotic twins. Proc Natl Acad Sci U S A. 2005 Jul 26;102(30):10604-9. Digital Object Identifier: 0500398102 [pii] 10.1073/pnas.0500398102. http://www.ncbi.nlm.nih.gov/entrez/query.fcgi?cmd=Retrieve&db=PubMed&dopt=Citation&list_uids=16009939

[49] Gordon L, Joo JH, Andronikos R, Ollikainen M, Wallace EM, Umstad MP, et al. Expression discordance of monozygotic twins at birth: effect of intrauterine environment and a possible mechanism for fetal programming. Epigenetics. 2011 May;6(5):579-92. Digital Object Identifier:

[50] Halder A, Jain M, Chaudhary I, Varma B. Chromosome 22q11.2 microdeletion in monozygotic twins with discordant phenotype and deletion size. Mol Cytogenet. 2012;5(1):13. Digital Object Identifier: 10.1186/1755-8166-5-13. http://www.ncbi.nlm.nih.gov/pubmed/22413934

[51] Javierre BM, Fernandez AF, Richter J, Al-Shahrour F, Martin-Subero JI, Rodriguez-Ubreva J, et al. Changes in the pattern of DNA methylation associate with twin discordance in systemic lupus erythematosus. Genome Research. 2010 February 1, 2010;20(2):170-9. Digital Object Identifier: 10.1101/gr.100289.109. http://genome.cshlp.org/content/20/2/170.abstract

[52] Maiti S, Kumar KHBG, Castellani CA, O'Reilly R, Singh SM. Ontogenetic De Novo Copy Number Variations (CNVs) as a Source of Genetic Individuality: Studies on Two Families with MZD Twins for Schizophrenia. PLoS ONE. 2011;6(3):e17125. Digital Object Identifier: http://dx.doi.org/10.1371%2Fjournal.pone.0017125

[53] Muqit MM, Larner AJ, Sweeney MG, Sewry C, Stinton VJ, Davis MB, et al. Multiple mitochondrial DNA deletions in monozygotic twins with OPMD. J Neurol Neurosurg Psychiatry. 2008 Jan;79(1):68-71. Digital Object Identifier: 10.1136/jnnp.2006.112250.

[54] Ollikainen M, Craig JM. Epigenetic discordance at imprinting control regions in twins. Epigenomics. 2011 Jun;3(3):295-306. Digital Object Identifier: 10.2217/epi.11.18.

[55] Stankiewicz P, Lupski JR. Structural variation in the human genome and its role in disease. Annu Rev Med. 2010;61:437-55. Digital Object Identifier: 10.1146/annurev-med-100708-204735.

[56] Wong AH, Gottesman, II, Petronis A. Phenotypic differences in genetically identical organisms: the epigenetic perspective. Hum Mol Genet. 2005 Apr 15;14 Spec No 1:R11-8. Digital Object Identifier: 14/suppl_1/R11 [pii] 10.1093/hmg/ddi116. http://www.ncbi.nlm.nih.gov/entrez/query.fcgi?cmd=Retrieve&db=PubMed&dopt=Citation&list_uids=15809262

[57] Holland J. Emergence: Perseus Publishing; 1999.

[58] Van Regenmortel M. Reductionism and the search for structure-function relationships in antibody molecules. J Mol Recognit. [Review]. 2002 Sep-Oct;15(5):240-7. Digital Object Identifier: 10.1002/jmr.584. http://www.ncbi.nlm.nih.gov/pubmed/12447900

[59] Gad S. Preface. In: Gad S, editor. Animal Models in Toxicology. Boca Rotan: CRC Press; 2007. p. 1-18.

[60] Calabrese EJ. Principles of Animal Extrapolation. Boca Rotan: CRC Press; 1991.

[61] Shah VP, Flynn GL, Guy RH, Maibach HI, Schaefer H, Skelly JP, et al. Workshop report on in vivo percutaneous penetration/absorption. Washington D.C., May 1-3, 1989. Skin Pharmacol. 1991;4(3):220-8. Digital Object Identifier: http://www.ncbi.nlm.nih.gov/entrez/query.fcgi?cmd=Retrieve&db=PubMed&dopt=Citation&list_uids=1685087

[62] Barber ED, Teetsel NM, Kolberg KF, Guest D. A comparative study of the rates of in vitro percutaneous absorption of eight chemicals using rat and human skin. Fundam

Appl Toxicol. 1992 Nov;19(4):493-7. Digital Object Identifier: http://www.ncbi.nlm.nih.gov/entrez/query.fcgi?cmd=Retrieve&db=PubMed&dopt=Citation&list_uids=1426706

[63] Scott RC, Batten PL, Clowes HM, Jones BK, Ramsey JD. Further validation of an in vitro method to reduce the need for in vivo studies for measuring the absorption of chemicals through rat skin. Fundam Appl Toxicol. 1992 Nov;19(4):484-92. Digital Object Identifier: http://www.ncbi.nlm.nih.gov/entrez/query.fcgi?cmd=Retrieve&db=PubMed&dopt=Citation&list_uids=1426705

[64] PLoS Press Release. Dalmatian bladder stones caused by gene that regulates uric acid in humans. http://wwweurekalertorg/pub_releases/2008-11/plos-dbs110408php. 2008(November 6). Digital Object Identifier:

[65] Mahmood I. Can absolute oral bioavailability in humans be predicted from animals? A comparison of allometry and different indirect methods. Drug Metabol Drug Interact. 2000;16(2):143-55. Digital Object Identifier: http://www.ncbi.nlm.nih.gov/entrez/query.fcgi?cmd=Retrieve&db=PubMed&dopt=Citation&list_uids=10962646

[66] Fox JG, Thibert P, Arnold DL, Krewski DR, Grice HC. Toxicology studies. II. The laboratory animal. Food Cosmet Toxicol. 1979 Dec;17(6):661-75. Digital Object Identifier: http://www.ncbi.nlm.nih.gov/entrez/query.fcgi?cmd=Retrieve&db=PubMed&dopt=Citation&list_uids=546701

[67] Paxton JW. The allometric approach for interspecies scaling of pharmacokinetics and toxicity of anti-cancer drugs. Clin Exp Pharmacol Physiol. 1995 Nov;22(11):851-4. Digital Object Identifier: http://www.ncbi.nlm.nih.gov/entrez/query.fcgi?cmd=Retrieve&db=PubMed&dopt=Citation&list_uids=8593743

[68] Parkinson C, Grasso P. The use of the dog in toxicity tests on pharmaceutical compounds. Hum Exp Toxicol. 1993 Mar;12(2):99-109. Digital Object Identifier: http://www.ncbi.nlm.nih.gov/entrez/query.fcgi?cmd=Retrieve&db=PubMed&dopt=Citation&list_uids=8096722

[69] Abelson PH. Exaggerated carcinogenicity of chemicals. Science. 1992 Jun 19;256(5064):1609. Digital Object Identifier: http://www.ncbi.nlm.nih.gov/entrez/query.fcgi?cmd=Retrieve&db=PubMed&dopt=Citation&list_uids=1609271

[70] Smith RL, Caldwell J. Drug metabolism in non-human primates. In: Parke DV, Smith RL, editors. Drug metabolism - from microbe to man. London: Taylor & Francis; 1977. p. 331-56.

[71] Walker RM, McElligott TF. Furosemide induced hepatotoxicity. J Pathol. 1981 Dec;135(4):301-14. Digital Object Identifier: 10.1002/path.1711350407. http://www.ncbi.nlm.nih.gov/entrez/query.fcgi?cmd=Retrieve&db=PubMed&dopt=Citation&list_uids=7328448

[72] Weatherall M. An end to the search for new drugs? Nature. 1982;296:387-90. Digital Object Identifier:

[73] Bonati M, Latini R, Tognoni G, Young JF, Garattini S. Interspecies comparison of in vivo caffeine pharmacokinetics in man, monkey, rabbit, rat, and mouse. Drug Metab Rev. 1984;15(7):1355-83. Digital Object Identifier: http://www.ncbi.nlm.nih.gov/entrez/query.fcgi?cmd=Retrieve&db=PubMed&dopt=Citation&list_uids=6543526

[74] Health Day. Hormone Lowers Glucose Levels in Mice. http://wwwhealthdaycom/Articleasp?AID=620987. 11/13/2008. Digital Object Identifier:

[75] BBC News. Window into cancer-spread secrets. 2008 [November 10].

[76] Caldwell J. Problems and opportunities in toxicity testing arising from species differences in xenobiotic metabolism. Toxicol Lett. 1992 Dec;64-65 Spec No:651-9. Digital Object Identifier: http://www.ncbi.nlm.nih.gov/entrez/query.fcgi?cmd=Retrieve&db=PubMed&dopt=Citation&list_uids=1471219

[77] Serrano D, Lazzeroni M, Zambon CF, Macis D, Maisonneuve P, Johansson H, et al. Efficacy of tamoxifen based on cytochrome P450 2D6, CYP2C19 and SULT1A1 genotype in the Italian Tamoxifen Prevention Trial. Pharmacogenomics J. 2011;11(2):100-7. Digital Object Identifier: http://dx.doi.org/10.1038/tpj.2010.17

[78] Sellers RS, Senese PB, Khan KN. Interspecies differences in the nephrotoxic response to cyclooxygenase inhibition. Drug Chem Toxicol. 2004 May;27(2):111-22. Digital Object Identifier: http://www.ncbi.nlm.nih.gov/entrez/query.fcgi?cmd=Retrieve&db=PubMed&dopt=Citation&list_uids=15198071

[79] Walton K, Dorne JL, Renwick AG. Species-specific uncertainty factors for compounds eliminated principally by renal excretion in humans. Food Chem Toxicol. 2004 Feb;42(2):261-74. Digital Object Identifier: S0278691503002722 [pii]. http://www.ncbi.nlm.nih.gov/entrez/query.fcgi?cmd=Retrieve&db=PubMed&dopt=Citation&list_uids=14667472

[80] Dixit R, Boelsterli U. Healthy animals and animal models of human disease(s) in safety assessment of human pharmaceuticals, including therapeutic antibodies. Drug Discovery Today. 2007;12(7-8):336-42. Digital Object Identifier:

[81] Hughes B. Industry concern over EU hepatotoxicity guidance. Nat Rev Drug Discov. 2008;7(9):719-. Digital Object Identifier: http://dx.doi.org/10.1038/nrd2677

[82] Weaver JL, Staten D, Swann J, Armstrong G, Bates M, Hastings KL. Detection of systemic hypersensitivity to drugs using standard guinea pig assays. Toxicology. 2003 Dec 1;193(3):203-17. Digital Object Identifier: S0300483X03002671 [pii]. http://www.ncbi.nlm.nih.gov/entrez/query.fcgi?cmd=Retrieve&db=PubMed&dopt=Citation&list_uids=14599760

[83] Force T, Kolaja KL. Cardiotoxicity of kinase inhibitors: the prediction and translation of preclinical models to clinical outcomes. Nat Rev Drug Discov. [10.1038/nrd3252]. 2011;10(2):111-26. Digital Object Identifier: http://dx.doi.org/10.1038/nrd3252

[84] Eason CT, Bonner FW, Parke DV. The importance of pharmacokinetic and receptor studies in drug safety evaluation. Regul Toxicol Pharmacol. 1990 Jun;11(3):288-307.

Digital Object Identifier: http://www.ncbi.nlm.nih.gov/entrez/query.fcgi?cmd=Retrieve&db=PubMed&dopt=Citation&list_uids=2196638

[85] Sankar U. The Delicate Toxicity Balance in Drug Discovery. The Scientist. 2005 August 1;19(15):32. Digital Object Identifier:

[86] Caponigro G, Sellers WR. Advances in the preclinical testing of cancer therapeutic hypotheses. Nat Rev Drug Discov. 2011 Mar;10(3):179-87. Digital Object Identifier: nrd3385 [pii] 10.1038/nrd3385. http://www.ncbi.nlm.nih.gov/entrez/query.fcgi?cmd=Retrieve&db=PubMed&dopt=Citation&list_uids=21358737

[87] Editors. In this issue. Nat Rev Drug Discov. [10.1038/nrd3411]. 2011;10(4):239-. Digital Object Identifier: http://dx.doi.org/10.1038/nrd3411

[88] Leaf C. Why we are losing the war on cancer. Fortune. 2004(March 9):77-92. Digital Object Identifier: http://money.cnn.com/magazines/fortune/fortune_archive/2004/03/22/365076/index.htm

[89] Park BK, Boobis A, Clarke S, Goldring CEP, Jones D, Kenna JG, et al. Managing the challenge of chemically reactive metabolites in drug development. Nat Rev Drug Discov. [10.1038/nrd3408]. 2011;10(4):292-306. Digital Object Identifier: http://dx.doi.org/10.1038/nrd3408

[90] Gad S. Model Selection and Scaling. In: Gad S, editor. Animal Models in Toxicology, Second Edition (Drug and Chemical Toxicology): Informa Healthcare; 2006. p. 831-62.

[91] Sarkar SK. Molecular imaging approaches. Drug Discovery World. 2009(Fall):33-8. Digital Object Identifier:

[92] Litchfield JT, Jr. Symposium on clinical drug evaluation and human pharmacology. XVI. Evaluation of the safety of new drugs by means of tests in animals. Clin Pharmacol Ther. 1962 Sep-Oct;3:665-72. Digital Object Identifier: http://www.ncbi.nlm.nih.gov/entrez/query.fcgi?cmd=Retrieve&db=PubMed&dopt=Citation&list_uids=14465857

[93] Suter K. What can be learned from case studies? The company approach. In: Lumley C, Walker S, editors. Animal Toxicity Studies: Their Relevance for Man. Lancaster: Quay; 1990. p. 71-8.

[94] Fourches D, Barnes JC, Day NC, Bradley P, Reed JZ, Tropsha A. Cheminformatics analysis of assertions mined from literature that describe drug-induced liver injury in different species. Chem Res Toxicol. 2010 Jan;23(1):171-83. Digital Object Identifier: 10.1021/tx900326k. http://www.ncbi.nlm.nih.gov/entrez/query.fcgi?cmd=Retrieve&db=PubMed&dopt=Citation&list_uids=20014752

[95] Sietsema WK. The absolute oral bioavailability of selected drugs. Int J Clin Pharmacol Ther Toxicol. 1989 Apr;27(4):179-211. Digital Object Identifier: http://www.ncbi.nlm.nih.gov/entrez/query.fcgi?cmd=Retrieve&db=PubMed&dopt=Citation&list_uids=2654032

[96] Fletcher AP. Drug safety tests and subsequent clinical experience. J R Soc Med. 1978 Sep;71(9):693-6. Digital Object Identifier: http://www.ncbi.nlm.nih.gov/entrez/query.fcgi?cmd=Retrieve&db=PubMed&dopt=Citation&list_uids=712750

[97] Lumley C. Clinical toxicity: could it have been predicted? Premarketing experience. In: Lumley C, Walker S, editors. Animal Toxicity Studies: Their Relevance for Man: Quay; 1990. p. 49-56.

[98] Spriet-Pourra C, Auriche M, (Eds). SCRIP Reports: PJB; 1994.

[99] Heywood R. Clinical Toxicity--Could it have been predicted? Post-marketing experience. In: CE Lumley, Walker S, editors. Animal Toxicity Studies: Their Relevance for Man. Lancaster: Quay; 1990. p. 57-67.

[100] Igarashi Y. Report from the Japanese Pharmaceutical Manufacturers Association 1994 Seiyakukyo data.

[101] Lin JH. Species similarities and differences in pharmacokinetics. Drug Metab Dispos. 1995 Oct;23(10):1008-21. Digital Object Identifier: http://www.ncbi.nlm.nih.gov/entrez/query.fcgi?cmd=Retrieve&db=PubMed&dopt=Citation&list_uids=8654187

[102] Garattini S. Toxic effects of chemicals: difficulties in extrapolating data from animals to man. Crit Rev Toxicol. 1985;16(1):1-29. Digital Object Identifier: http://www.ncbi.nlm.nih.gov/entrez/query.fcgi?cmd=Retrieve&db=PubMed&dopt=Citation&list_uids=3910353

[103] Heywood R. Target organ toxicity II. Toxicol Lett. 1983 Aug;18(1-2):83-8. Digital Object Identifier: 0378-4274(83)90075-9 [pii]. http://www.ncbi.nlm.nih.gov/entrez/query.fcgi?cmd=Retrieve&db=PubMed&dopt=Citation&list_uids=6623552

[104] Wall RJ, Shani M. Are animal models as good as we think? Theriogenology. 2008 Jan 1;69(1):2-9. Digital Object Identifier: S0093-691X(07)00598-5 [pii] 10.1016/j.theriogenology.2007.09.030. http://www.ncbi.nlm.nih.gov/entrez/query.fcgi?cmd=Retrieve&db=PubMed&dopt=Citation&list_uids=17988725

[105] Markou A, Chiamulera C, Geyer MA, Tricklebank M, Steckler T. Removing obstacles in neuroscience drug discovery: the future path for animal models. Neuropsychopharmacology : official publication of the American College of Neuropsychopharmacology. 2009 Jan;34(1):74-89. Digital Object Identifier: 10.1038/npp.2008.173. http://www.ncbi.nlm.nih.gov/pubmed/18830240

[106] Mullane K, Williams M. Translational semantics and infrastructure: another search for the emperor's new clothes? Drug Discovery Today 2012;17(9/10):459-68. Digital Object Identifier:

[107] Rice J. Animal models: Not close enough. Nature. [10.1038/nature11102]. 2012;484(7393):S9-S. Digital Object Identifier: http://dx.doi.org/10.1038/nature11102

[108] Cook N, Jodrell DI, Tuveson DA. Predictive in vivo animal models and translation to clinical trials. Drug Discovery Today. 2012;17(5/6):253-60. Digital Object Identifier:

[109] Johnson JI, Decker S, Zaharevitz D, Rubinstein LV, Venditti JM, Schepartz S, et al. Relationships between drug activity in NCI preclinical in vitro and in vivo models and early clinical trials. Br J Cancer. 2001 May 18;84(10):1424-31. Digital Object Identifier: 10.1054/bjoc.2001.1796 S0007092001917963 [pii]. http://www.ncbi.nlm.nih.gov/entrez/query.fcgi?cmd=Retrieve&db=PubMed&dopt=Citation&list_uids=11355958

[110] Suggitt M, Bibby MC. 50 years of preclinical anticancer drug screening: empirical to target-driven approaches. Clinical cancer research : an official journal of the American Association for Cancer Research. [Research Support, Non-U.S. Gov't Review]. 2005 Feb 1;11(3):971-81. Digital Object Identifier: http://www.ncbi.nlm.nih.gov/pubmed/15709162

[111] Salsburg D. The lifetime feeding study in mice and rats--an examination of its validity as a bioassay for human carcinogens. Fundam Appl Toxicol. 1983 Jan-Feb;3(1):63-7. Digital Object Identifier: http://www.ncbi.nlm.nih.gov/entrez/query.fcgi?cmd=Retrieve&db=PubMed&dopt=Citation&list_uids=6884625

[112] Tomatis L, Agthe C, Bartsch H, Huff J, Montesano R, Saracci R, et al. Evaluation of the carcinogenicity of chemicals: a review of the Monograph Program of the International Agency for Research on Cancer (1971 to 1977). Cancer Res. 1978 Apr;38(4):877-85. Digital Object Identifier: http://www.ncbi.nlm.nih.gov/entrez/query.fcgi?cmd=Retrieve&db=PubMed&dopt=Citation&list_uids=346205

[113] Reuters. U.S. to develop chip that tests if a drug is toxic. Reuters; 2011 [updated September 16; cited 2011 October 6]; Available from: http://www.msnbc.msn.com/id/44554007/ns/health-health_care/ -.To5AMnPaixF.

[114] Gura T. Cancer Models: Systems for identifying new drugs are often faulty. Science. 1997 Nov 7;278(5340):1041-2. Digital Object Identifier: http://www.ncbi.nlm.nih.gov/entrez/query.fcgi?cmd=Retrieve&db=PubMed&dopt=Citation&list_uids=9381203

[115] Björquist P, Sartipy P. Raimund Strehl and Johan Hyllner. Human ES cell derived functional cells as tools in drug discovery. Drug Discovery World. 2007(Winter):17-24. Digital Object Identifier:

[116] FDA. FDA Issues Advice to Make Earliest Stages Of Clinical Drug Development More Efficient. FDA; 2006 [updated June 18, 2009; cited 2010 March 7]; FDA News Release]. Available from: http://www.fda.gov/NewsEvents/Newsroom/PressAnnouncements/2006/ucm108576.htm.

[117] Zielinska E. Building a better mouse. The Scientist. 2010 April 1;24(4):34-8. Digital Object Identifier:

[118] DiMasi JA, Hansen RW, Grabowski HG. The price of innovation: new estimates of drug development costs. J Health Econ. 2003 Mar;22(2):151-85. Digital Object Identifier: S0167-6296(02)00126-1 [pii] 10.1016/S0167-6296(02)00126-1. http://www.ncbi.nlm.nih.gov/entrez/query.fcgi?cmd=Retrieve&db=PubMed&dopt=Citation&list_uids=12606142

[119] Kola I, Landis J. Can the pharmaceutical industry reduce attrition rates? Nat Rev Drug Discov. 2004 Aug;3(8):711-5. Digital Object Identifier: 10.1038/nrd1470 nrd1470 [pii]. http://www.ncbi.nlm.nih.gov/entrez/query.fcgi?cmd=Retrieve&db=PubMed&dopt=Citation&list_uids=15286737

[120] Shaffer C. Safety Through Sequencing. Drug Discovery & Development 2012 [updated January 1, 2012; cited 2012 January 30]; Available from: http://www.dddmag.com/article-Safety-Through-Sequencing-12412.aspx?et_cid=2450547&et_rid=45518461&linkid=http%3a%2f%2fwww.dddmag.com%2farticle-Safety-Through-Sequencing-12412.aspx.

[121] Paul SM, Mytelka DS, Dunwiddie CT, Persinger CC, Munos BH, Lindborg SR, et al. How to improve R&D productivity: the pharmaceutical industry's grand challenge. Nat Rev Drug Discov. 2010 Mar;9(3):203-14. Digital Object Identifier: nrd3078 [pii] 10.1038/nrd3078. http://www.ncbi.nlm.nih.gov/entrez/query.fcgi?cmd=Retrieve&db=PubMed&dopt=Citation&list_uids=20168317

[122] Cressey D. Traditional drug-discovery model ripe for reform. Nature. 2011 Mar 3;471(7336):17-8. Digital Object Identifier: 471017a [pii] 10.1038/471017a. http://www.ncbi.nlm.nih.gov/entrez/query.fcgi?cmd=Retrieve&db=PubMed&dopt=Citation&list_uids=21368796

[123] Giri S, Bader A. Foundation review: Improved preclinical safety assessment using micro-BAL devices: the potential impact on human discovery and drug attrition. Drug Discovery Today. 2011;16(9/10):382-97. Digital Object Identifier:

[124] Unknown. Drug Discovery & Development. 2002(November):35. Digital Object Identifier:

[125] Roy ASA. Stifling New Cures: The True Cost of Lengthy Clinical Drug Trials. New York: Manhattan Institute for Policy Research2012 March

[126] Makarova SI. Human N-acetyltransferases and drug-induced hepatotoxicity. Current drug metabolism. [Review]. 2008 Jul;9(6):538-45. Digital Object Identifier: http://www.ncbi.nlm.nih.gov/pubmed/18680474

[127] Mullard A. Marc Kirschner. Nat Rev Drug Discov. [10.1038/nrd3613]. 2011;10(12): 894-. Digital Object Identifier: http://dx.doi.org/10.1038/nrd3613

[128] Alonso-Zaldivar R. Earlier Drug Testing on Humans OKd. Los Angeles: LA Times; 2006 [updated January 13; cited 2010 March 8]; Available from: http://articles.latimes.com/2006/jan/13/nation/na-fda13.

[129] Waldman M. Drive for drugs leads to baby clinical trials. Nature. 2006 Mar 23;440(7083):406-7. Digital Object Identifier: 440406a [pii] 10.1038/440406a. http://www.ncbi.nlm.nih.gov/entrez/query.fcgi?cmd=Retrieve&db=PubMed&dopt=Citation&list_uids=16554774

[130] Lappin G, Garner RC. Big physics, small doses: the use of AMS and PET in human microdosing of development drugs. Nat Rev Drug Discov. 2003 Mar;2(3):233-40. Dig-

ital Object Identifier: 10.1038/nrd1037 nrd1037 [pii]. http://www.ncbi.nlm.nih.gov/entrez/query.fcgi?cmd=Retrieve&db=PubMed&dopt=Citation&list_uids=12612650

[131] Lappin G, Garner RC. The utility of microdosing over the past 5 years. Expert Opinion on Drug Metabolism & Toxicology. [Review]. 2008 Dec;4(12):1499-506. Digital Object Identifier: 10.1517/17425250802531767. http://www.ncbi.nlm.nih.gov/pubmed/19040326

[132] Lappin G, Kuhnz W, Jochemsen R, Kneer J, Chaudhary A, Oosterhuis B, et al. Use of microdosing to predict pharmacokinetics at the therapeutic dose: experience with 5 drugs. Clin Pharmacol Ther. 2006 Sep;80(3):203-15. Digital Object Identifier: S0009-9236(06)00200-1 [pii] 10.1016/j.clpt.2006.05.008. http://www.ncbi.nlm.nih.gov/entrez/query.fcgi?cmd=Retrieve&db=PubMed&dopt=Citation&list_uids=16952487

[133] Gill DM. Bacterial toxins: a table of lethal amounts. Microbiol Rev. [Review]. 1982 Mar;46(1):86-94. Digital Object Identifier: http://www.ncbi.nlm.nih.gov/pubmed/6806598

[134] National Institute of Occupational Safety and Health. Registry of Toxic Effects of Chemical Substances (R-TECS). Cincinnati: National Institute of Occupational Safety and Health; 1996.

[135] Cohen AF. Developing drug prototypes: pharmacology replaces safety and tolerability? Nat Rev Drug Discov. 2010 Nov;9(11):856-65. Digital Object Identifier: nrd3227 [pii] 10.1038/nrd3227. http://www.ncbi.nlm.nih.gov/entrez/query.fcgi?cmd=Retrieve&db=PubMed&dopt=Citation&list_uids=20847743

[136] ATSDR. Cancer Fact Sheet. Atlanta: CDC. Agency for Toxic Substances & Disease Registry; 2002 [updated August 30, 2002; cited 2012 May 22]; Available from: http://www.atsdr.cdc.gov/com/cancer-fs.html.

[137] Shah RR. Pharmacogenetics in drug regulation: promise, potential and pitfalls. Philos Trans R Soc Lond B Biol Sci. 2005 Aug 29;360(1460):1617-38. Digital Object Identifier: 3VFVUVCNBUK20M3Q [pii] 10.1098/rstb.2005.1693. http://www.ncbi.nlm.nih.gov/entrez/query.fcgi?cmd=Retrieve&db=PubMed&dopt=Citation&list_uids=16096112

[138] Roses AD. Pharmacogenetics and the practice of medicine. Nature. 2000 Jun 15;405(6788):857-65. Digital Object Identifier: 10.1038/35015728. http://www.ncbi.nlm.nih.gov/entrez/query.fcgi?cmd=Retrieve&db=PubMed&dopt=Citation&list_uids=10866212

[139] Angst MS, Chu LF, Tingle MS, Shafer SL, Clark JD, Drover DR. No evidence for the development of acute tolerance to analgesic, respiratory depressant and sedative opioid effects in humans. Pain. 2009 Mar;142(1-2):17-26. Digital Object Identifier: 10.1016/j.pain.2008.11.001. http://www.ncbi.nlm.nih.gov/pubmed/19135798

[140] Dolin SJ, Cashman JN. Tolerability of acute postoperative pain management: nausea, vomiting, sedation, pruritus, and urinary retention. Evidence from published data.

British journal of anaesthesia. [Review]. 2005 Nov;95(5):584-91. Digital Object Identifier: 10.1093/bja/aei227. http://www.ncbi.nlm.nih.gov/pubmed/16169893

[141] Yucesoy B, Johnson VJ, Fluharty K, Kashon ML, Slaven JE, Wilson NW, et al. Influence of cytokine gene variations on immunization to childhood vaccines. Vaccine. 2009 Nov 23;27(50):6991-7. Digital Object Identifier: S0264-410X(09)01423-6 [pii] 10.1016/j.vaccine.2009.09.076. http://www.ncbi.nlm.nih.gov/entrez/query.fcgi?cmd=Retrieve&db=PubMed&dopt=Citation&list_uids=19819209

[142] King C. Personalised vaccines could protect all children New Scientist. 2009 December 5(2737):11. Digital Object Identifier:

[143] Willyard C. Blue's clues. Nat Med. 2007 Nov;13(11):1272-3. Digital Object Identifier: nm1107-1272 [pii] 10.1038/nm1107-1272. http://www.ncbi.nlm.nih.gov/entrez/query.fcgi?cmd=Retrieve&db=PubMed&dopt=Citation&list_uids=17987010

[144] Canto JG, Rogers WJ, Goldberg RJ, Peterson ED, Wenger NK, Vaccarino V, et al. Association of Age and Sex With Myocardial Infarction Symptom Presentation and In-Hospital Mortality. JAMA: The Journal of the American Medical Association. 2012 February 22/29, 2012;307(8):813-22. Digital Object Identifier: 10.1001/jama.2012.199. http://jama.ama-assn.org/content/307/8/813.abstract

[145] Holden C. Sex and the suffering brain. Science. 2005 Jun 10;308(5728):1574. Digital Object Identifier: 308/5728/1574 [pii] 10.1126/science.308.5728.1574. http://www.ncbi.nlm.nih.gov/entrez/query.fcgi?cmd=Retrieve&db=PubMed&dopt=Citation&list_uids=15947170

[146] Kaiser J. Gender in the pharmacy: does it matter? Science. 2005 Jun 10;308(5728):1572. Digital Object Identifier: 308/5728/1572 [pii] 10.1126/science.308.5728.1572. http://www.ncbi.nlm.nih.gov/entrez/query.fcgi?cmd=Retrieve&db=PubMed&dopt=Citation&list_uids=15947169

[147] Klein S, Huber S. Sex differences in susceptibility to viral infection. In: Klein S, Roberts C, editors. Sex hormones and immunity to infection. Berlin: Springer-Verlag; 2010. p. 93-122.

[148] Simon V. Wanted: women in clinical trials. Science. 2005 Jun 10;308(5728):1517. Digital Object Identifier: 308/5728/1517 [pii] 10.1126/science.1115616. http://www.ncbi.nlm.nih.gov/entrez/query.fcgi?cmd=Retrieve&db=PubMed&dopt=Citation&list_uids=15947140

[149] Wald C, Wu C. Of Mice and Women: The Bias in Animal Models. Science. 2010;327(5973):1571-2. Digital Object Identifier:

[150] Willyard C. HIV gender clues emerge. Nat Med. 2009 Aug;15(8):830. Digital Object Identifier: nm0809-830b [pii] 10.1038/nm0809-830b. http://www.ncbi.nlm.nih.gov/entrez/query.fcgi?cmd=Retrieve&db=PubMed&dopt=Citation&list_uids=19661976

[151] Cheung DS, Warman ML, Mulliken JB. Hemangioma in twins. Ann Plast Surg. 1997 Mar;38(3):269-74. Digital Object Identifier: http://www.ncbi.nlm.nih.gov/entrez/query.fcgi?cmd=Retrieve&db=PubMed&dopt=Citation&list_uids=9088466

[152] Couzin J. Cancer research. Probing the roots of race and cancer. Science. 2007 Feb 2;315(5812):592-4. Digital Object Identifier: 315/5812/592 [pii] 10.1126/science.315.5812.592. http://www.ncbi.nlm.nih.gov/entrez/query.fcgi?cmd=Retrieve&db=PubMed&dopt=Citation&list_uids=17272699

[153] Gregor Z, Joffe L. Senile macular changes in the black African. Br J Ophthalmol. 1978 Aug;62(8):547-50. Digital Object Identifier: http://www.ncbi.nlm.nih.gov/entrez/query.fcgi?cmd=Retrieve&db=PubMed&dopt=Citation&list_uids=687553

[154] Haiman CA, Stram DO, Wilkens LR, Pike MC, Kolonel LN, Henderson BE, et al. Ethnic and racial differences in the smoking-related risk of lung cancer. N Engl J Med. 2006 Jan 26;354(4):333-42. Digital Object Identifier: 354/4/333 [pii] 10.1056/NEJMoa033250. http://www.ncbi.nlm.nih.gov/entrez/query.fcgi?cmd=Retrieve&db=PubMed&dopt=Citation&list_uids=16436765

[155] Kalow W. Interethnic variation of drug metabolism. Trends in Pharmacological Sciences. [Review]. 1991 Mar;12(3):102-7. Digital Object Identifier: http://www.ncbi.nlm.nih.gov/pubmed/2053186

[156] Kopp JB, Nelson GW, Sampath K, Johnson RC, Genovese G, An P, et al. APOL1 Genetic Variants in Focal Segmental Glomerulosclerosis and HIV-Associated Nephropathy. Journal of the American Society of Nephrology. 2011 October 13, 2011. Digital Object Identifier: 10.1681/asn.2011040388. http://jasn.asnjournals.org/content/early/2011/10/06/ASN.2011040388.abstract

[157] Spielman RS, Bastone LA, Burdick JT, Morley M, Ewens WJ, Cheung VG. Common genetic variants account for differences in gene expression among ethnic groups. Nat Genet. 2007 Feb;39(2):226-31. Digital Object Identifier: ng1955 [pii] 10.1038/ng1955. http://www.ncbi.nlm.nih.gov/entrez/query.fcgi?cmd=Retrieve&db=PubMed&dopt=Citation&list_uids=17206142

[158] Stamer UM, Stuber F. The pharmacogenetics of analgesia. Expert Opin Pharmacother. 2007 Oct;8(14):2235-45. Digital Object Identifier: 10.1517/14656566.8.14.2235. http://www.ncbi.nlm.nih.gov/entrez/query.fcgi?cmd=Retrieve&db=PubMed&dopt=Citation&list_uids=17927480

[159] Wilke RA, Dolan ME. Genetics and Variable Drug Response. JAMA: The Journal of the American Medical Association. 2011 July 20, 2011;306(3):306-7. Digital Object Identifier: 10.1001/jama.2011.998. http://jama.ama-assn.org/content/306/3/306.short

[160] HealthDay. Gene Sequences May Make You Unique. HealthDay_News; 2010 [updated March 18; cited 2010 March 18]; Available from: http://health.yahoo.com/news/healthday/genesequencesmaymakeyouunique.html.

[161] Kasowski M, Grubert F, Heffelfinger C, Hariharan M, Asabere A, Waszak SM, et al. Variation in Transcription Factor Binding Among Humans. Science. 2010 Mar 18;328(5975):232-5. Digital Object Identifier: science.1183621 [pii] 10.1126/science.1183621. http://www.ncbi.nlm.nih.gov/entrez/query.fcgi?cmd=Retrieve&db=PubMed&dopt=Citation&list_uids=20299548

[162] Herzig M, Christofori G. Recent advances in cancer research: mouse models of tumorigenesis. Biochim Biophys Acta. 2002 Jun 21;1602(2):97-113. Digital Object Identifier: S0304419X02000392 [pii]. http://www.ncbi.nlm.nih.gov/entrez/query.fcgi?cmd=Retrieve&db=PubMed&dopt=Citation&list_uids=12020798

[163] Ingram DK, Jucker M. Developing mouse models of aging: a consideration of strain differences in age-related behavioral and neural parameters. Neurobiol Aging. 1999 Mar-Apr;20(2):137-45. Digital Object Identifier: S0197458099000330 [pii]. http://www.ncbi.nlm.nih.gov/entrez/query.fcgi?cmd=Retrieve&db=PubMed&dopt=Citation&list_uids=10537023

[164] Raineri I, Carlson EJ, Gacayan R, Carra S, Oberley TD, Huang TT, et al. Strain-dependent high-level expression of a transgene for manganese superoxide dismutase is associated with growth retardation and decreased fertility. Free Radic Biol Med. 2001 Oct 15;31(8):1018-30. Digital Object Identifier: S0891584901006864 [pii]. http://www.ncbi.nlm.nih.gov/entrez/query.fcgi?cmd=Retrieve&db=PubMed&dopt=Citation&list_uids=11595386

[165] Hunter K, Welch DR, Liu ET. Genetic background is an important determinant of metastatic potential. Nat Genet. 2003 May;34(1):23-4; author reply 5. Digital Object Identifier: 10.1038/ng0503-23b ng0503-23b [pii]. http://www.ncbi.nlm.nih.gov/entrez/query.fcgi?cmd=Retrieve&db=PubMed&dopt=Citation&list_uids=12721549

[166] Thein SL. Genetic modifiers of beta-thalassemia. Haematologica. 2005 May;90(5):649-60. Digital Object Identifier: http://www.ncbi.nlm.nih.gov/entrez/query.fcgi?cmd=Retrieve&db=PubMed&dopt=Citation&list_uids=15921380

[167] Agarwal S, Moorchung N. Modifier genes and oligogenic disease. J Nippon Med Sch. 2005 Dec;72(6):326-34. Digital Object Identifier: JST.JSTAGE/jnms/72.326 [pii]. http://www.ncbi.nlm.nih.gov/entrez/query.fcgi?cmd=Retrieve&db=PubMed&dopt=Citation&list_uids=16415512

[168] Friedman A, Perrimon N. Genetic screening for signal transduction in the era of network biology. Cell. 2007 Jan 26;128(2):225-31. Digital Object Identifier: S0092-8674(07)00063-3 [pii] 10.1016/j.cell.2007.01.007. http://www.ncbi.nlm.nih.gov/entrez/query.fcgi?cmd=Retrieve&db=PubMed&dopt=Citation&list_uids=17254958

[169] Editorial. Deconstructing Genetic Contributions to Autoimmunity in Mouse Models. PLoS Biology. 2004 August 01, 2004;2(8):e220. Digital Object Identifier: http://dx.doi.org/10.1371%2Fjournal.pbio.0020220

[170] Weiss ST, McLeod HL, Flockhart DA, Dolan ME, Benowitz NL, Johnson JA, et al. Creating and evaluating genetic tests predictive of drug response. Nat Rev Drug Dis-

cov. 2008 Jul;7(7):568-74. Digital Object Identifier: nrd2520 [pii] 10.1038/nrd2520. http://www.ncbi.nlm.nih.gov/entrez/query.fcgi?cmd=Retrieve&db=PubMed&dopt=Citation&list_uids=18587383

[171] Dolgin E. Big pharma moves from 'blockbusters' to 'niche busters'. Nat Med. [10.1038/nm0810-837a]. 2010;16(8):837-. Digital Object Identifier: http://dx.doi.org/10.1038/nm0810-837a

[172] Herscu P, Hoover TA, Randolph AG. Clinical prediction rules: new opportunities for pharma. Drug Discov Today. 2009 Dec;14(23-24):1143-9. Digital Object Identifier: S1359-6446(09)00341-9 [pii] 10.1016/j.drudis.2009.09.012. http://www.ncbi.nlm.nih.gov/entrez/query.fcgi?cmd=Retrieve&db=PubMed&dopt=Citation&list_uids=19853059

[173] The Medical Letter. Invader UGT1A1 Molecular Assay for Irinotecan Toxicity. The Medical Letter. 2006 May 8;48(1234):39-40. Digital Object Identifier:

[174] Hudson KL. Genomics, Health Care, and Society. New England Journal of Medicine. 2011;365(11):1033-41. Digital Object Identifier: doi:10.1056/NEJMra1010517. http://www.nejm.org/doi/full/10.1056/NEJMra1010517

[175] Hughes AR, Spreen WR, Mosteller M, Warren LL, Lai EH, Brothers CH, et al. Pharmacogenetics of hypersensitivity to abacavir: from PGx hypothesis to confirmation to clinical utility. Pharmacogenomics J. 2008 Dec;8(6):365-74. Digital Object Identifier: tpj20083 [pii] 10.1038/tpj.2008.3. http://www.ncbi.nlm.nih.gov/entrez/query.fcgi?cmd=Retrieve&db=PubMed&dopt=Citation&list_uids=18332899

[176] Blair E. Predictive tests and personalised medicine. Drug Discovery World. 2009(Fall):27-31. Digital Object Identifier:

[177] PMC. Personalized Medicine. Personalized Medicine Coalition; 2006 [cited 2006 October 30]; Available from: http://www.ageofpersonalizedmedicine.org/personalized_medicine/today_case.asp.

Chapter 7

Renal Transporters and Biomarkers in Safety Assessment

P.D. Ward, D. La and J.E. McDuffie

Additional information is available at the end of the chapter

http://dx.doi.org/10.5772/54857

1. Introduction

Understanding the effect of renal transporters on the distribution of drugs, metabolites, and endogenous compounds (e.g., biomarkers for renal toxicity and physiological regulators) are important in safety assessment studies [1]. Drugs (and their metabolites) that preferentially distribute into the kidney may have a greater potential to induce renal toxicity because these compounds may accumulate in the cells surrounding/forming the renal tubules. This disposition may not be deduced by simply sampling plasma; therefore, sampling kidney tissue in addition to plasma is important for measuring concentrations of drugs when renal toxicity is observed in animals. In human safety assessment, sampling of kidney is not generally feasible; therefore, the utility of qualified tissue-, serum- and/or urine-specific biomarkers may help to extrapolate between animal tissue and human exposures.

This chapter will review the role of renal transporters and biomarkers in the safety assessment of drug candidates. Membrane permeability and types of drug transporters will be introduced with focus on specific renal transporters. Examples of cause-effect relationships between renal transporters and toxicity will be discussed. The effect of drugs on the ability of renal transporters to regulate the disposition of endogenous compounds involved in maintaining homeostasis will be discussed. In addition, a case example on the effect of a proprietary drug candidate on a classical biomarker of renal safety will be highlighted where an increase of this biomarker via inhibition of a renal transporter was determined to be benign and not the consequence of renal toxicity. Finally, we will highlight the recent qualification of novel diagnostic renal urinary biomarkers that outperform the traditional renal biomarkers, serum creatinine (sCr) and/or blood urea nitrogen (BUN) in monitoring renal injury in preclinical (rat) studies. We will also highlight use of selected novel renal biomarkers in rat and dog studies with the paradigm renal toxicant, cisplatin.

2. Transport through cellular barriers

Molecules cross cellular barriers by three main pathways: (1) passive diffusion across the cell membranes; (2) passive diffusion between adjacent cells; and (3) carrier-mediated transport (Fig. 1). Lipophilic molecules cross the cells membrane by transcellular diffusion. By contrast, hydrophilic molecules that are not recognized by a carrier cannot partition into the hydrophobic membrane and thus traverse the epithelial barrier via the paracellular pathway. Hormones and certain immune system molecules can utilize membrane invaginations for transport across the cell (e.g. via caveolae). All other compounds must interact with carrier proteins, either in a facilitated manner (down the concentration gradient) or via "active" transport, potentially against a concentration gradient. The driving force to allow active transport may include the use of ATP hydrolysis, pH gradients, or electrogenic properties of the cell. [2]

Transporters depicted in Pathway ④ (Fig. 1) efflux compounds from cell into the lumen or blood and are thought to act as a cellular defender to prevent xenobiotics from either entering the cells or endogenous waste products from accumulating in the cells. These types of transporters are referred to as efflux transporters. With respect to pharmaceutical compounds, clinically relevant transporters are members of the ATP-binding cassette (ABC) superfamily membrane bound transporters [3]. P-glycoprotein (P-gp) is the most well characterized ABC transporter [4, 5]. Other efflux transporters such as multidrug resistance-associated protein (MRP) members in proximal tubular cells function as an extrusion pump for organic anions from the apical membrane, especially large and hydrophobic organic anions such as glutathione and glucuronide conjugates [6].

Transporters depicted in Pathway ③ (Fig. 1) facilitate transport of nutrients (e.g., amino acids and glucose) and drugs into cells. These types of transporters are referred to as uptake or influx transporters. For nutrients, uptake transporters are essential for reabsorbing glucose from the tubule lumen into the systemic circulation. The importance of these types of transporters and the impact of interrupting their function on safety assessment will be further discussed in Section 5.

For pharmaceutical compounds, members of the Solute Carrier (SLC) superfamily of membrane transport proteins (depicted in Pathway ⑤, transport an extraordinarily diverse set of solutes, including both charged and uncharged organic molecules as well as inorganic ions) have wide implications on human physiology, pathology, and in multiple therapeutic areas [7]. Examples of SLC transporters (Fig. 2) include organic cation transporters (OCT) and organic anion transporters (OAT). Renal transporters (e.g., OAT and OCT) allow the entry of drugs (with low passive transcellular permeability) through the basolateral membrane into the tubule cells, which leads to elimination of the drug into urine by transport of the drug through the apical membrane by either SLC or efflux transporters (i.e., tubular secretion). Interestingly, SLC transporters expressed on the apical or luminal membrane (e.g., novel organic cation transporters (OCTN) and OAT4) may also play a role in tubular reabsorption, process by which compounds are removed from the tubular fluid and transported into the blood [8].

http://dx.doi.org/10.5772/54857

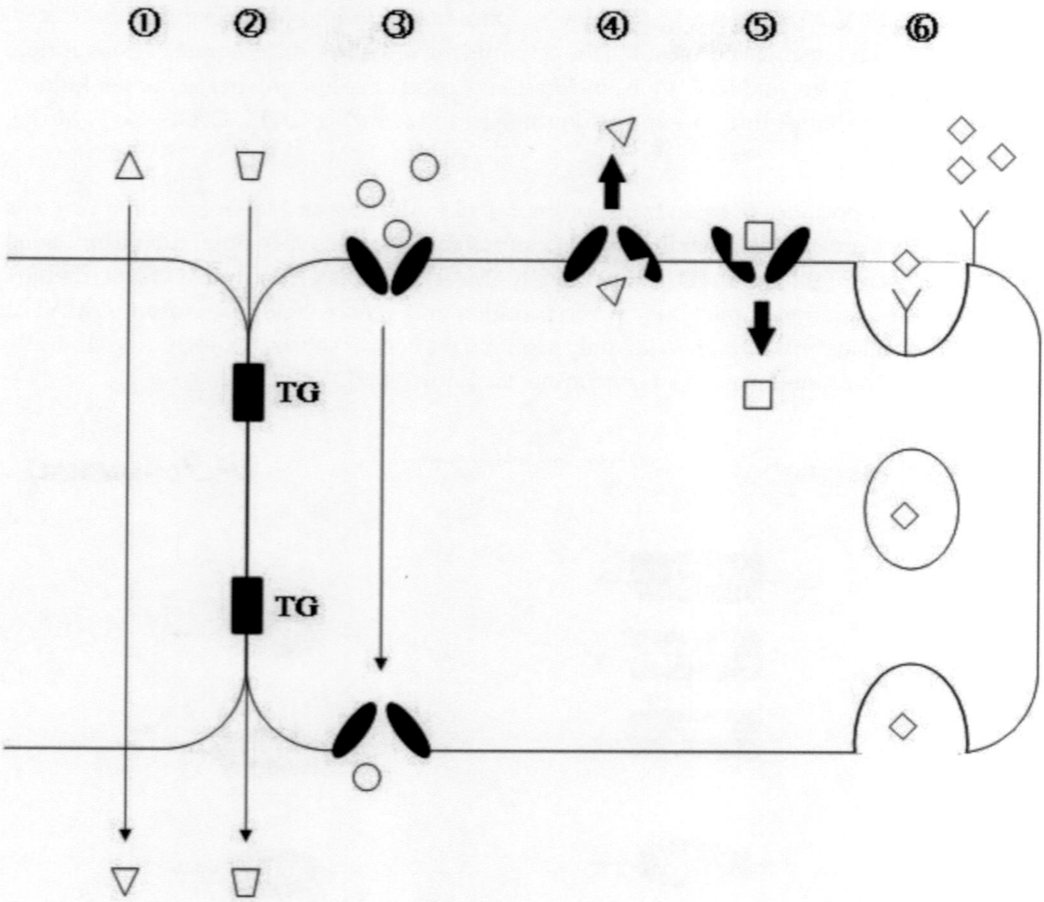

Figure 1. Routes of translocation through cellular barriers. ① Lipid soluble compounds can permeate through the epithelium by simple passive diffusion (transcellular route). ②Small molecular weight compounds such as CO_2 can permeate through the tight junctions (TG) between cells (paracellular route). ③Facilitative transport (e.g., uptake of amino acids) occurs via a transport carrier down the concentration gradient of the solute. ④Transport can also occur via a carrier, but against the concentration gradient of the solute. In the case of efflux transporters such as P-glycoprotein (P-gp), ATP-hydrolysis is the driving force for this transport. ⑤Uptake carriers such as the organic anion or organic cation transporters can also transport substances against a concentration gradient. The driving force is dependent on the particular transporter but can be pH-dependent or electrogenic. ⑥Some hormones are transported through the epithelium via receptor-mediated transcytosis. The ligand binds to a cell surface receptor, which cause an invagination in the membrane. This invagination is internalized and carried to the opposite membrane where the ligand is then released ([2]; reproduced with permission).

3. Drug transporters in the kidney

The kidney is responsible for clearance of many drugs including polar hydrophilic compounds such as ß-lactam antibiotics and non-steroidal anti-inflammatory drugs [9]. Polar compounds may be actively taken up by the proximal tubule cells through a variety of transporters including OCT2, OAT1 and 3 (Fig. 2, Table 1). Once taken up into the proximal tubule cells, compounds generally must efflux out of the cells into the urine by a different set of transporters including MRP2, P-gp, and MRP4 (i.e., facilitation of tubular secretion). In the human kidney, the order of transporter mRNA expression (highest to lowest) is OAT1, OAT3, P-gp, MRP2, and OCT2 [10].

Recently, the importance of renal transporters called multidrug and toxin extrusion proteins (MATE), which are expressed in the apical (luminal) membrane of proximal tubule epithelial cells, have been highlighted [11]. Functionally, MATEs act as efflux transporters, thereby mediating the excretion of metabolic waste products and xenobiotics. Two isoforms, MATE1 and 2, have been identified, and, so far, only a limited number of substrates, including clinically used drugs such as metformin and cimetidine, are known [12].

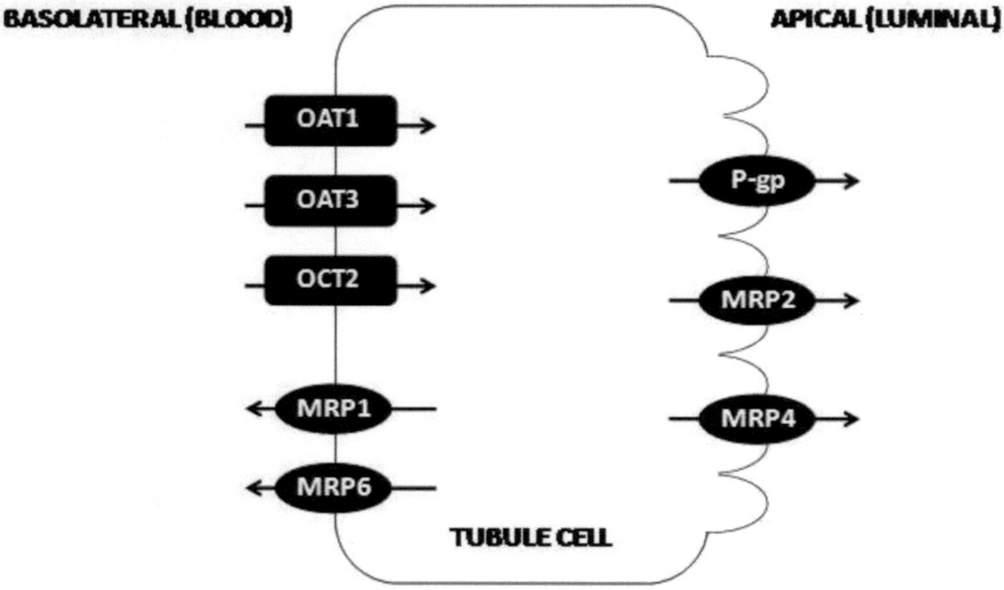

Figure 2. Select drug transporters located in the kidney predicted to play a role in drug distribution and elimination. Influx transporters located on the basolateral or blood side of the kidney tubule cells include the organic anion transporters OAT1 and 3, and the organic cation transporter OCT2. Efflux transporters located on the basolateral side include multiple members of the multidrug resistance protein family such as MRP1 and MRP6. Efflux transporters located on the apical or luminal side of the tubule membrane which pump drugs from the interior of the tubule cell into the tubular fluid include P-gp, MRP2 and MRP4 ([2]; reproduced with permission).

Compounds may be reabsorbed from the tubular fluid back into the tubule cells or cleared from the body. The interplay between various transporters located on the basolateral (blood) or apical (luminal) side dictates the overall renal clearance of a compound. As with the liver, renal transporters can therefore be a site of potential drug-drug interactions (DDI). Inhibition of the basolateral transporters (by the primary compound, metabolites, or a co-administered compound) can lead to increased exposure of the drug and longer half-lives in the

http://dx.doi.org/10.5772/54857

systemic circulation. Inhibition of renal uptake of some drugs may actually induce toxicity by inhibiting their renal excretion. For example, severe methotrexate toxicity due to an increase in serum concentrations was observed in patients after co-administration with probenecid which inhibited OAT1 and MRP, and consequently the tubular secretion of methotrexate [13, 14]. Inhibition of the luminal efflux transporters, again by either the compound itself or a co-administered drug, can also cause an increase in systemic exposure if the basolateral transporters are able to transport the compound back into the systemic circulation. Alternatively, inhibition of the luminal efflux transporters can cause a compound to be "trapped" in the cell which may lead to renal toxicity [2].

Protein/Gene	Substrates	Inhibitors	References
OCT2/SLC22A2	cimetidine, metformin, MPP+, quinine TEA	cimetidine, clonidine, procainamide, quinine	[15, 16]
OAT1/SLC22A6	adefovir, para-aminohippurate, furosemide	furosemide, indomethacin, probenecid, urate	[17, 18]
OAT3/SLC22A8	benzylpenicillin, furosemide, methotrexate, pravastatin	gemfibrozil, indomethacin, probenecid, salicylate	[17, 19]
P-gp/ABCB1	digoxin, daunorubicin, doxorubicin, fexofenadine, irinotecan, paclitaxel, quinidine, saquinavir, verapamil	cyclosporine A, elacridar, quinidine, valspodar, verapamil	[4, 5, 20, 21]
MRP1/ABCC1	daunorubicin, etoposide, methotrexate, glutathione, glucuronide and sulfate conjugates, vincristine	delavirdine, efavirenz, MK571, probenecid	[6, 20]
MRP2/ABCC2	Similar to MRP1, cisplatin, methotrexate	delavirdine, efavirenz, MK571, probenecid	[20, 22, 23]
MRP4/ABCC4	adefovir, azidothymidine monophosphate, prostaglandins, methotrexate	indomethacin, ketoprofen	[24, 25]

Table 1. Substrates and inhibitors of select renal transporters ([2]; partially reproduced with permission)

4. Importance of plasma sampling and understanding drug disposition in renal tissue during safety assessment

Compound-induced toxicities can be better extrapolated from animals to humans when these comparisons are based on toxicokinetics instead of dose alone [26]. For example, the safety margin that is based on the ratio of the animal exposure at the no observed adverse effect level (NOAEL) to human exposure at the efficacious dose is a key predictor of human safety risk. To calculate this safety margin, the animal and human exposure is determined by analyzing drug and metabolite(s) concentrations in plasma, which is the most practical and widely accepted way of assessing this risk. However, most safety issues are not due to drug plasma concentration but due to concentration of drug in various organs/tissues.

Sampling plasma and extrapolating this exposure to organs or tissues assumes that 1) concentration of drug in plasma is in equilibrium with concentrations in tissues, 2) changes in plasma drug concentrations reflect changes in tissue drug concentrations over time, and 3) distribution of drug and its metabolites are not affected by cells (e.g., drug transporters and enzymes) that protect many of these tissues [27]. Drug transport into tissues may not be a passive process and may depend on drug transporters, and thus these assumptions may result in an inaccurate assessment of target organ exposure to drug and/or metabolites. Even without a drug being a substrate for a drug transporter, lysosomal trapping of weak bases (e.g., liver and lung) or accumulation in membranes (e.g., muscle) can occur that can subsequently give rise to preferential distribution of the drug and its metabolites. For more details, refer to http://www.intechopen.com/books/toxicity-and-drug-testing/toxicokinetics-and-organ-specific-toxicity [27].

If the compound enters tubular cells via uptake transporters (e.g. OCT2, OAT1, OAT3), but not effluxed (into luminal fluid or urine), very high compound concentrations can occur in the renal cells/tissue. A convincing cause-effect relationship exists between uptake of renal toxicants via transporters and associated renal toxicity where co-administration of probenecid (inhibits renal uptake of organic anions) or either cimetidine or imatinib (inhibits renal uptake of organic cations) may reduce renal toxicity (by limiting uptake). For example, co-administration of cisplatin with imatinib prevents cisplatin-induced renal toxicity by inhibiting influx via OCT2 [28]. Another example is co-administration of cephaloridine with probenecid lowers the potential risk of cephaloridine-induced renal toxicity by inhibiting the OAT1-mediated transport of cephaloridine into the proximal tubule cell [29].

Influx transporter OAT1 (minor contribution by OAT3) is involved in the renal safety of acyclic nucleotide phosphonates (adefovir, cidofovir, and tenofovir), which are eliminated predominantly into the urine [30-32]. The dose-limiting toxicity for acyclic nucleotide phosphonates is renal failure, particularly for adefovir and cidofovir which may accumulate in the kidney [33, 34]. Patients treated with tenofovir exhibit a lower incidence of renal dysfunction at doses used to treat HIV compared to adefovir and cidofovir [35, 36]. In vitro studies showed that cells expressing human OAT1 showed enhanced toxicity to adefovir and cidofovir [500-fold) compared to cells that do not express OAT1 [37]. Unlike adefovir and cidofovir, tenofovir is less nephrotoxic to OAT1-expressing cells [38]. Additional in vitro studies demonstrated that OAT1 inhibitors such as nonsteroidal anti-inflammatory drugs, protect OAT1-expressing cells from adefovir- and cidofovir-induced cytotoxicity by preventing their cellular accumulation [39].

Efflux transporters in the kidney also play a potential role in the safety of a drug by pumping the drug out of the tubule cell and into the blood or urine (tubular fluid) and preventing the accumulation of the drug in the tubule cell. For example, the efflux transporters, MRPs, may be another crucial factor in the renal accumulation of acyclic nucleotide analogs (in addition to the uptake) and subsequent nephrotoxicity. Interestingly, renal toxicity in patients is observed with tenofovir when co-administered with an inhibitor of MRP2, ritonavir [40]. However, tenofovir is also a substrate for MRP4 that may not be inhibited by ritonavir [41, 42]. Other members of the MRP family (MRP5 and 8) may also be involved in the transport of acyclic nucleotide analogs [43]. Transport of adefovir and cidofovir was not observed in the membrane vesicles expressing human MRP2 and BCRP; furthermore, transport of adefovir and tenofovir but not cidofovir was observed only in the membrane vesicles expressing MRP4 [41]. To support these in vitro observations, the kidney accumulation of adefovir and tenofovir was significantly greater in Mrp4 knockout mice; however, there was no change in the kinetic parameters of cidofovir in these mice [41].

Another example of the relationship between efflux transporters and renal safety is MATE and platinum drugs. MATE can effectively mediate the transport of oxaliplatin, but not that of cisplatin [44]. Interestingly, oxaliplatin is effectively transported into renal proximal tubular cells by OCT2 but does not accumulate due to MATE-mediated renal extrusion, which may be the reason that oxaliplatin is much less nephrotoxic than cisplatin. Therefore, the interplay between renal OCTs and MATEs may influence the pharmacokinetics of platinum compounds and may critically determine the severity of platinum-associated adverse events [45].

This idea of reducing tubule exposure or even renal tissue half-life and consequently increasing the safety of drugs is also emphasized by studies investigating differences in renal safety of bisphophonates. In a rat model, zoledronic acid, but not ibandronate, induces progressive renal toxicity [46]. Ibandronate has a terminal renal tissue half-life of 24 days [47], whereas the renal tissue half-life of zoledronic acid (150–200 days) does not allow enough time for repair of renal damage [48]. Renal excretion is the only route of elimination of bisphosphonates. Interestingly, studies in rats demonstrated that alendronate is actively secreted by an uncharacterized renal transport system, and not by the anionic or cationic renal transport systems [49].

Understanding the tissue distribution and the substrate specificity for drug transporters can significantly aid safety assessment. In addition, this increased understanding can support the development of drugs with improved safety [1, 27] and/or a different route of administration that avoids distribution to the organ(s) where the compound-induced toxicity occurs. For example, an aerosolized form of [^{14}C]-cidofovir (dose-limiting toxicity is nephrotoxicity) administered to mice (via inhalation) results in the prolonged retention of radiolabeled drug in the lungs (site of initial viral replication) at levels exceeding those in the kidneys [34]. In contrast, subcutaneous injection produces much higher concentrations of [^{14}C]-cidofovir in the kidneys compared to the lungs [34]. Possibly in the future, the disposition of drug candidates may be directed by targeting specific drug transporters in organs like the kidney to significantly improve the renal safety of the drug candidate.

5. Importance of renal transporters in the regulation of homeostasis

Renal transporters regulate disposition of endogenous compounds that control homeostasis of a physiological system. Therefore, alteration in the activity of renal transporters by drugs may be a method to treat disease but also unexpected changes to the activity of these transporters may induce adverse effects. For example, Na+-dependent dicarboxylate transporters and OATs are involved in the disposition of dicarboxylates which are important regulators of the renovascular system; therefore, these renal transporters may play an important role in the maintenance of blood pressure [50]. Another example is the role of renal transporters in the regulation of serum uric acid levels where renal transporters of uric acid like GLUT9 (SLC2A9) may be a target for treatment of gout [51].

Recently, renal glucose transport has become a very active target for drug development. The kidney reabsorbs 99% of the glucose that filters through the renal glomeruli [52]. Approximately 90% of the glucose is reabsorbed by the low affinity, high capacity sodium-dependent glucose cotransporter (SGLT) 2 in the proximal tubules. The remaining glucose is reabsorbed by the high affinity, low capacity transporter, SGLT1 (expressed in the segment 3 of the proximal tubule). Co-transport with sodium enables movement of glucose by SGLTs against a concentration gradient, with the sodium gradient maintained by the Na+/K+ ATPase pump. Individuals with SGLT2 mutations (e.g., familial renal glucosuria or FRG) have persistent yet benign renal glucosuria [53]. Similar to the effect observed with FRG, novel drugs are being developed to reduce glucose reabsorption by inhibiting SGLT2. One such example, dapagliflozin is a selective SGLT2 inhibitor that is being developed for the treatment of type 2 diabetes mellitus, a disorder characterized by elevated blood glucose [54]. In diabetic rat models, dapagliflozin has been shown to decrease serum glucose concomitant with glycosuria. Similar effects have been observed in clinical trials with decreased hemoglobin A1c, fasting plasma glucose, postprandial glucose, and body weight in patients with type 2 diabetes.

6. Importance of renal drug transporters in the disposition of a classical biomarker in renal safety assessment

Creatinine is a breakdown product of creatine phosphate in muscle that is cleared by glomerular filtration and tubular secretion, and is routinely used as a diagnostic biomarker of renal function. For example, sCr can be used to estimate creatinine clearance which is then used to calculate glomerular filtration rate (GFR). Generally, a doubling of sCr suggests a 50% reduction in GFR.

Yet, sCr measurement as an indicator of compound-induced renal toxicity is often unreliable as sCr levels can be altered by changes in the levels of muscle mass and/or dietary protein. For example, sCr levels are often less reliable for detecting impaired GFR in the elderly, females, those with chronic illness associated with muscle wasting, African Americans, amputees, and vegans; various equations can be used to adjust for some of these factors to obtain a more reliable estimation of GFR [55, 56].

Creatinine is actively secreted by organic cation transporters including OCT2 and MATE which results in an overestimation of GFR by up to 40% [57-60]. For example, a drug that inhibits OCT2 can cause an increase in sCr levels independent of renal impairment [61]. Increased sCr levels in such cases typically stabilize over time and are not considered clinically relevant.

http://dx.doi.org/10.5772/54857

sCr increases due to OCT2 and MATE inhibition show a characteristic temporal pattern. When a drug is administered over several days, creatinine levels increase quickly, reach a plateau, and return to baseline levels shortly after drug discontinuation. This pattern is illustrated in the following case example from a clinical study with Compound A (Fig. 3). Subjects were administered placebo or one of three dose levels of Compound A daily for 2 weeks. sCr levels were unchanged for the placebo group, but mild, dose-dependent increases were observed for subjects receiving Compound A. Increases were observed at the first post-treatment time point, and increased levels were maintained during the 2-week treatment period. sCr levels decreased once treatment was discontinued. In nonclinical studies (rat and monkey) with Compound A, there was no evidence of renal injury associated with sCr increases even when elevated sCr levels were maintained for durations as long as 9 months. The time course and magnitude of the sCr changes observed with Compound A are consistent with transporter inhibition and have been observed for marketed drugs, such as cimetidine and trimethoprim. For cimetidine, maximum inhibition of sCr secretion occurs within 24 hours after administration and sCr levels return to baseline several days after discontinuation of dosing [62].

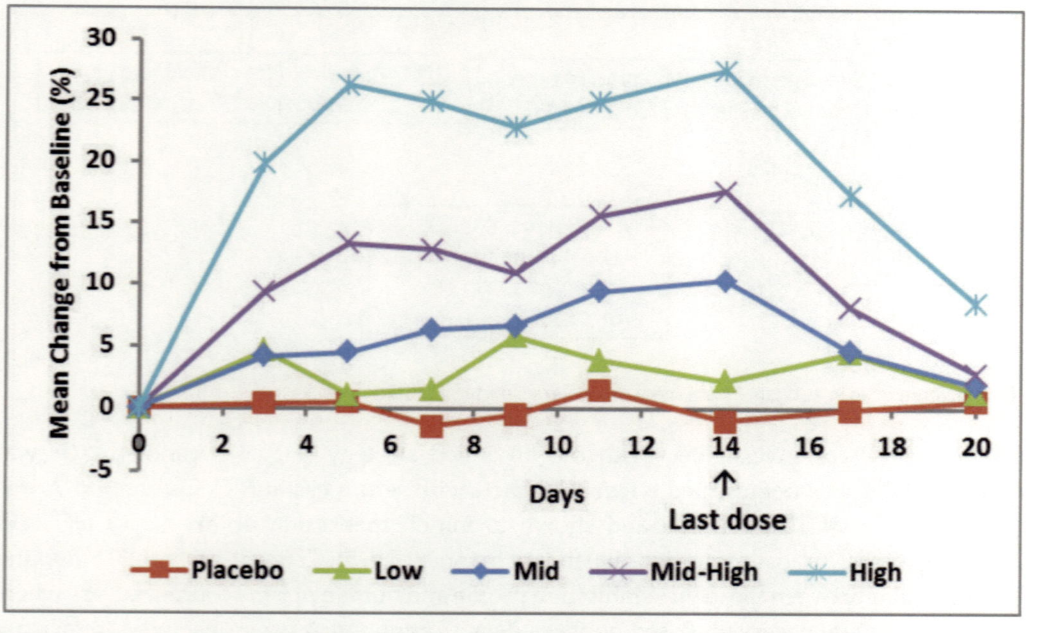

Figure 3. Temporal pattern of sCr changes in human subjects following 14 days oral administration of Compound A.

A proposed strategy for investigating increased sCr levels when inhibition of renal transporter(s) is suspected is provided in Fig. 4. First, GFR should be determined with an alternative method (e.g., measurement of serum levels of cystatin C) to rule out renal impairment as a cause for the creatinine increase. Serum cystatin C is a more accurate biomarker for GFR estimation because it is filtered in the glomeruli, but not secreted by renal transporters [55]. Other methods such as inulin [63] or radioisotopes also are available, but are impractical clinically as these methods can be costly and time-consuming and may delay clinical intervention. If the GFR measured with an alternative method remains suppressed, potential renal injury can be investigated with various biomarkers (see Section 7). If GFR is not affected, then OCT2 or MATE inhibition can be explored with an in vitro study. An IC_{50} in the range of clinically relevant concentrations would support inhibition of renal transporters as the mechanism for the sCr increase. Other mechanisms such as changes in sCr production (e.g., diet, disease status) would need to be explored if the sCr increase is not explained by inhibition of renal transporters.

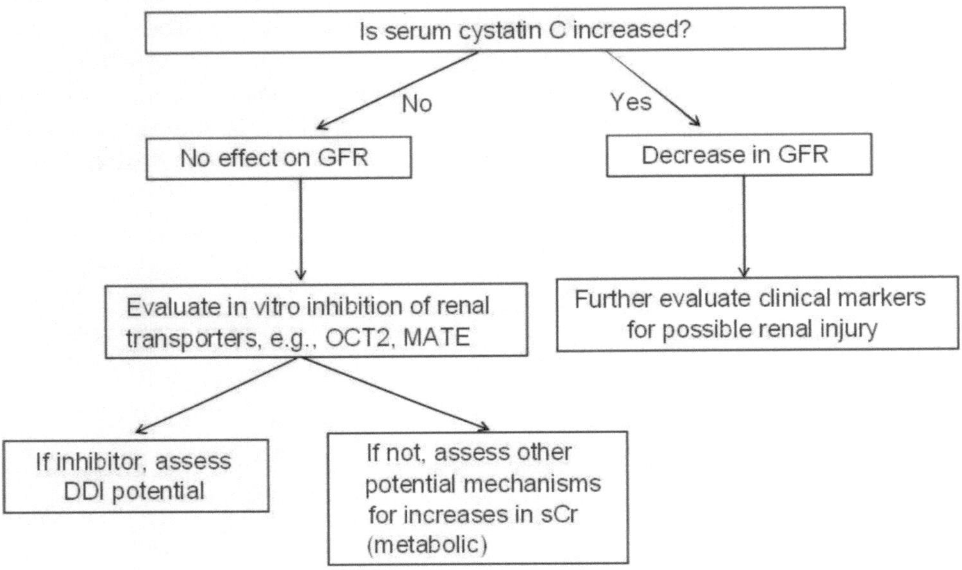

Figure 4. Strategy to investigate involvement of renal transporters in sCr changes.

Compound A was investigated with the described strategy (Fig. 4). Although sCr was increased, GFR was not affected when calculated with serum cystatin C. Compound A was then tested for OCT2 inhibition and shown to inhibit metformin uptake into CHO cells expressing OCT2 in a concentration-dependent manner (Fig. 5). Concentrations of Compound A were similar between the in vitro inhibition profile and human plasma concentrations where sCr increases were observed. Based on these data, Compound A was considered to increase sCr levels by inhibiting tubular secretion of creatinine via OCT2.

Similar to OCT2, elevation of sCr by a drug can also occur with the inhibition of MATE transporters. For example, pyrimethamine, a potent inhibitor of MATE transporters and a weak inhibitor of OCT2 [64], increased sCr within 28 h from 81 +/- 14 to 102 +/- 16 μM (P = 0.002) in the healthy volunteers [65]. Therefore, inhibition of MATE transporters should also be considered to be a potential mechanism when increased levels of sCr are clinically-associated with drug administration.

http://dx.doi.org/10.5772/54857

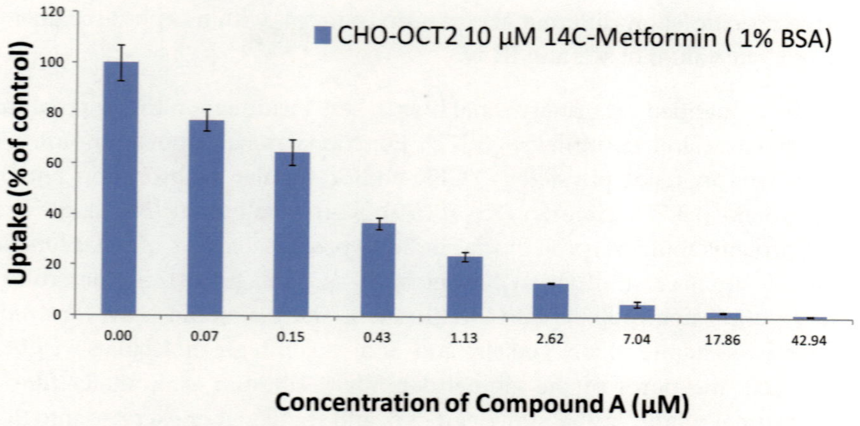

Figure 5. Inhibition of metformin uptake into CHO cells expressing OCT2 by Compound A. With CHO cells, stably transfected with cDNA encoding for OCT2, transport of a prototypical substrate of OCT2, metformin (10 μM, 1 min) was determined in the presence and absence of various concentrations of Compound A.

7. Importance of biomarkers in renal safety assessment

While the aforementioned examples in this chapter show that concentrations of drug and/or metabolites in tissues provide greater predictivity for toxicity compared to plasma, routine tissue sampling is not generally feasible in clinical safety assessments. Biomarkers are important tools in renal safety assessment because they can provide early and non-invasive indication of compound-induced toxicities. Regulatory agencies (i.e., United States Food & Drug Administration, FDA; European Medicines Agency, EMA and/or Japanese Pharmaceuticals & Medical Devices Agency, PMDA) have recognized the need for novel, qualified, translational renal biomarkers [66-68]. Traditional renal biomarkers, sCr and BUN, used in both preclinical and clinical settings lack both specificity and sensitivity. For example, increases in sCr and BUN levels may reflect alteration in GFR that can occur with or without renal tubular pathology and increases in sCr and BUN are measureable 2-3 days after significant loss of renal function because the kidney has a huge functional reserve [69, 70]. Increased sCr may be predictive of kidney injury only when nearly half of the functional nephron capacity has been lost and the kidneys are unable to regulate fluid and electrolyte homeostasis [71]. sCr may also be elevated due to physiologic states unrelated to compound-induced nephrotoxicity such as dehydration and muscle damage [68, 72].

To date, eight urinary rat renal biomarkers have been qualified by the Critical Path Institute's Predictive Safety Testing Consortium (PSTC), Nephrotoxicity Working Group [66, 67] and the International Life Sciences Institute-Health and Environmental Safety Institute (ILSI-HESI), Biomarkers of Nephrotoxicity Project Group [68] for monitoring compound-induced, progressive renal injury in rats. The qualified rat renal biomarkers include urinary markers: kidney injury molecule-1 (KIM-1), albumin, total protein, ß2-microalbumin, cystatin C, clusterin, trefoil factor-3 (TFF-3) and renal papillary antigen-1 (RPA-1). These novel biomarkers are highly sensitive, specific (show differential expression patterns within nephron segments), and add to the diagnostic values of sCr and BUN.

The utility of these qualified rat urinary renal biomarkers include monitoring renal function, tissue injury response and tissue leakage [72]. Functional renal biomarkers are used for monitoring changes in renal physiology, GFR and/or tubular reabsorption and include urinary total protein [73-77], albumin [75, 78, 79], ß2-microalbumin [80], and cystatin C. High levels of proteins in urine (proteinuria) indicate progressive loss of renal function and alterations of the glomerular filtration barrier such as damage to the glomerular podocytes or leakage of plasma proteins into the filtrate. Urinary albumin is synthesized in the liver, circulates in systemic blood vessels, and is a major high molecular weight serum protein larger than the pores of the glomerular filter. Albumin is normally filtered and absorbed by proximal tubule epithelium, degraded, and reutilized or excreted into the urine; therefore, the appearance of albumin in urine represents injury to the glomerular basement membrane [72]. Glomerular injury with subsequent impairment of tubular reabsorption may be detected by urinary levels of ß2-microalbumin and cystatin C; which appear to be more reliable than traditional renal biomarkers, sCr and BUN [67]. The gene for cystatin C is expressed in all nucleated cells and bears the characteristics of a housekeeping gene; therefore, cystatin C production rate is assumed to remain constant, a characteristic which lends to its utility in the clinic as an endogenous marker of GFR [80]. ß2-microalbumin is produced by mononulear cells which limits use as a GFR marker.

Urinary total protein, urinary albumin, urinary ß2-microalbumin and urinary cystatin C are qualified for use in GLP rat studies to assess potential glomerular changes and/or impaired tubular reabsorption [67]. When compound-induced tubular injury or glomerular alterations have been identified in rat studies, urinary total protein, urinary albumin, urinary β2-microglobulin and urinary cystatin C can be used as bridging biomarkers to monitor kidney safety in clinical settings.

Renal tissue injury response biomarkers that have been qualified for monitoring compound-induced renal injury in the rat include urinary KIM-1, urinary clusterin, urinary RPA-1 and urinary TFF-3. Urinary KIM-1, also referred to as T-cell immunoglobulin mucin-1 (TIM-1) or hepatitis A virus cellular receptor-1 (HAVCR-1) is expressed primarily but not exclusively in proximal tubular epithelial cells and lymphocytes [81, 82]. KIM-1 mRNA and subsequently KIM-1 protein is expressed during de-differentiation of proximal tubular epithelial cells. KIM-1 has been reported to function as a receptor in the phagocytosis of apoptotic tubule epithelial cells [82]. When KIM-1 protein is cleaved, the ectodomain is shed into the urine and is stable at room temperature for several hours. KIM-1 has specificity and sensitivity for use as a urinary biomarker to monitor compound-induced proximal tubular injury in rats. Similar KIM-1 characteristics observed in the rat have been demonstrated in humans; and the cleaved ectodomain of KIM-1 can be detected in the urine of patients with acute tubular necrosis; therefore, urinary KIM-1 is also considered qualified as a clinical bridging biomarker to monitor kidney safety in clinical studies on a "case-by-case" basis following the identification of tubular injury in rats [82].

Early detection and sensitivity of urinary KIM-1 as a biomarker of renal tubular injury were demonstrated with a model of cisplatin-induced acute kidney injury (AKI) in male Sprague Dawley rats treated for 1, 3, 5, 7, or 14 days at 1 mg/kg/day [83]. As early as 1 day after cisplatin treatment, positive KIM-1 immunostaining, observed in the outer medulla of the kidney, indicated the onset of proximal tubular injury in the absence of functional changes. After 3 days of treatment, KIM-1 protein levels in urine increased more than 20-fold concurrently with tubular basophilia. After 5 days, sCr and BUN levels were elevated concurrently with tubular degeneration. Cisplatin-induced increases in urinary and renal KIM-1 protein levels were detected prior to changes in BUN, demonstrating the sensitivity of KIM-1 as a diagnostic tool for detection of compound-induced proximal tubular injury in rats.

In another study in male Beagle dogs, KIM-1 was identified as a renal tissue injury response marker (author's unpublished data). Animals were intravenously administered cisplatin [0.75 mg/kg/day for up to 5 days) and humanely euthanized when sCr levels were ≥1.9 mg/dL, indicating significant loss of GFR. AKI was histologically characterized by tubule dilatation, vacuolization, degeneration, regeneration, and interstitial inflammation. Increased sCr was not observed until approximately day 16 (Fig. 6], while increased urinary KIM-1 mRNA levels were detected as early as Day 2 and were highly predictive of cisplatin-induced renal tissue injury. KIM-1 protein expression was detected in the injured proximal tubular epithelial cells (degenerated, vacuolized and dilated tubules) or regenerated proximal tubular epithelial cells (tubular basophilia), primarily in the S2 segment correlated with histomorphologic changes (Fig. 7). Neither urinary KIM-1 mRNA by quantitative polymerase chain reaction analysis nor renal KIM-1 protein expression with immunostaining in canines with compound-induced AKI has been previously reported.

Another renal injury biomarker, clusterin, exists as a secreted isoform or a nuclear isoform, although only the 80 kDa glycosylated secreted isoform is constitutively expressed during early stages of renal development and later in response to injury to proximal and distal tubules, papillae, glomeruli, and collecting ducts [72, 81, 84, 85]. Secreted clusterin is believed to be anti-apoptotic, and involved in lipid recycling, cell aggregation and cell attachment. Urinary clusterin levels correlate with the severity of tubular damage [84]. In male Wistar rats, clusterin mRNA was markedly induced and immunostaining demonstrated clusterin primarily in tubules in the cortex and medulla following administration of puromycin aminonucleoside (15 mg/100 g body weight, subcutaneously). Clusterin may differentiate between glomerular and tubular injuries [84]. In a model of cisplatin-induced AKI in male Sprague Dawley rats, urinary clusterin measurements were detected prior to changes in BUN [83]. Positive clusterin immunostaining accurately correlated with the histopathologic findings. Urinary clusterin has not been approved for clinical use [82].

Induction of RPA-1 expression correlates with immunoreactivity of inducible nitric oxide synthase (iNOS) and nitrotyrosine. Thus, RPA-1 is believed to be increased in the cytoplasm of intact cells of the collecting duct epithelium and proximal tubule epithelium following compound-induced injury to nephron segments as a result of iNOS-dependent signal transduction pathways [72, 86]. Rat renal RPA-1 is highly expressed in the epithelial cells in medullary (papilla) and cortical collecting ducts and in the medullary loop of Henle. In the rat,

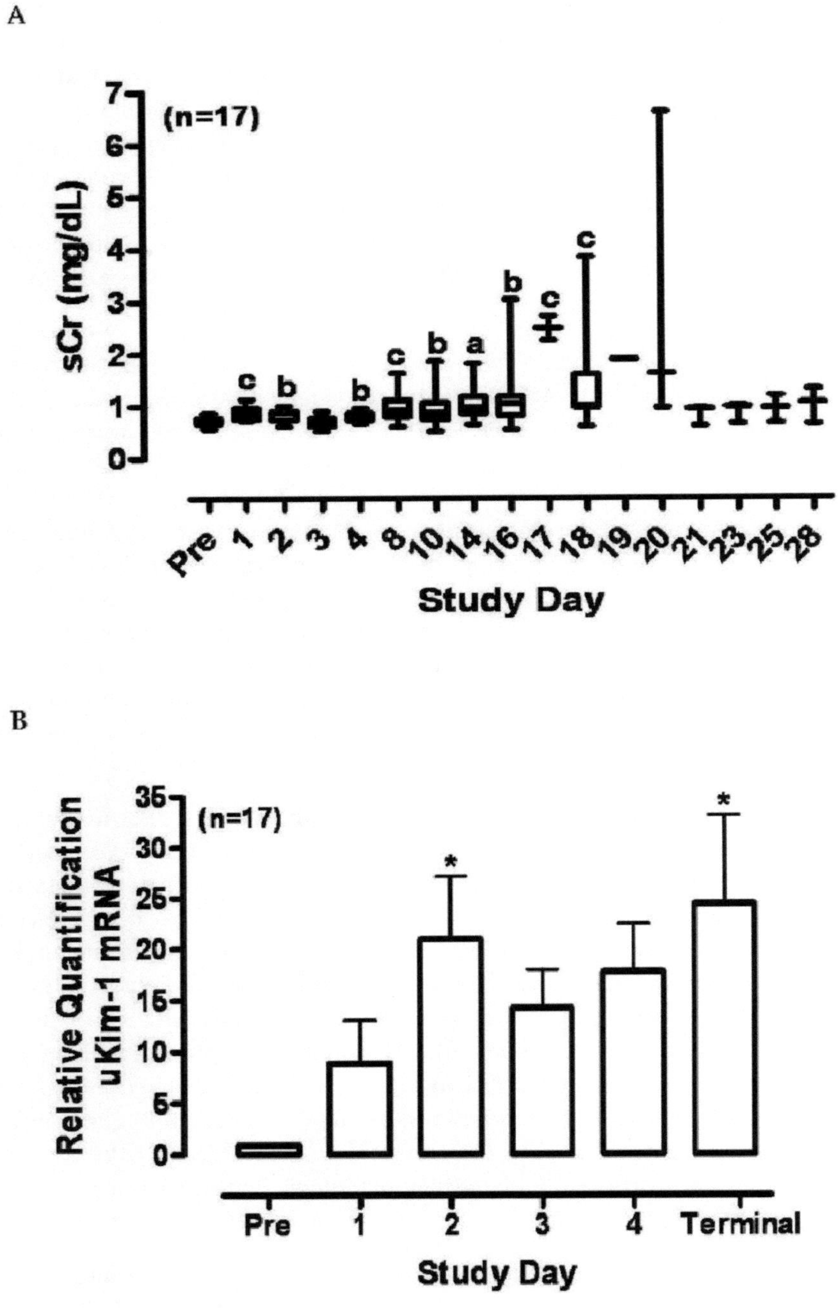

Figure 6. sCr and urinary KIM-1 (uKIM-1] mRNA measurements in dogs with cisplatin-induced AKI. (A) sCr increased significantly in one dog on day 16. (B) Relative quantification of uKIM-1 mRNA levels in dogs with cisplatin-induced AKI. Data are means ± SEM; a indicates $P<0.001$, b indicates $P<0.01$, and c and * indicate $P<0.05$ relative to predose (Pre) values.

http://dx.doi.org/10.5772/54857

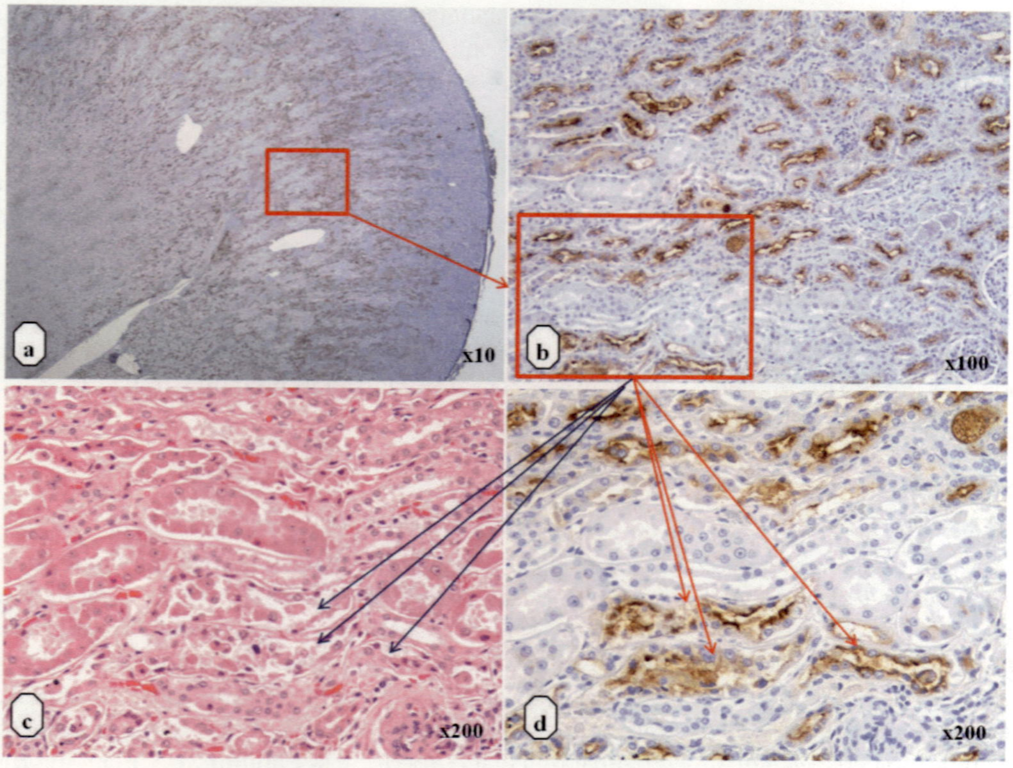

Figure 7. Representative hematoxylin and eosin-staining in a cisplatin-treated dog indicating tubular degeneration in proximal tubules (c); representative cytoplasmic renal KIM-1 immunostaining in S2 segment proximal tubular epithelial cells (a, b and d).

urinary RPA-1 is the qualified diagnostic marker of choice for monitoring compound-induced progressive renal papillary necrosis [50] and recovery [72]. TFF-3 is expressed in tubules of the outer stripe of the outer medulla; urinary TFF3 protein levels are markedly reduced in response to renal tubular injury [79]; however, TFF-3 may not outperform BUN and/or sCr to detect kidney injury in rats [79]. Neither urinary RPA-1 nor urinary TFF-3 [79] has been qualified for clinical use to date.

Tissue leakage markers: glutathione-S-transferase alpha (α-GST), glutathione-S-transferase-mu (mu-GST/GSTYb1), and N-acetyl-β-D-glucosaminidase (NAG) are released from cells upon structural damage to proximal tubular epithelium (rat α-GST) and distal tubular epithelium (rat mu-GST) and reflect primarily tubular cell necrosis in various animal models [83, 87, 88] and humans [89] where compound induced kidney injury was evident. Yet, α-GST, mu-GST, and NAG have not been qualified; and their translational characteristics have not been well defined to date.

In conclusion, the importance of biomarkers in renal safety assessment have been described with emphasis on those biomarkers that have been qualified in rats and on a case-by-case basis in the clinical setting [67]. Other potentially translational biomarkers of kidney injury have been reported and are under consideration for qualification [90-92]. In addition, biomarkers specific to a condition or disease are available. For example, erythropoietin (EPO) which is produced primarily by fibroblast-like cortical interstitial cells in the kidney and functions to prevent apoptosis of early erythroid precursor cells can be used as a biomarker for various conditions of anemia [93], secondary forms of polycythemia [94], and abuse of erythropoiesis-stimulating agents by athletes [95]. Another example is ferritin, a ubiquitous intracellular protein that functions to store iron in a non-toxic form [96]. Serum ferritin levels correlate with total body iron stores and is often used along with other iron tests as a biomarker for determination of endogenous iron stores to aid diagnosis of disease including but not limited to iron deficiency anemia and acute renal failure [97] in patients with nephrohotic proteinuria likely due to non-specific hepatic protein synthesis to compensate for loss of iron-binding transferrin [98].

8. Conclusions

Increased understanding of the effect of renal transporters on the distribution of a drug will enhance safety assessment. Limiting the accumulation and/or distribution of a compound to the kidney through selective interaction with renal transporters will potentially identify safer drugs. Renal transporters also can be exploited as potential targets for therapeutic agents by affecting the disposition of endogenous substrates. In the case of sCr, potential inhibition of renal transporters can limit its utility as a safety biomarker. Whereas data are available for the relationship between 8 qualified biomarkers that outperform sCr and/or BUN in monitoring compound-induced renal injury in rats, the translation from rats to humans is limited by the availability of qualified human biomarkers. Efforts are in progress to further assess the translatability of urinary biomarkers in higher species including canines, non-human primates and humans.

Acknowledgements

We would like to thank Maarten Huisman for his contribution to OCT2 inhibition study. The support of dog renal biomarker studies from Marciano Sablad, Antonio Guy, Jennifer Vegas, Lynn Varacallo, Jing Ying Ma, Anton Bittner, Jingjin Gao, and Manisha Sonee is greatly appreciated. We would also like to thank Shannon Dallas, Manisha Sonee, and Sandra Snook for their thorough review of this chapter

Author details

P.D. Ward, D. La and J.E. McDuffie

Janssen Research & Development, L.L.C, USA

http://dx.doi.org/10.5772/54857

References

[1] Ward P. Importance of drug transporters in pharmacokinetics and drug safety. Toxicol Mech Methods. 2008;18(1):1-10.

[2] Dallas S, Ward P. Drug Transporters and ADME. In: Swarbrick J, editor. Encyclopedia of Pharmaceutical Technology. 4th ed. New York: Informa Healthcare; in press.

[3] Jones PM, George AM. The ABC transporter structure and mechanism: perspectives on recent research. Cell Mol Life Sci. 2004 Mar;61(6):682-99.

[4] Lin JH. Drug-drug interaction mediated by inhibition and induction of P-glycoprotein. Adv Drug Deliv Rev. 2003 Jan 21;55(1):53-81.

[5] Lin JH, Yamazaki M. Role of P-glycoprotein in pharmacokinetics: clinical implications. Clin Pharmacokinet. 2003;42(1):59-98.

[6] Borst P, Evers R, Kool M, Wijnholds J. A family of drug transporters: the multidrug resistance-associated proteins. J Natl Cancer Inst. 2000 Aug 16;92(16):1295-302.

[7] Hediger MA, Romero MF, Peng JB, Rolfs A, Takanaga H, Bruford EA. The ABCs of solute carriers: physiological, pathological and therapeutic implications of human membrane transport proteinsIntroduction. Pflugers Arch. 2004 Feb;447(5):465-8.

[8] Giacomini KM, Sugiyama Y. Membrane Transporters and Drug Response. In: Brunton LL, editor. Goodman & Gilman's The Pharmacological Basis of Therapeutics. 12th ed: McGraw-Hill; 2011.

[9] Anzai N, Endou H. Drug transport in the kidney. In: You G, Morris M, editors. Drug transporters, molecular characterization and Role in Drug Disposition: John Wiley and Sons; 2007.

[10] Hilgendorf C, Ahlin G, Seithel A, Artursson P, Ungell AL, Karlsson J. Expression of thirty-six drug transporter genes in human intestine, liver, kidney, and organotypic cell lines. Drug Metab Dispos. 2007 Aug;35(8):1333-40.

[11] Moriyama Y, Hiasa M, Matsumoto T, Omote H. Multidrug and toxic compound extrusion (MATE)-type proteins as anchor transporters for the excretion of metabolic waste products and xenobiotics. Xenobiotica. 2008 Jul;38(7-8):1107-18.

[12] Damme K, Nies AT, Schaeffeler E, Schwab M. Mammalian MATE (SLC47A) transport proteins: impact on efflux of endogenous substrates and xenobiotics. Drug Metab Rev. 2011 Nov;43(4):499-523.

[13] Nozaki Y, Kusuhara H, Kondo T, Iwaki M, Shiroyanagi Y, Nakayama H, et al. Species difference in the inhibitory effect of nonsteroidal anti-inflammatory drugs on the uptake of methotrexate by human kidney slices. J Pharmacol Exp Ther. 2007 Sep; 322(3):1162-70.

[14] Uwai Y, Saito H, Inui K. Interaction between methotrexate and nonsteroidal anti-inflammatory drugs in organic anion transporter. Eur J Pharmacol. 2000 Dec 1;409(1): 31-6.

[15] Fujita T, Urban TJ, Leabman MK, Fujita K, Giacomini KM. Transport of drugs in the kidney by the human organic cation transporter, OCT2 and its genetic variants. J Pharm Sci. 2006 Jan;95(1):25-36.

[16] Koepsell H, Lips K, Volk C. Polyspecific organic cation transporters: structure, function, physiological roles, and biopharmaceutical implications. Pharm Res. 2007 Jul; 24(7):1227-51.

[17] Muller F, Fromm MF. Transporter-mediated drug-drug interactions. Pharmacogenomics. 2011 Jul;12(7):1017-37.

[18] Van Aubel RA, Masereeuw R, Russel FG. Molecular pharmacology of renal organic anion transporters. Am J Physiol Renal Physiol. 2000 Aug;279(2):F216-32.

[19] Rizwan AN, Burckhardt G. Organic anion transporters of the SLC22 family: biopharmaceutical, physiological, and pathological roles. Pharm Res. 2007 Mar;24(3):450-70.

[20] Weiss J, Theile D, Ketabi-Kiyanvash N, Lindenmaier H, Haefeli WE. Inhibition of MRP1/ABCC1, MRP2/ABCC2, and MRP3/ABCC3 by nucleoside, nucleotide, and non-nucleoside reverse transcriptase inhibitors. Drug Metab Dispos. 2007 Mar;35(3): 340-4.

[21] Marchetti S, Mazzanti R, Beijnen JH, Schellens JH. Concise review: Clinical relevance of drug drug and herb drug interactions mediated by the ABC transporter ABCB1 (MDR1, P-glycoprotein). Oncologist. 2007 Aug;12(8):927-41.

[22] Cui Y, Konig J, Buchholz JK, Spring H, Leier I, Keppler D. Drug resistance and ATP-dependent conjugate transport mediated by the apical multidrug resistance protein, MRP2, permanently expressed in human and canine cells. Mol Pharmacol. 1999 May; 55(5):929-37.

[23] Suzuki H, Sugiyama Y. Excretion of GSSG and glutathione conjugates mediated by MRP1 and cMOAT/MRP2. Semin Liver Dis. 1998;18(4):359-76.

[24] Reid G, Wielinga P, Zelcer N, De Haas M, Van Deemter L, Wijnholds J, et al. Characterization of the transport of nucleoside analog drugs by the human multidrug resistance proteins MRP4 and MRP5. Mol Pharmacol. 2003 May;63(5):1094-103.

[25] Reid G, Wielinga P, Zelcer N, van der Heijden I, Kuil A, de Haas M, et al. The human multidrug resistance protein MRP4 functions as a prostaglandin efflux transporter and is inhibited by nonsteroidal antiinflammatory drugs. Proc Natl Acad Sci U S A. 2003 Aug 5;100(16):9244-9.

[26] Dixit R, Ward P. Use of Classical Pharmacokinetic Evaluations in Drug Development and Safety Assessment. In: Lipscomb JC, Ohanian EV, editors. Toxicokinetics and Risk Assessment. New York, NY: Informa Healthcare USA Inc.; 2007. p. 95-122.

[27] Ward PD. Toxicokinetics and Organ-Specific Toxicity. In: Acree W, editor. Toxicity and Drug Testing: Intech; 2012.

[28] Tanihara Y, Masuda S, Katsura T, Inui K. Protective effect of concomitant administration of imatinib on cisplatin-induced nephrotoxicity focusing on renal organic cation transporter OCT2. Biochem Pharmacol. 2009 Nov 1;78(9):1263-71.

[29] Anzai N, Endou H. Renal drug transporters and nephrotoxicity. AATEX. 2007;14(Special Issue):447-52.

[30] Cihlar T, Lin DC, Pritchard JB, Fuller MD, Mendel DB, Sweet DH. The antiviral nucleotide analogs cidofovir and adefovir are novel substrates for human and rat renal organic anion transporter 1. Mol Pharmacol. 1999 Sep;56(3):570-80.

[31] Cundy KC. Clinical pharmacokinetics of the antiviral nucleotide analogues cidofovir and adefovir. Clin Pharmacokinet. 1999 Feb;36(2):127-43.

[32] Uwai Y, Ida H, Tsuji Y, Katsura T, Inui K. Renal transport of adefovir, cidofovir, and tenofovir by SLC22A family members (hOAT1, hOAT3, and hOCT2). Pharm Res. 2007 Apr;24(4):811-5.

[33] Naesens L, Balzarini J, De Clercq E. Pharmacokinetics in mice of the anti-retrovirus agent 9-(2-phosphonylmethoxyethyl)adenine. Drug Metab Dispos. 1992 Sep-Oct; 20(5):747-52.

[34] Roy CJ, Baker R, Washburn K, Bray M. Aerosolized cidofovir is retained in the respiratory tract and protects mice against intranasal cowpox virus challenge. Antimicrob Agents Chemother. 2003 Sep;47(9):2933-7.

[35] Gallant JE, Parish MA, Keruly JC, Moore RD. Changes in renal function associated with tenofovir disoproxil fumarate treatment, compared with nucleoside reverse-transcriptase inhibitor treatment. Clin Infect Dis. 2005 Apr 15;40(8):1194-8.

[36] Roling J, Schmid H, Fischereder M, Draenert R, Goebel FD. HIV-associated renal diseases and highly active antiretroviral therapy-induced nephropathy. Clin Infect Dis. 2006 May 15;42(10):1488-95.

[37] Ho ES, Lin DC, Mendel DB, Cihlar T. Cytotoxicity of antiviral nucleotides adefovir and cidofovir is induced by the expression of human renal organic anion transporter 1. J Am Soc Nephrol. 2000 Mar;11(3):383-93.

[38] Cihlar T, Ho ES, Lin DC, Mulato AS. Human renal organic anion transporter 1 (hOAT1) and its role in the nephrotoxicity of antiviral nucleotide analogs. Nucleosides Nucleotides Nucleic Acids. 2001 Apr-Jul;20(4-7):641-8.

[39] Mulato AS, Ho ES, Cihlar T. Nonsteroidal anti-inflammatory drugs efficiently reduce the transport and cytotoxicity of adefovir mediated by the human renal organic anion transporter 1. J Pharmacol Exp Ther. 2000 Oct;295(1):10-5.

[40] Peyriere H, Reynes J, Rouanet I, Daniel N, de Boever CM, Mauboussin JM, et al. Renal tubular dysfunction associated with tenofovir therapy: report of 7 cases. J Acquir Immune Defic Syndr. 2004 Mar 1;35(3):269-73.

[41] Imaoka T, Kusuhara H, Adachi M, Schuetz JD, Takeuchi K, Sugiyama Y. Functional involvement of multidrug resistance-associated protein 4 (MRP4/ABCC4) in the renal elimination of the antiviral drugs adefovir and tenofovir. Mol Pharmacol. 2007 Feb; 71(2):619-27.

[42] Madeddu G, Bonfanti P, De Socio GV, Carradori S, Grosso C, Marconi P, et al. Tenofovir renal safety in HIV-infected patients: results from the SCOLTA Project. Biomed Pharmacother. 2008 Jan;62(1):6-11.

[43] Borst P, Balzarini J, Ono N, Reid G, de Vries H, Wielinga P, et al. The potential impact of drug transporters on nucleoside-analog-based antiviral chemotherapy. Antiviral Res. 2004 Apr;62(1):1-7.

[44] Yokoo S, Yonezawa A, Masuda S, Fukatsu A, Katsura T, Inui K. Differential contribution of organic cation transporters, OCT2 and MATE1, in platinum agent-induced nephrotoxicity. Biochem Pharmacol. 2007 Aug 1;74(3):477-87.

[45] Burger H, Loos WJ, Eechoute K, Verweij J, Mathijssen RH, Wiemer EA. Drug transporters of platinum-based anticancer agents and their clinical significance. Drug Resist Updat. 2011 Feb;14(1):22-34.

[46] Pfister T, Atzpodien E, Bauss F. The renal effects of minimally nephrotoxic doses of ibandronate and zoledronate following single and intermittent intravenous administration in rats. Toxicology. 2003 Sep 30;191(2-3):159-67.

[47] Bauss F, Russell RG. Ibandronate in osteoporosis: preclinical data and rationale for intermittent dosing. Osteoporos Int. 2004 Jun;15(6):423-33.

[48] Body JJ, Pfister T, Bauss F. Preclinical perspectives on bisphosphonate renal safety. Oncologist. 2005;10 Suppl 1:3-7.

[49] Lin JH. Bisphosphonates: a review of their pharmacokinetic properties. Bone. 1996 Feb;18(2):75-85.

[50] Anzai N, Kanai Y, Endou H. Organic anion transporter family: current knowledge. J Pharmacol Sci. 2006;100(5):411-26.

[51] Caulfield MJ, Munroe PB, O'Neill D, Witkowska K, Charchar FJ, Doblado M, et al. SLC2A9 is a high-capacity urate transporter in humans. PLoS Med. 2008 Oct 7;5(10):e197.

[52] Wood IS, Trayhurn P. Glucose transporters (GLUT and SGLT): expanded families of sugar transport proteins. Br J Nutr. 2003 Jan;89(1):3-9.

[53] Santer R, Kinner M, Lassen CL, Schneppenheim R, Eggert P, Bald M, et al. Molecular analysis of the SGLT2 gene in patients with renal glucosuria. J Am Soc Nephrol. 2003 Nov;14(11):2873-82.

[54] Chao EC. A paradigm shift in diabetes therapy--dapagliflozin and other SGLT2 inhibitors. Discov Med. 2011 Mar;11(58):255-63.

[55] Dharnidharka VR, Kwon C, Stevens G. Serum cystatin C is superior to serum creatinine as a marker of kidney function: a meta-analysis. Am J Kidney Dis. 2002 Aug; 40(2):221-6.

[56] Roos JF, Doust J, Tett SE, Kirkpatrick CM. Diagnostic accuracy of cystatin C compared to serum creatinine for the estimation of renal dysfunction in adults and children--a meta-analysis. Clin Biochem. 2007 Mar;40(5-6):383-91.

[57] Breyer MD, Qi Z. Better nephrology for mice--and man. Kidney Int. 2010 Mar;77(6): 487-9.

[58] Imamura Y, Murayama N, Okudaira N, Kurihara A, Okazaki O, Izumi T, et al. Prediction of fluoroquinolone-induced elevation in serum creatinine levels: a case of drug-endogenous substance interaction involving the inhibition of renal secretion. Clin Pharmacol Ther. 2011 Jan;89(1):81-8.

[59] Sarapa N, Wickremasingha P, Ge N, Weitzman R, Fuellhart M, Yen C, et al. Lack of effect of DX-619, a novel des-fluoro(6)-quinolone, on glomerular filtration rate measured by serum clearance of cold iohexol. Antimicrob Agents Chemother. 2007 Jun; 51(6):1912-7.

[60] Tett SE, Kirkpatrick CM, Gross AS, McLachlan AJ. Principles and clinical application of assessing alterations in renal elimination pathways. Clin Pharmacokinet. 2003;42(14):1193-211.

[61] Kastrup J, Petersen P, Bartram R, Hansen JM. The effect of trimethoprim on serum creatinine. Br J Urol. 1985 Jun;57(3):265-8.

[62] van Acker BA, Koomen GC, Koopman MG, de Waart DR, Arisz L. Creatinine clearance during cimetidine administration for measurement of glomerular filtration rate. Lancet. 1992 Nov 28;340(8831):1326-9.

[63] Nakata J, Ohsawa I, Onda K, Tanimoto M, Kusaba G, Takeda Y, et al. Risk of Overestimation of Kidney Function Using GFR-Estimating Equations in Patients with Low Inulin Clearance. J Clin Lab Anal. 2012;26(4):248-53.

[64] Ito S, Kusuhara H, Kuroiwa Y, Wu C, Moriyama Y, Inoue K, et al. Potent and specific inhibition of mMate1-mediated efflux of type I organic cations in the liver and kidney by pyrimethamine. J Pharmacol Exp Ther. 2010 Apr;333(1):341-50.

[65] Opravil M, Keusch G, Luthy R. Pyrimethamine inhibits renal secretion of creatinine. Antimicrob Agents Chemother. 1993 May;37(5):1056-60.

[66] Dennis E, Walker E, Baker A, Lundstrom G, King N, Short K. Predictive Safety Testing Consortium. http://c-pathorg/pstccfm#Milestones.

[67] Dieterle F, Sistare F, Goodsaid F, Papaluca M, Ozer JS, Webb CP, et al. Renal biomarker qualification submission: a dialog between the FDA-EMEA and Predictive Safety Testing Consortium. Nat Biotechnol. 2010 May;28(5):455-62.

[68] Harpur E, Ennulat D, Hoffman D, Betton G, Gautier JC, Riefke B, et al. Biological qualification of biomarkers of chemical-induced renal toxicity in two strains of male rat. Toxicol Sci. 2011 Aug;122(2):235-52.

[69] Andreoli CM, Andreoli MT, Kloek CE, Ahuero AE, Vavvas D, Durand ML. Low rate of endophthalmitis in a large series of open globe injuries. Am J Ophthalmol. 2009 Apr;147(4):601-8 e2.

[70] Gautier JC, Riefke B, Walter J, Kurth P, Mylecraine L, Guilpin V, et al. Evaluation of novel biomarkers of nephrotoxicity in two strains of rat treated with Cisplatin. Toxicol Pathol. 2012 Oct;38(6):943-56.

[71] Bonventre JV, Vaidya VS, Schmouder R, Feig P, Dieterle F. Next-generation biomarkers for detecting kidney toxicity. Nat Biotechnol. 2010 May;28(5):436-40.

[72] Rouse RL, Zhang J, Stewart SR, Rosenzweig BA, Espandiari P, Sadrieh NK. Comparative profile of commercially available urinary biomarkers in preclinical drug-induced kidney injury and recovery in rats. Kidney Int. 2012 Jun;79(11):1186-97.

[73] Guder WG, Hofmann W. Markers for the diagnosis and monitoring of renal tubular lesions. Clin Nephrol. 1992;38 Suppl 1:S3-7.

[74] Herget-Rosenthal S, Poppen D, Husing J, Marggraf G, Pietruck F, Jakob HG, et al. Prognostic value of tubular proteinuria and enzymuria in nonoliguric acute tubular necrosis. Clin Chem. 2004 Mar;50(3):552-8.

[75] Peterson PA, Evrin PE, Berggard I. Differentiation of glomerular, tubular, and normal proteinuria: determinations of urinary excretion of beta-2-macroglobulin, albumin, and total protein. J Clin Invest. 1969 Jul;48(7):1189-98.

[76] Schmid H, Henger A, Cohen CD, Frach K, Grone HJ, Schlondorff D, et al. Gene expression profiles of podocyte-associated molecules as diagnostic markers in acquired proteinuric diseases. J Am Soc Nephrol. 2003 Nov;14(11):2958-66.

[77] Zomas A, Anagnostopoulos N, Dimopoulos MA. Successful treatment of multiple myeloma relapsing after high-dose therapy and autologous transplantation with thalidomide as a single agent. Bone Marrow Transplant. 2000 Jun;25(12):1319-20.

[78] Greive KA, Nikolic-Paterson DJ, Guimaraes MA, Nikolovski J, Pratt LM, Mu W, et al. Glomerular permselectivity factors are not responsible for the increase in fractional clearance of albumin in rat glomerulonephritis. Am J Pathol. 2001 Sep;159(3):1159-70.

[79] Yu Y, Jin H, Holder D, Ozer JS, Villarreal S, Shughrue P, et al. Urinary biomarkers trefoil factor 3 and albumin enable early detection of kidney tubular injury. Nat Biotechnol. 2010 May;28(5):470-7.

[80] Bokenkamp A, van Wijk JA, Lentze MJ, Stoffel-Wagner B. Effect of corticosteroid therapy on serum cystatin C and beta2-microglobulin concentrations. Clin Chem. 2002 Jul;48(7):1123-6.

[81] Rosenberg ME, Silkensen J. Clusterin and the kidney. Exp Nephrol. 1995 Jan-Feb;3(1): 9-14.

[82] Vaidya VS, Ozer JS, Dieterle F, Collings FB, Ramirez V, Troth S, et al. Kidney injury molecule-1 outperforms traditional biomarkers of kidney injury in preclinical biomarker qualification studies. Nat Biotechnol. 2010 May;28(5):478-85.

[83] Vinken P, Starckx S, Barale-Thomas E, Looszova A, Sonee M, Goeminne N, et al. Tissue Kim-1 and Urinary Clusterin as Early Indicators of Cisplatin-Induced Acute Kidney Injury in Rats. Toxicol Pathol. 2012 May 11.

[84] Correa-Rotter R, Ibarra-Rubio ME, Schwochau G, Cruz C, Silkensen JR, Pedraza-Chaverri J, et al. Induction of clusterin in tubules of nephrotic rats. J Am Soc Nephrol. 1998 Jan;9(1):33-7.

[85] Hidaka S, Kranzlin B, Gretz N, Witzgall R. Urinary clusterin levels in the rat correlate with the severity of tubular damage and may help to differentiate between glomerular and tubular injuries. Cell Tissue Res. 2002 Dec;310(3):289-96.

[86] Zhang J, Goering PL, Espandiari P, Shaw M, Bonventre JV, Vaidya VS, et al. Differences in immunolocalization of Kim-1, RPA-1, and RPA-2 in kidneys of gentamicin-, cisplatin-, and valproic acid-treated rats: potential role of iNOS and nitrotyrosine. Toxicol Pathol. 2009 Aug;37(5):629-43.

[87] Pinches M, Betts C, Bickerton S, Burdett L, Thomas H, Derbyshire N, et al. Evaluation of novel renal biomarkers with a cisplatin model of kidney injury: gender and dosage differences. Toxicol Pathol. 2012 Apr;40(3):522-33.

[88] Sasaki D, Yamada A, Umeno H, Kurihara H, Nakatsuji S, Fujihira S, et al. Comparison of the course of biomarker changes and kidney injury in a rat model of drug-induced acute kidney injury. Biomarkers. 2011 Nov;16(7):553-66.

[89] Westhuyzen J, Endre ZH, Reece G, Reith DM, Saltissi D, Morgan TJ. Measurement of tubular enzymuria facilitates early detection of acute renal impairment in the intensive care unit. Nephrol Dial Transplant. 2003 Mar;18(3):543-51.

[90] Adiyanti S, Loho T. Acute Kidney Injury (AKI) Biomarker. Acta Medica Indonesiana. 2008;44(3):246-55.

[91] Mehta RL, Kellum JA, Shah SV, Molitoris BA, Ronco C, Warnock DG, et al. Acute Kidney Injury Network: report of an initiative to improve outcomes in acute kidney injury. Crit Care. 2007;11(2):R31.

[92] Xie HG, Wang SK, Cao CC, Harpur E. Qualified kidney biomarkers and their potential significance in drug safety evaluation and prediction. Pharmacol Ther. 2012 Sep 25.

[93] Jelkmann W. Biosimilar recombinant human erythropoietins ("epoetins") and future erythropoiesis-stimulating treatments. Expert Opin Biol Ther. 2012 May;12(5):581-92.

[94] Lasne F, Martin L, Crepin N, de Ceaurriz J. Detection of isoelectric profiles of erythropoietin in urine: differentiation of natural and administered recombinant hormones. Anal Biochem. 2002 Dec 15;311(2):119-26.

[95] Pottgiesser T, Schumacher YO. Biomarker monitoring in sports doping control. Bioanalysis. 2012 Jun;4(10):1245-53.

[96] Goswami B, Tayal D, Mallika V. Ferritin: A multidimensional bio marker. The Internet Journal of Laboratory Medicine 2009;3(2):http://www.ispub.com:80/journal/the-internet-journal-of-laboratory-medicine/volume-3-number-2/ferritin-a-multidimensional-bio-marker.html

[97] Mavromatidis K, Fytil C, Kynigopoulou P, Fragia T, Sombolos K. Serum ferritin levels are increased in patients with acute renal failure. Clin Nephrol. 1998 May;49(5): 296-8.

[98] Branten AJ, Swinkels DW, Klasen IS, Wetzels JF. Serum ferritin levels are increased in patients with glomerular diseases and proteinuria. Nephrol Dial Transplant. 2004 Nov;19(11):2754-60.

Chapter 8

Autophagy: A Possible Defense Mechanism in Parkinson's Disease?

Rosa A. González-Polo, Rubén Gómez-Sánchez,
Lydia Sánchez-Erviti, José M Bravo-San Pedro,
Elisa Pizarro-Estrella, Mireia Niso-Santano and
José M. Fuentes

Additional information is available at the end of the chapter

http://dx.doi.org/10.5772/54851

1. Introduction

Growing evidence supports an active role for deregulated macroautophagy (autophagic stress) in neuronal cell death and neurodegenerative diseases, as Parkinson's disease (PD). The exact etiology of PD is currently unknown, but it seems clear that its pathogenesis is a multifactorial process. The detection of genetic alterations may be useful as a biomarker of early molecular diagnosis, but it is also important to know and identify changes at the molecular level, more frequent in cases of Parkinsonism. In this sense, the phenomenon of autophagic cell death, described in the normal nervous system, could be the result of a pathological process, such as those related to neurodegenerative diseases. Autophagy is an intracellular catabolic mechanism mediated by lysosomes, which is responsible for most of the degradation and recycling of cytoplasmic components and intracellular organelles dysfunctional or damaged. For a long time, it is unknown why the aggregation of proteins and developmental neurotoxicity are given in a later period of life, even in familial forms of the disease, where the mutant protein is present throughout life in the individual. It has been shown that genetic ablation of autophagy induces neurodegeneration and accumulation of ubiquitinated proteins. In addition, some genetic mutations that cause neurodegenerative diseases directly affect proteolytic systems responsible for the degradation of the mutant protein. In this paper, we analyze the possible neuroprotective role that autophagy-inducing substances can have on the mechanism and development of PD.

2. Contents

2.1. The role of autophagy in PD – Importance of oxidative stress

PD is a progressive neurodegenerative disorder characterized by slow movements (bradykinesia), poverty of movements (hypokinesia), resting tremor and rigidity. PD is characterized pathologically by the loss of dopaminergic neurons in the *substantia nigra pars compacta* and the presence of Lewy bodies (LB), which are intra-cytoplasmic inclusions containing high levels of alpha-synuclein protein. Combined with the ubiquitous alpha-synuclein aggregates in PD brains the finding of mutations and multiplications of the alpha-synuclein gene in familial forms of PD add to the importance of alpha-synuclein to PD pathology. Recent observations have suggested that alpha-synuclein can be directly transmitted from pathological affected neurons to healthy unaffected neurons. This is consistent with the Braak staging of PD pathology which suggests there is a progression of LB pathology from the brainstem to the cortex consistent with the pathological propagation along specific neural pathways. The release of alpha-synuclein from cells and the transfer of an aggregated form of alpha-synuclein to neighboring cells have been demonstrated in vitro and in vivo and is potentially an important step in the progression of PD pathology. While these processes are poorly understood, exosomes have been associated with the release and transfer of prion protein via a novel processing pathway that involves the N-terminal modification of PrP and selection of distinct PrP glycoforms for incorporation into these vesicles and there is increasing evidence that alpha-synuclein is also released from cells in exosomes. Lysosomal dysfunction increases alpha-synuclein release and transmission mediated by exosomes in cell models.

While the primary cause of PD in the majority of patients is not known, the number of genetic causes and risk factors are gradually increasing and are beginning to highlight important pathogenetic pathways. The role of mitochondrial dysfunction in PD is supported by the ability of the mitochondrial toxins MPTP (1-methyl-4-phenylpyridinium) and rotenone to target the dopaminergic neurons and more recently by PTEN-induced kinase 1 (PINK1) and parkin, which are mutated in PD and have a role in regulating mitochondrial integrity. Oxidative stress and damage are important observations in PD brains and are common observations in various genetic and toxin models of PD. Protein turnover pathways have been implicated in PD, initially involving the proteasomal system and more recently autophagy and the lysosomal pathways. The *G2019S* mutation of leucine-rich repeat kinase 2 (LRRK2) is a relatively common cause of PD, and recessive mutations of the lysosomal enzyme glucocerebrosidase-1 (GBA-1) have recently been identified as one of the most important genetic risk factors for PD although the disease mechanisms have not yet been elucidated.

Autophagy is a catabolic pathway for destruction and turnover of long-live proteins and organelles in lysosomes. Autophagy contributes to degradation of damaged long-live proteins and organelles and the normal turn-over of these components, moreover is up-regulated in response to external stressors as starvation and oxidative stress. In mammalian cells autophagy comprises three separate pathways: macroautophagy, microautophagy and chaperone-mediated autophagy (CMA).

http://dx.doi.org/10.5772/54851

Macroautophagy involves the de novo formation of double membrane vacuoles, autophagosomes originated from mitochondria and/or plasma membrane. Autophagosomes fuse with lysosomes to deliver cytoplasmic contents including misfolded or aggregated proteins and organelles for digestion and recycling of amino acids. Macroautophagy is regulated at molecular level by proteins of the Atg family, which form dynamic complexes involved in the assembly, docking and degradation of the autophagosome. The serine/threonine kinase mTOR (mammalian target of rapamicyn) is a key mediator of macroautophagy upregulation under starvation, this protein regulates cell cycle progression, protein synthesis and cell growth. Activated mTOR promotes protein synthesis and inhibits catabolism by decreasing macroautophagy in a mechanism mediated by Atg13 phosphorylation that modulates Atg1 activity. During starvation mTOR is inactivated resulting in hypophosphorylation of Atg13 and stimulation of Atg1-Atg13 complexes required for induction of autophagy.

Microautophagy involves lysosomal pinocytosis of cytoplasmic contents and is involved in the turnover of long half-life cytosolic proteins. However, the underlying process is poorly understood in mammalian cells.

It is important to note that both macro and microautophagy are highly conserved process that occurs in same manner in all cells. In this sense most of the knowledge of autophagy was first described in yeast.

CMA is a selective autophagic pathway dependent upon the protein chaperone hsc70 and its binding to LAMP-2A (Lysosomal-associated membrane protein 2A), a lysosomal surface receptor. A highly specific subset of cytosolic proteins with a KFREQ motif are recognized by the hsc70 chaperone and internalized for degradation by Lysosomal-associated membrane protein 2A LAMP-2A lysosomal membrane receptors. The substrate protein is unfolded by the complex and is translocated to the lysosome with the help of a lysosomal chaperone (lys-hsc70).

Recent reports identified a increase in autophagic vacuoles, decrease in macroautophagy and CMA proteins in PD brain areas affected by the neurodegenerative process, which might have a direct impact in alpha-synuclein levels as this protein in degraded in lysosomes mainly by CMA. The increase cytosolic alpha-synuclein levels favours the modification of alpha-synuclein and formation of oligomers, fibrils and aggregates. Indeed, CMA is important in the removal of oxidized and altered proteins during conditions of mild oxidative stress, and blockage of CMA resulted in increased intracellular levels of oxidized and aggregate proteins. Conversely the pathological environment in PD may lead to alpha-synuclein post-translational modifications (e.g. nitration, oxidation, dopamine adducts), or oligomeric or fibrilar formations which may not be degraded by CMA and may even inhibit CMA promoting aggregation. Moreover, mutations in PINK1 and parkin proteins, associated with PD, affect the remove of damaged mitochondria by lysosomes (mitophagy). Finally, other genetic mutations associated with PD, as ATP13A2 and LRRK2, affect autophagy and lysosomal function, reinforcing the involvement of autophagic function in PD.

Several studies described an increase in markers related with oxidative stress as protein nitration and lipid peroxidation in LB. Additional findings described a decrease in several defense antioxidant molecules in PD including the thiol-reducing agent glutathione (GSH) and the glutathione peroxidase activity. This increase in reactive oxygen species (ROS) levels involves an increased oxidized alteration of proteins as alpha-synuclein resulting in increasing protein misfolding and impaired degradation, which might cause the accumulation of toxic soluble oligomers or insoluble aggregates.

Mitochondria are the main source of ROS involved in oxidative stress and its role in PD is highlighted by the toxic animal models (MPTP, 6-hydroxydopamine (6-OHDA), rotenone) and the mutation in PINK1, parkin and DJ-1, involved in mitochondrial function and turnover, is related with early onset PD. When oxidative processes clearly contribute to the pathology and progression of PD the initiation of this cascade is probably secondary to other causes.

2.2. Toxic stress inducers related to PD

MPTP. In the early 1980s, a group of young drug abusers from Northern California developed a parkinsonian syndrome clinically indistinguishable from PD caused by the intravenous injection of a synthetic analog of demerol. Chemical analysis of this synthetic drug showed that it contained around 3% of MPTP. Post-mortem investigations clearly confirm the lesion of the substantia nigra MPTP was thus considered as a powerful drug to induce nigral degeneration both rodent and primate models of PD. Since that time, a number of environmental toxicants have been associated with PD etiology including metals, solvents, and pesticides. Epidemiologic and toxicological studies suggest a consistent correlation between pesticide exposure and PD. MPTP is a lipophilic toxin that rapidly crosses the blood-brain barrier. Inside the brain, MPTP is oxidized to an unstable intermediary 1-methyl-4-phenyl-2,3-dihydroxipyridinium ($MPDP^+$) via the action of monoamine oxidase B (MAO-B). MPDP then undergoes spontaneous oxidation to the active toxic 1-methyl-4-phenylpiridinium (MPP^+). Following its release into the extracellular space, MPP^+ is taken up by the dopamine transporter (DAT), the amino acid transporter cationic or glutamate transporter. Once inside the cell, cytoplasmatic MPP^+ can trigger the production of ROS, which may contribute to its overall neurotoxicity. However, the majority of MPP^+ is transported into the mitochondria of dopaminergic neurons, where it disrupts oxidative phosphorylation by inhibiting complex I activity. The inhibition of mitochondrial electron transport chain causes an acute ATP deficiency, loss of mitochondrial membrane potential, alterations of intracellular calcium levels and increase ROS production, particularly superoxide. Finally, MPP^+ induces the activation of cell death signaling pathways such as c-jun N-terminal kinase (JNK), p38 mitogen activated kinase and Bax Moreover MPTP interact with familial PD gene products. It has reported that MPTP triggers an upregulation of alpha-synuclein and is accompanied by PD-like modifications of alpha-synuclein, including its aggregation, nitration and phosphorylation and modifies parkin solubility causing Parkin aggregation.

Rotenone. Rotenone is an non mutagenic active agent of many pesticides and a well-characterized, high affinity specific inhibitor of complex I of the mitochondrial respiratory chain which emerged in the 90's as a potential parkinsonian environmental toxin. Because it is highly lipophilic, it crosses biological membranes easily and apparently independent of specific transport system (unlike MPP^+), and it gets into the brain very quickly, where accumulates within

http://dx.doi.org/10.5772/54851

mitochondria and inhibits complex I. Despite this complex I inhibition, rotenone caused selective degeneration of the nigrostriatal dopaminergic pathway, selective striatal oxidative damage, and formation of ubiquitin- and alpha-synuclein positive inclusions in nigral cells, which were similar to the LB of PD. Furthermore, rotenone activates both mitochondrial and endoplasmic dependent caspases that induces apoptosis. Additionally, increased oxidative stress, ubiquitin accumulation, proteasomal inhibition and inflammation, all have been observed in response to rotenone exposure. Rotenone has also been reported to induce caspase independent cell death, accumulation of alpha-synuclein, parkin aggregation and oxidation mitochondrial of thioredoxin. Rotenone and MPTP share the same principle mechanism of action and their toxic effects are quite similar. The toxicity of both compounds is linked with glial cell activation. Microglial activation is exhibited in the rotenone rat model of Parkinsonism, occurring prior to evidence of dopaminergic cell loss.

6-OHDA. 6-OHDA was the first chemical compound discovered with specific neurotoxic effects on catecholaminergic pathways. 6-OHDA is one of the most common neurotoxins used to experimentally model nigral degeneration in vitro as well as in vivo. 6-OHDA is a hydroxylate analogue of the natural dopamine that induces degeneration of dopaminergic neurons in the nigrostriatal tract and is commonly used to model dopaminergic degeneration both *in vitro* and *in vivo*. 6-OHDA is taken up into dopaminergic neurons via the dopamine transporter although it shows high affinity for the noradrenaline transporter. Consequently, 6-OHDA can produce specific degeneration of catecholaminergic neurons. Interestingly, 6-OHDA can be formed from dopamine by non-enzymatic hydroxylation in presence of Fe^{2+} and H_2O_2. The mechanism of action of 6-OHDA is related to its pro-oxidant properties. Once in the neuron, 6-OHDA accumulates in the cytosol and readily oxidizes to form ROS, mostly hydrogen peroxide and paraquinone to reduce striatal levels of antioxidant enzymes and to elevate levels of iron in the system nervous. As an additional mechanism, 6-OHDA can accumulate in the mitochondria where interacts directly with complexes I and IV of the mitochondrial respiratory chain causing respiratory inhibition and oxidative stress. Moreover, oxidized proteins by 6-OHDA induce ER stress and upregulation of the unfolded protein response (UPR), which regulates protein translation, protein folding and protein degradation. Like dopamine and other related compounds, 6-OHDA can be metabolized by monoamine oxidase to generate ROS. However, pretreatment with MAO inhibitors enhances the toxicity of 6-OHDA, offering evidence against the contributions of MAO-dependent ROS sources in the neurotoxic process. The 6-OHDA model has been extensively used ever since and is still the most widely used tool for replicating a PD-like loss of dopaminergic neurons in the *substantia nigra pars compacta*.

Paraquat. The potent herbicide paraquat (PQ, N,N'-dimethyl-1,4,4'-bipiridinium) was first identified as a prototypic non mutagenic neurotoxin due to shares structural similarities to MPP^+, the active metabolite of MPTP. PQ is highly effective, fast-acting and non-selective herbicide widely used herbicide in the world. PQ has been banned or restricted by Environmental Protection Agency (EPA) in some countries (United States and European Union) but it still widely used in developing countries. Because of its use as a pesticide, the possibility that this herbicide could be an environmental contributor to the etiology of PD has received a great deal attention. Furthermore, epidemiological studies have suggested an increased incidence of PD associated with PQ exposure, raising the possibility that PQ could be an environmental parkinsonian toxin. It has been reported several cases of lethal poisoning resulting from ingestion or skin contact and this is the main route of exposure of workers from prolonged contact. Experimental studies using PQ showed that acute exposure to this pesticide had deleterious effects on lung, liver and kidney, whereas chronic PQ exposure induced Parkinsonism. However, significant damage to the brain is reported in individuals who died from PQ intoxication despite the fact that the ability of PQ to cross the blood-brain barrier spontaneously is limited. Being a charged molecule, PQ enters the brain via the neutral amino acid transporter before Na^+-dependent uptake into cells occurs. Based of its structural similarities to MPP^+, the mechanism of action of PQ was initially thought to be through selective complex I inhibition. However, complex I blockade does not appear to play a significant role in PQ induced neurotoxicity because this toxin has low affinity to mitochondrial complex I and only at high doses. Interestingly, complex III of mitochondrial respiratory chain is involved in the formation of PQ-induced ROS in the brain. At the cytosolic levels, PQ causes cellular toxicity via redox cycling. PQ dication (PQ^{2+}) accepts an electron from a reductant to form PQ monocation (PQ^+), which then rapidly reacts with O_2^- to produce the superoxide radical (O_2^-) and regenerate PQ^{2+}. The formation of O_2^- initiates a series of chain reactions that lead to the generation of ROS. Moreover, PQ produces depletion of reducing equivalents (NADPH and GSH), due to increased oxidation, resulting in the disruption of important biochemical processes. Therefore oxidative stress arises if antioxidant mechanisms to detoxify ROS generated are compromised resulting in DNA, protein and lipid oxidation, ROS is involved in the mechanism by which PQ induces dopaminergic cell death through the activation of proapoptotic signaling pathways. PQ can trigger the sequential activation of JNK, c-Jun and caspase 3 both *in vitro* and *in vivo*, induces cytochrome c release and caspase 9 activation, which are preceded by activation of pro-apoptotic Bax and Bak. PQ neurotoxicity has also been reported to require ER stress associated with the activation of the inositol-requiring enzyme 1 (IRE1), apoptosis signal regulating kinase 1 (ASK1) and JNK. Moreover, repeated exposures of mice to the herbicide PQ increase in brain levels of alpha-synuclein and decrease the endogenous levels of DJ-1 *in vitro* experiments.

2.3. Enhancers of autophagy as neuroprotectors in PD

Autophagy is involved in stress-induced adaptation as well as cellular development, differentiation and survival. Regulation of autophagy determines the fate of cells in multiple organs. One of the main concerns of autophagic regulation is the significance of cell-type or tissue specificity. Specifically, neurons could be vulnerable to an accumulation of abnormal components such as cytosolic proteins or organelles that are damaged regarding their post-mitotic nature. Therefore, the regulation of neuronal autophagy in a healthy or diseased environment is most likely context-dependent. Neurons differ from other cell types in that they are post-mitotic and highly dependent on the endo-lysosomal pathway for active signaling in the axons and dendrites. Due to these features, neurons require effective protein degradation as a quality control for cell survival, especially under disease conditions for the removal of toxic components. Any alteration of protein degradation can cause the accumulation of abnormal proteins, leading to cellular toxicity and ultimately neurodegeneration. In this sense, increasing evidences suggest that auto-

http://dx.doi.org/10.5772/54851

phagic deregulation causes accumulation of abnormal proteins or damaged organelles, which is a characteristic of chronic neurodegenerative conditions, such as PD. A viable therapeutic strategy might be to reduce the accumulation of the toxic protein in the cytoplasm. Indeed, promoting the clearance of aggregate-prone proteins via pharmacological induction of autophagy has proved to be a useful mechanism for protecting cells against the toxic effects of these proteins. An additional benefit of autophagy upregulation in models of neurodegenerative diseases is that it seems to protect cells against apoptotic insults. Some evidence also indicates that autophagy might protect cells against necrotic cell death, although this mechanism has not been studied in the context of neurodegeneration. Therapeutic approaches that promote autophagy could, therefore, have two beneficial effects in the context of neurodegenerative diseases; first, they might improve the removal of toxic aggregate-prone proteins from neurons, and second, they could protect neurons from apoptosis.

Autophagy enhancers can be classified in two groups, mTOR dependent and mTOR independent. For this review we will focus in the second.

Which have effect over mTOR dependent autophagy. The very first known drug identified as an autophagy inducer by mTOR pathway is rapamycin, which was already in clinical use for other indications. Rapamycin is a lipophilic macrolide antibiotic originally used as an immunosuppressant. In mammalian cells, rapamycin inhibits the kinase activity of mTOR by forming a complex with the immunophilin FK506-binding protein of 12 kDa (FKBP12). Rapamycin acts specifically on the mTORC1 complex that suppresses autophagy when active.

Which have effect over mTOR independent autophagy. A growing number of little molecules has been show as autophagy inductors by a non canonical (mTOR dependent) pathway. Most of these substances are molecules used for other pharmacological purposes and indications including neurological diseases. We can highlight resveratrol, lithium, trehalose and carbazepine (CBZ).

Resveratrol. Resveratrol (3,5,4-trihydroxystilbene), a type of natural phenol and a phytoalexin, is produced naturally by grapes, mulber-ries, and certain nuts when under attack by pathogens. This powerful anti-oxidant possesses a broad range of bio-logical effects such as neuroprotection, anti-inflammation, and anti-cancer. It especially attenuates neurodegeneration in animal models of Alzheimer's disease and PD associated with the neuronal accumulation of β-amyloid and alpha-synuclein, respectively. These therapeutic benefits of resveratrol in neuronal disorders are associated with activation of autophagy. A recent study showed that resveratrol protects against rotenone-mediated neurotoxicity in cellular models of PD by autophagy induction. Recently has been described that suppression of AMPK and/or SIRT1 caused decrease of protein level of LC3-II, indicating that AMPK and/or SIRT1 are required in resveratrol mediated autophagy induction. Moreover, suppression of AMPK caused inhibition of SIRT1 activity and attenuated protective effects of resveratrol on rotenone-induced apoptosis, suggesting that AMPK-SIRT1-autophagy pathway plays an important role in the neuroprotection by resveratrol on PD cellular models.

Lithium. For more than 60 years, lithium has been the standard pharmacological treatment for bipolar disorder (BD), a chronic mental illness characterized by cycling between moods of mania and depression. However, in the last two decades the role of lithium as an effective neuroprotector has emerged. Thus, Lithium treatment inhibits the activation of caspase-3 in a PI3K-dependent manner and prevents 6-OHDA and MPP^+-induced neuronal death. Lithium's ability to deplete free inositol and subsequently decrease IP3 levels was recently identified as a novel route (independent of mTOR) for inducing autophagy. In this sense, in animal models, therapeutic concentrations of lithium have been shown to facilitate clearance of the mutant form of alpha-synuclein, an autophagy substrate. These protective effects suggest that lithium may have substantial therapeutic potential in the treatment of PD.

Trehalose. Trehalose is a nonreducing disaccharide found in organisms from bacteria to plants, including yeast, fungi, and invertebrates. It protects the integrity of cells against various stresses like heat, dehydration, cold, desiccation, and oxidation by preventing protein denaturation, and it is the sugar in the hemolymph of invertebrates. The majority of the protecting properties of trehalose were discovered in yeast ; however, it also has beneficial effects in mammals where it is not endogenously synthesized. In this sense has been recently identified trehalose as a mTOR-independent autophagy enhancer. Although the exact mechanism by which this drug promotes autophagy is unknown, trehalose at a relatively low concentration disaggregates existent A53T-alpha-synuclein protofibrils and fibrils into random coil or soluble β-sheet conformers, and trehalose at a higher concentration inhibits the formation of A53T alpha-synuclein fibrils. In addition, by stabilizing the partially unfolded protein or activating autophagy in an mTOR independent manner, trehalose accelerates the clearance of the aggregate-prone proteins in various neurodegenerative disorders including polyglutamine in the R6/2 mouse model of Huntington disease, beta-amyloid in Alzheimer's disease, and alpha-synuclein in PD. Finally, trehalose also protected cells against several proapoptotic insults.

Carbamazepine. Carbamazepine (CBZ) is an anticonvulsant and mood-stabilizing drug used primarily in the treatment of epilepsy and bipolar disorder, as well as certain neuralgias. The mechanism of action of CBZ and its derivatives is relatively well understood, voltage-gated sodium channels or potentiation of gamma-aminobutyric acid receptors are implicated. However new effects for CBZ has been described in the last years. Thus, CBZ has been implicated with autophagy induction through inhibition of inositol synthesis, which decreases intracellular levels of IP3. Consistent with a role for inositol depletion in autophagy regulation, CBZ significantly reduced EGFP-HDQ74 aggregates and attenuated polyglutamine toxicity in COS-7 cells and enhanced clearance of A30P alpha-synuclein. CBZ also significantly ameliorated rotenone-induced damage in SH-SY5Y cells, by inhibiting the ROS production and inhibiting neuronal apoptosis, and especially for the clearance of malfunction organelles by autophagy induction.

http://dx.doi.org/10.5772/54851

3. Conclusions and future perspectives

Future studies may focus on identifying specific molecules that modulate each step in the autophagy pathway. Small molecules and pharmacologic agents that can more selectively modulate certain aspects of autophagic stress may also help usher in the first wave of disease-specific therapies. Ideally, small molecule regulators would affect only certain aspects or targets of the autophagy pathway, since global inhibition or enhancement of protein turnover could be problematic. In situations with substantial aggregation, however, a global induction of autophagy may be required provided this does not outstrip the degradative capacity of the aged or diseased cell. Promoting expression of biomolecules required for both induction and clearance of autophagosomes may serve to prevent potential autophagic stress. To determine the mechanism of the possible neuroprotective role of autophagy in PD would provide, eventually, the design of therapeutic interventions (drugs or cell therapy) for treatment of patients affected by this disease.

4. Funding sources

Dr. Rosa A. González-Polo received research support from ISCIII (Ministerio de Economía y Competitividad, Spain (CP0800010, PI11/0040) and FUNDESALUD (PRIS11014). Dr. José M. Fuentes received research support from the ISCIII (Ministerio de Economía y Competitividad, Spain (PI12/02280), FUNDESALUD (PRIS11019), CIBERNED (CB06/05/004) and Consejería, Economía, Comercio e Innovación, Junta de Extremadura (GRU10054). Mireia Niso-Santano was supported as a postdoctoral researcher by the University of Extremadura. Rosa A. González-Polo was supported by a "Miguel Servet" contract (ISCIII, Ministerio de Economía y Competitividad, Spain). Elisa Pizarro-Estrella is supported by a predoctoral contract from CIBERNED. Jose M Bravo San-Pedro and Ruben Gómez-Sánchez are beneficiaries to fellowship from Univesity of Extremadura and Minister of Economia y Competitividad respectively.

Abbreviations

The following abbreviations were used in this paper:

PD, Parkinson´s disease; CBZ, carbamazepine; LB, Lewy bodies; LAMP-2A, Lysosomal-associated membrane protein 2A; LRRK2, Leucine-rich repeat kinase 2; PINK1, PTEN-induced kinase 1; CMA, chaperone-mediated autophagy; mTOR, mammalian target of rapamicyn; FKBP12, FK506-binding protein of 12 kDa; AMPK, 5'-adenosine monophosphate-activated protein kinase; MPP^+, 1-methyl-4-phenylpyridinium; MPTP, 1-methyl-4-phenyl-1,2,3,6-tetrahydropyridine; PQ, paraquat; *Atg*, autophagy genes; ROS, reactive oxygen species; BP, bipolar disorder; LC3, microtubule-associated protein light chain 3; GBA-1, glucocerebrosidase; MAO-B, monoamine oxidase B; DAT, dopamine transporter; JNK, c-jun N-terminal kinase JNK; 6-

OHDA, 6-Hydroxydopamine; UPR, unfolded protein response; IRE1, inositol-requiring enzyme 1; ASK1, apoptosis signal regulating kinase 1; GSH, glutathione

Author details

Rosa A. González-Polo[1], Rubén Gómez-Sánchez[1], Lydia Sánchez-Erviti[2], José M Bravo-San Pedro[1], Elisa Pizarro-Estrella[1], Mireia Niso-Santano[1,3] and José M. Fuentes[1]

*Address all correspondence to: jfuentes@unex.es, rosapolo@unex.es

1 Centro de Investigación Biomédica en Red sobre Enfermedades Neurodegenerativas (CIBERNED). Departamento de Bioquímica y Biología Molecular y Genética, E. Enfermería y T.O., Universidad de Extremadura, CP 10003, Cáceres, España

2 Department of Clinical Neuroscience, UCL Institute of Neurology, London, UK

3 INSERM, U848, Institut Gustave Roussy, Université Paris Sud, Paris, France

References

[1] Rodriguez-Oroz, M.C., et al., Initial clinical manifestations of Parkinson's disease: features and pathophysiological mechanisms. Lancet Neurol, 2009. 8(12): p. 1128-39.

[2] Spillantini, M.G., et al., Alpha-synuclein in Lewy bodies. Nature, 1997. 388(6645): p. 839-40.

[3] Polymeropoulos, M.H., et al., Mutation in the alpha-synuclein gene identified in families with Parkinson's disease. Science, 1997. 276(5321): p. 2045-7.

[4] Kruger, R., et al., Ala30Pro mutation in the gene encoding alpha-synuclein in Parkinson's disease. Nat Genet, 1998. 18(2): p. 106-8.

[5] Singleton, A.B., et al., alpha-Synuclein locus triplication causes Parkinson's disease. Science, 2003. 302(5646): p. 841.

[6] Li, J.Y., et al., Lewy bodies in grafted neurons in subjects with Parkinson's disease suggest host-to-graft disease propagation. Nat Med, 2008. 14(5): p. 501-3.

[7] Kordower, J.H., et al., Lewy body-like pathology in long-term embryonic nigral transplants in Parkinson's disease. Nat Med, 2008. 14(5): p. 504-6.

[8] Braak, H., et al., Staging of brain pathology related to sporadic Parkinson's disease. Neurobiol Aging, 2003. 24(2): p. 197-211.

[9] Lee, H.J., S. Patel, and S.J. Lee, Intravesicular localization and exocytosis of alpha-synuclein and its aggregates. J Neurosci, 2005. 25(25): p. 6016-24.

[10] Desplats, P., et al., Inclusion formation and neuronal cell death through neuron-to-neuron transmission of alpha-synuclein. Proc Natl Acad Sci U S A, 2009. 106(31): p. 13010-5.

[11] Vella, L.J., et al., Packaging of prions into exosomes is associated with a novel pathway of PrP processing. J Pathol, 2007. 211(5): p. 582-90.

[12] Alvarez-Erviti, L., et al., Lysosomal dysfunction increases exosome-mediated alpha-synuclein release and transmission. Neurobiol Dis, 2011. 42(3): p. 360-7.

[13] Emmanouilidou, E., et al., Cell-produced alpha-synuclein is secreted in a calcium-dependent manner by exosomes and impacts neuronal survival. J Neurosci, 2010. 30(20): p. 6838-51.

[14] Schapira, A.H., et al., Mitochondrial complex I deficiency in Parkinson's disease. J Neurochem, 1990. 54(3): p. 823-7.

[15] Mizuno, Y., et al., Inhibition of ATP synthesis by 1-methyl-4-phenylpyridinium ion (MPP+) in isolated mitochondria from mouse brains. Neurosci Lett, 1987. 81(1-2): p. 204-8.

[16] Sherer, T.B., et al., Mechanism of toxicity in rotenone models of Parkinson's disease. J Neurosci, 2003. 23(34): p. 10756-64.

[17] Valente, E.M., et al., Hereditary early-onset Parkinson's disease caused by mutations in PINK1. Science, 2004. 304(5674): p. 1158-60.

[18] Kitada, T., et al., Mutations in the parkin gene cause autosomal recessive juvenile parkinsonism. Nature, 1998. 392(6676): p. 605-8.

[19] Matsuda, N., et al., PINK1 stabilized by mitochondrial depolarization recruits Parkin to damaged mitochondria and activates latent Parkin for mitophagy. J Cell Biol, 2010. 189(2): p. 211-21.

[20] Owen, A.D., et al., Oxidative stress and Parkinson's disease. Ann N Y Acad Sci, 1996. 786: p. 217-23.

[21] Kachergus, J., et al., Identification of a novel LRRK2 mutation linked to autosomal dominant parkinsonism: evidence of a common founder across European populations. Am J Hum Genet, 2005. 76(4): p. 672-80.

[22] Goker-Alpan, O., et al., Glucocerebrosidase mutations are an important risk factor for Lewy body disorders. Neurology, 2006. 67(5): p. 908-10.

[23] Neumann, J., et al., Glucocerebrosidase mutations in clinical and pathologically proven Parkinson's disease. Brain, 2009. 132(Pt 7): p. 1783-94.

[24] Yang, Z. and D.J. Klionsky, Eaten alive: a history of macroautophagy. Nat Cell Biol, 2010. 12(9): p. 814-22.

[25] Olson, T.S. and J.F. Dice, Regulation of protein degradation rates in eukaryotes. Curr Opin Cell Biol, 1989. 1(6): p. 1194-200.

[26] Mortimore, G.E. and A.R. Poso, Intracellular protein catabolism and its control during nutrient deprivation and supply. Annu Rev Nutr, 1987. 7: p. 539-64.

[27] Kiffin, R., et al., Activation of chaperone-mediated autophagy during oxidative stress. Mol Biol Cell, 2004. 15(11): p. 4829-40.

[28] Cadwell, K., et al., A key role for autophagy and the autophagy gene Atg16l1 in mouse and human intestinal Paneth cells. Nature, 2008. 456(7219): p. 259-63.

[29] Li, W., Q. Yang, and Z. Mao, Chaperone-mediated autophagy: machinery, regulation and biological consequences. Cell Mol Life Sci, 2011. 68(5): p. 749-63.

[30] Hailey, D.W., et al., Mitochondria supply membranes for autophagosome biogenesis during starvation. Cell, 2010. 141(4): p. 656-67.

[31] Ravikumar, B., et al., Plasma membrane contributes to the formation of pre-autophagosomal structures. Nat Cell Biol, 2010. 12(8): p. 747-57.

[32] Ravikumar, B., et al., Mammalian macroautophagy at a glance. J Cell Sci, 2009. 122(Pt 11): p. 1707-11.

[33] Xie, Z. and D.J. Klionsky, Autophagosome formation: core machinery and adaptations. Nat Cell Biol, 2007. 9(10): p. 1102-9.

[34] Dennis, P.B., S. Fumagalli, and G. Thomas, Target of rapamycin (TOR): balancing the opposing forces of protein synthesis and degradation. Curr Opin Genet Dev, 1999. 9(1): p. 49-54.

[35] Hosokawa, N., et al., Nutrient-dependent mTORC1 association with the ULK1-Atg13-FIP200 complex required for autophagy. Mol Biol Cell, 2009. 20(7): p. 1981-91.

[36] Scott, S.V., et al., Apg13p and Vac8p are part of a complex of phosphoproteins that are required for cytoplasm to vacuole targeting. J Biol Chem, 2000. 275(33): p. 25840-9.

[37] Mijaljica, D., M. Prescott, and R.J. Devenish, Microautophagy in mammalian cells: revisiting a 40-year-old conundrum. Autophagy, 2011. 7(7): p. 673-82.

[38] Chiang, H.L., et al., A role for a 70-kilodalton heat shock protein in lysosomal degradation of intracellular proteins. Science, 1989. 246(4928): p. 382-5.

[39] Cuervo, A.M. and J.F. Dice, A receptor for the selective uptake and degradation of proteins by lysosomes. Science, 1996. 273(5274): p. 501-3.

[40] Anglade, P., et al., Apoptosis and autophagy in nigral neurons of patients with Parkinson's disease. Histol Histopathol, 1997. 12(1): p. 25-31.

[41] Dehay, B., et al., Pathogenic lysosomal depletion in Parkinson's disease. J Neurosci, 2010. 30(37): p. 12535-44.

[42] Alvarez-Erviti, L., et al., Chaperone-mediated autophagy markers in Parkinson disease brains. Arch Neurol, 2010. 67(12): p. 1464-72.

[43] Cuervo, A.M., et al., Impaired degradation of mutant alpha-synuclein by chaperone-mediated autophagy. Science, 2004. 305(5688): p. 1292-5.

[44] Mak, S.K., et al., Lysosomal degradation of alpha-synuclein in vivo. J Biol Chem, 2010. 285(18): p. 13621-9.

[45] Martinez-Vicente, M., et al., Dopamine-modified alpha-synuclein blocks chaperone-mediated autophagy. J Clin Invest, 2008. 118(2): p. 777-88.

[46] Narendra, D., et al., Parkin is recruited selectively to impaired mitochondria and promotes their autophagy. J Cell Biol, 2008. 183(5): p. 795-803.

[47] Narendra, D.P., et al., PINK1 is selectively stabilized on impaired mitochondria to activate Parkin. PLoS Biol, 2010. 8(1): p. e1000298.

[48] Dehay, B., et al., Loss of P-type ATPase ATP13A2/PARK9 function induces general lysosomal deficiency and leads to Parkinson disease neurodegeneration. Proc Natl Acad Sci U S A, 2012. 109(24): p. 9611-6.

[49] Sanchez-Danes, A., et al., Disease-specific phenotypes in dopamine neurons from human iPS-based models of genetic and sporadic Parkinson's disease. EMBO Mol Med, 2012. 4(5): p. 380-95.

[50] Bravo-San Pedro, J.M., et al., The LRRK2 G2019S mutant exacerbates basal autophagy through activation of the MEK/ERK pathway. Cell Mol Life Sci, 2012.

[51] Good, P.F., et al., Protein nitration in Parkinson's disease. J Neuropathol Exp Neurol, 1998. 57(4): p. 338-42.

[52] Dexter, D.T., et al., Basal lipid peroxidation in substantia nigra is increased in Parkinson's disease. J Neurochem, 1989. 52(2): p. 381-9.

[53] Dexter, D.T., et al., Increased levels of lipid hydroperoxides in the parkinsonian substantia nigra: an HPLC and ESR study. Mov Disord, 1994. 9(1): p. 92-7.

[54] Perry, T.L., D.V. Godin, and S. Hansen, Parkinson's disease: a disorder due to nigral glutathione deficiency? Neurosci Lett, 1982. 33(3): p. 305-10.

[55] Kish, S.J., C. Morito, and O. Hornykiewicz, Glutathione peroxidase activity in Parkinson's disease brain. Neurosci Lett, 1985. 58(3): p. 343-6.

[56] Yamin, G., V.N. Uversky, and A.L. Fink, Nitration inhibits fibrillation of human alpha-synuclein in vitro by formation of soluble oligomers. FEBS Lett, 2003. 542(1-3): p. 147-52.

[57] Paxinou, E., et al., Induction of alpha-synuclein aggregation by intracellular nitrative insult. J Neurosci, 2001. 21(20): p. 8053-61.

[58] Langston, J.W. and P.A. Ballard, Jr., Parkinson's disease in a chemist working with 1-methyl-4-phenyl-1,2,5,6-tetrahydropyridine. N Engl J Med, 1983. 309(5): p. 310.

[59] Davis, G.C., et al., Chronic Parkinsonism secondary to intravenous injection of meperidine analogues. Psychiatry Res, 1979. 1(3): p. 249-54.

[60] Riachi, N.J., J.C. LaManna, and S.I. Harik, Entry of 1-methyl-4-phenyl-1,2,3,6-tetrahydropyridine into the rat brain. J Pharmacol Exp Ther, 1989. 249(3): p. 744-8.

[61] Chiba, K., A. Trevor, and N. Castagnoli, Jr., Metabolism of the neurotoxic tertiary amine, MPTP, by brain monoamine oxidase. Biochem Biophys Res Commun, 1984. 120(2): p. 574-8.

[62] Javitch, J.A., et al., Parkinsonism-inducing neurotoxin, N-methyl-4-phenyl-1,2,3,6 -tetrahydropyridine: uptake of the metabolite N-methyl-4-phenylpyridine by dopamine neurons explains selective toxicity. Proc Natl Acad Sci U S A, 1985. 82(7): p. 2173-7.

[63] Gonzalez-Polo, R.A., et al., Mechanisms of MPP(+) incorporation into cerebellar granule cells. Brain Res Bull, 2001. 56(2): p. 119-23.

[64] Sheldon, A.L. and M.B. Robinson, The role of glutamate transporters in neurodegenerative diseases and potential opportunities for intervention. Neurochem Int, 2007. 51(6-7): p. 333-55.

[65] Nicklas, W.J., I. Vyas, and R.E. Heikkila, Inhibition of NADH-linked oxidation in brain mitochondria by 1-methyl-4-phenyl-pyridine, a metabolite of the neurotoxin, 1-methyl-4-phenyl-1,2,5,6-tetrahydropyridine. Life Sci, 1985. 36(26): p. 2503-8.

[66] Di Monte, D., et al., 1-Methyl-4-phenyl-1,2,3,6-tetrahydropyridine (MPTP) and 1-methyl-4-phenylpyridine (MPP+) cause rapid ATP depletion in isolated hepatocytes. Biochem Biophys Res Commun, 1986. 137(1): p. 310-5.

[67] Saporito, M.S., B.A. Thomas, and R.W. Scott, MPTP activates c-Jun NH(2)-terminal kinase (JNK) and its upstream regulatory kinase MKK4 in nigrostriatal neurons in vivo. J Neurochem, 2000. 75(3): p. 1200-8.

[68] Karunakaran, S., et al., Selective activation of p38 mitogen-activated protein kinase in dopaminergic neurons of substantia nigra leads to nuclear translocation of p53 in 1-methyl-4-phenyl-1,2,3,6-tetrahydropyridine-treated mice. J Neurosci, 2008. 28(47): p. 12500-9.

[69] Hassouna, I., et al., Increase in bax expression in substantia nigra following 1-methyl-4-phenyl-1,2,3,6-tetrahydropyridine (MPTP) treatment of mice. Neurosci Lett, 1996. 204(1-2): p. 85-8.

[70] Vila, M., et al., Bax ablation prevents dopaminergic neurodegeneration in the 1-methyl-4-phenyl-1,2,3,6-tetrahydropyridine mouse model of Parkinson's disease. Proc Natl Acad Sci U S A, 2001. 98(5): p. 2837-42.

[71] McCormack, A.L., et al., Pathologic modifications of alpha-synuclein in 1-methyl-4-phenyl-1,2,3,6-tetrahydropyridine (MPTP)-treated squirrel monkeys. J Neuropathol Exp Neurol, 2008. 67(8): p. 793-802.

[72] Wang, C., et al., Stress-induced alterations in parkin solubility promote parkin aggregation and compromise parkin's protective function. Hum Mol Genet, 2005. 14(24): p. 3885-97.

[73] Talpade, D.J., et al., In vivo labeling of mitochondrial complex I (NADH:ubiquinone oxidoreductase) in rat brain using [(3)H]dihydrorotenone. J Neurochem, 2000. 75(6): p. 2611-21.

[74] Chung, W.G., C.L. Miranda, and C.S. Maier, Epigallocatechin gallate (EGCG) potentiates the cytotoxicity of rotenone in neuroblastoma SH-SY5Y cells. Brain Res, 2007. 1176: p. 133-42.

[75] Wang, X.F., et al., Inhibitory effects of pesticides on proteasome activity: implication in Parkinson's disease. Neurobiol Dis, 2006. 23(1): p. 198-205.

[76] Sherer, T.B., et al., An in vitro model of Parkinson's disease: linking mitochondrial impairment to altered alpha-synuclein metabolism and oxidative damage. J Neurosci, 2002. 22(16): p. 7006-15.

[77] Jonsson, G. and C. Sachs, Actions of 6-hydroxydopamine quinones on catecholamine neurons. J Neurochem, 1975. 25(4): p. 509-16.

[78] Ungerstedt, U., 6-Hydroxy-dopamine induced degeneration of central monoamine neurons. Eur J Pharmacol, 1968. 5(1): p. 107-10.

[79] Blum, D., et al., Molecular pathways involved in the neurotoxicity of 6-OHDA, dopamine and MPTP: contribution to the apoptotic theory in Parkinson's disease. Prog Neurobiol, 2001. 65(2): p. 135-72.

[80] Luthman, J., et al., Selective lesion of central dopamine or noradrenaline neuron systems in the neonatal rat: motor behavior and monoamine alterations at adult stage. Behav Brain Res, 1989. 33(3): p. 267-77.

[81] Kienzl, E., et al., The role of transition metals in the pathogenesis of Parkinson's disease. J Neurol Sci, 1995. 134 Suppl: p. 69-78.

[82] Linert, W., et al., Dopamine, 6-hydroxydopamine, iron, and dioxygen--their mutual interactions and possible implication in the development of Parkinson's disease. Biochim Biophys Acta, 1996. 1316(3): p. 160-8.

[83] Deumens, R., A. Blokland, and J. Prickaerts, Modeling Parkinson's disease in rats: an evaluation of 6-OHDA lesions of the nigrostriatal pathway. Exp Neurol, 2002. 175(2): p. 303-17.

[84] Blandini, F., M.T. Armentero, and E. Martignoni, The 6-hydroxydopamine model: news from the past. Parkinsonism Relat Disord, 2008. 14 Suppl 2: p. S124-9.

[85] Oestreicher, E., et al., Degeneration of nigrostriatal dopaminergic neurons increases iron within the substantia nigra: a histochemical and neurochemical study. Brain Res, 1994. 660(1): p. 8-18.

[86] Glinka, Y., M. Gassen, and M.B. Youdim, Mechanism of 6-hydroxydopamine neurotoxicity. J Neural Transm Suppl, 1997. 50: p. 55-66.

[87] Holtz, W.A., et al., Oxidative stress-triggered unfolded protein response is upstream of intrinsic cell death evoked by parkinsonian mimetics. J Neurochem, 2006. 99(1): p. 54-69.

[88] Ryu, E.J., et al., Endoplasmic reticulum stress and the unfolded protein response in cellular models of Parkinson's disease. J Neurosci, 2002. 22(24): p. 10690-8.

[89] Drechsel, D.A. and M. Patel, Role of reactive oxygen species in the neurotoxicity of environmental agents implicated in Parkinson's disease. Free Radic Biol Med, 2008. 44(11): p. 1873-86.

[90] Cannon, J.R. and J.T. Greenamyre, Neurotoxic in vivo models of Parkinson's disease recent advances. Prog Brain Res, 2010. 184: p. 17-33.

[91] Liou, H.H., et al., Environmental risk factors and Parkinson's disease: a case-control study in Taiwan. Neurology, 1997. 48(6): p. 1583-8.

[92] Smith, J.G., Paraquat poisoning by skin absorption: a review. Hum Toxicol, 1988. 7(1): p. 15-9.

[93] Dinis-Oliveira, R.J., et al., Paraquat exposure as an etiological factor of Parkinson's disease. Neurotoxicology, 2006. 27(6): p. 1110-22.

[94] Grant, H., P.L. Lantos, and C. Parkinson, Cerebral damage in paraquat poisoning. Histopathology, 1980. 4(2): p. 185-95.

[95] Shimizu, K., et al., Carrier-mediated processes in blood--brain barrier penetration and neural uptake of paraquat. Brain Res, 2001. 906(1-2): p. 135-42.

[96] Richardson, J.R., et al., Paraquat neurotoxicity is distinct from that of MPTP and rotenone. Toxicol Sci, 2005. 88(1): p. 193-201.

[97] Castello, P.R., D.A. Drechsel, and M. Patel, Mitochondria are a major source of paraquat-induced reactive oxygen species production in the brain. J Biol Chem, 2007. 282(19): p. 14186-93.

[98] Miller, G.W., Paraquat: the red herring of Parkinson's disease research. Toxicol Sci, 2007. 100(1): p. 1-2.

[99] Moretto, A. and C. Colosio, Biochemical and toxicological evidence of neurological effects of pesticides: the example of Parkinson's disease. Neurotoxicology, 2011. 32(4): p. 383-91.

[100] Bus, J.S. and J.E. Gibson, Paraquat: model for oxidant-initiated toxicity. Environ Health Perspect, 1984. 55: p. 37-46.

[101] Ryter, S.W., et al., Mechanisms of cell death in oxidative stress. Antioxid Redox Signal, 2007. 9(1): p. 49-89.

[102] West, J.D. and L.J. Marnett, Endogenous reactive intermediates as modulators of cell signaling and cell death. Chem Res Toxicol, 2006. 19(2): p. 173-94.

[103] Peng, J., et al., The herbicide paraquat induces dopaminergic nigral apoptosis through sustained activation of the JNK pathway. J Biol Chem, 2004. 279(31): p. 32626-32.

[104] Niso-Santano, M., et al., Low concentrations of paraquat induces early activation of extracellular signal-regulated kinase 1/2, protein kinase B, and c-Jun N-terminal kinase 1/2 pathways: role of c-Jun N-terminal kinase in paraquat-induced cell death. Toxicol Sci, 2006. 92(2): p. 507-15.

[105] Fei, Q., et al., Paraquat neurotoxicity is mediated by a Bak-dependent mechanism. J Biol Chem, 2008. 283(6): p. 3357-64.

[106] Gonzalez-Polo, R.A., et al., Paraquat-induced apoptotic cell death in cerebellar granule cells. Brain Res, 2004. 1011(2): p. 170-6.

[107] Yang, W. and E. Tiffany-Castiglioni, Paraquat-induced apoptosis in human neuroblastoma SH-SY5Y cells: involvement of p53 and mitochondria. J Toxicol Environ Health A, 2008. 71(4): p. 289-99.

[108] Yang, W., et al., Paraquat activates the IRE1/ASK1/JNK cascade associated with apoptosis in human neuroblastoma SH-SY5Y cells. Toxicol Lett, 2009. 191(2-3): p. 203-10.

[109] Niso-Santano, M., et al., Activation of apoptosis signal-regulating kinase 1 is a key factor in paraquat-induced cell death: modulation by the Nrf2/Trx axis. Free Radic Biol Med, 2010. 48(10): p. 1370-81.

[110] Manning-Bog, A.B., et al., The herbicide paraquat causes up-regulation and aggregation of alpha-synuclein in mice: paraquat and alpha-synuclein. J Biol Chem, 2002. 277(3): p. 1641-4.

[111] Gonzalez-Polo, R., et al., Silencing DJ-1 reveals its contribution in paraquat-induced autophagy. J Neurochem, 2009. 109(3): p. 889-98.

[112] Fleming, A., et al., Chemical modulators of autophagy as biological probes and potential therapeutics. Nat Chem Biol, 2011. 7(1): p. 9-17.

[113] Ravikumar, B., et al., Inhibition of mTOR induces autophagy and reduces toxicity of polyglutamine expansions in fly and mouse models of Huntington disease. Nat Genet, 2004. 36(6): p. 585-95.

[114] Ravikumar, B., et al., Rapamycin pre-treatment protects against apoptosis. Hum Mol Genet, 2006. 15(7): p. 1209-16.

[115] Kim, D.H., et al., mTOR interacts with raptor to form a nutrient-sensitive complex that signals to the cell growth machinery. Cell, 2002. 110(2): p. 163-75.

[116] Sarbassov, D.D., et al., Prolonged rapamycin treatment inhibits mTORC2 assembly and Akt/PKB. Mol Cell, 2006. 22(2): p. 159-68.

[117] Walle, T., Bioavailability of resveratrol. Ann N Y Acad Sci, 2011. 1215: p. 9-15.

[118] Richard, T., et al., Neuroprotective properties of resveratrol and derivatives. Ann N Y Acad Sci, 2011. 1215: p. 103-8.

[119] Tili, E. and J.J. Michaille, Resveratrol, MicroRNAs, Inflammation, and Cancer. J Nucleic Acids, 2011. 2011: p. 102431.

[120] Vingtdeux, V., et al., AMP-activated protein kinase signaling activation by resveratrol modulates amyloid-beta peptide metabolism. J Biol Chem, 2010. 285(12): p. 9100-13.

[121] Wu, Y., et al., Resveratrol-activated AMPK/SIRT1/autophagy in cellular models of Parkinson's disease. Neurosignals, 2011. 19(3): p. 163-74.

[122] Manji, H.K. and R.H. Lenox, Lithium: a molecular transducer of mood-stabilization in the treatment of bipolar disorder. Neuropsychopharmacology, 1998. 19(3): p. 161-6.

[123] King, T.D., G.N. Bijur, and R.S. Jope, Caspase-3 activation induced by inhibition of mitochondrial complex I is facilitated by glycogen synthase kinase-3beta and attenuated by lithium. Brain Res, 2001. 919(1): p. 106-14.

[124] Chen, G., et al., Glycogen synthase kinase 3beta (GSK3beta) mediates 6-hydroxydopamine-induced neuronal death. FASEB J, 2004. 18(10): p. 1162-4.

[125] Sarkar, S., et al., Lithium induces autophagy by inhibiting inositol monophosphatase. J Cell Biol, 2005. 170(7): p. 1101-11.

[126] Sarkar, S. and D.C. Rubinsztein, Inositol and IP3 levels regulate autophagy: biology and therapeutic speculations. Autophagy, 2006. 2(2): p. 132-4.

[127] Chen, Q. and G.G. Haddad, Role of trehalose phosphate synthase and trehalose during hypoxia: from flies to mammals. J Exp Biol, 2004. 207(Pt 18): p. 3125-9.

[128] Kandror, O., et al., Yeast adapt to near-freezing temperatures by STRE/Msn2,4-dependent induction of trehalose synthesis and certain molecular chaperones. Mol Cell, 2004. 13(6): p. 771-81.

[129] Yu, W.B., et al., Trehalose inhibits fibrillation of A53T mutant alpha-synuclein and disaggregates existing fibrils. Arch Biochem Biophys, 2012. 523(2): p. 144-50.

[130] Sarkar, S., et al., Trehalose, a novel mTOR-independent autophagy enhancer, accelerates the clearance of mutant huntingtin and alpha-synuclein. J Biol Chem, 2007. 282(8): p. 5641-52.

[131] Casarejos, M.J., et al., The accumulation of neurotoxic proteins, induced by proteasome inhibition, is reverted by trehalose, an enhancer of autophagy, in human neuroblastoma cells. Neurochem Int, 2011. 58(4): p. 512-20.

[132] Kruger, U., et al., Autophagic degradation of tau in primary neurons and its enhancement by trehalose. Neurobiol Aging, 2011.

[133] Chen, W., et al., Trehalose protects against ocular surface disorders in experimental murine dry eye through suppression of apoptosis. Exp Eye Res, 2009. 89(3): p. 311-8.

[134] Granger, P., et al., Modulation of the gamma-aminobutyric acid type A receptor by the antiepileptic drugs carbamazepine and phenytoin. Mol Pharmacol, 1995. 47(6): p. 1189-96.

http://dx.doi.org/10.5772/54851

[135] Xiong, N., et al., Potential autophagy enhancers attenuate rotenone-induced toxicity in SH-SY5Y. Neuroscience, 2011. 199: p. 292-302.

Chapter 9

Physiologically Based Pharmacokinetic Modeling: A Tool for Understanding ADMET Properties and Extrapolating to Human

Micaela B. Reddy, Harvey J. Clewell III,
Thierry Lave and Melvin E. Andersen

Additional information is available at the end of the chapter

http://dx.doi.org/10.5772/54965

1. Introduction

Physiologically based pharmacokinetic (PBPK) models differ from classical PK models in that they include specific compartments for tissues involved in exposure, toxicity, biotransformation and clearance processes connected by blood flow (Figure 1). Compartments and blood flows are described using physiologically meaningful parameters, which allows for interspecies extrapolation by altering the physiological parameters appropriately [1]. A key benefit to PBPK models is that factors influencing the absorption, distribution, metabolism, and elimination of a compound can be incorporated into a PBPK model in a mechanistic, meaningful way, if a mechanism is understood and sufficient data are available. This mechanistic aspect is supported by physiological parameters influencing absorption (e.g., pH values and transit times through various sections of the GI tract), distribution (e.g., tissue volumes and composition), metabolism (e.g., expression levels of various hepatic enzymes and transporters involved with metabolic elimination), and elimination (e.g., glomerular filtration rate and expression levels of transporters in the kidneys involved with renal elimination), which can be explicitly incorporated in the PBPK model.

Because the models have a mechanistic basis, extrapolation to situations differing from the conditions of the data used to calibrate the model is justifiable [2]. The mechanistic basis allows PBPK models to be used to determine if results from different experimental designs are consistent, and to explore possible mechanisms responsible for unexpected or unusual data. PBPK modeling has been used to great effect for interspecies extrapolation, both among animal models [3] and for predicting human PK based on animal data [4-5].

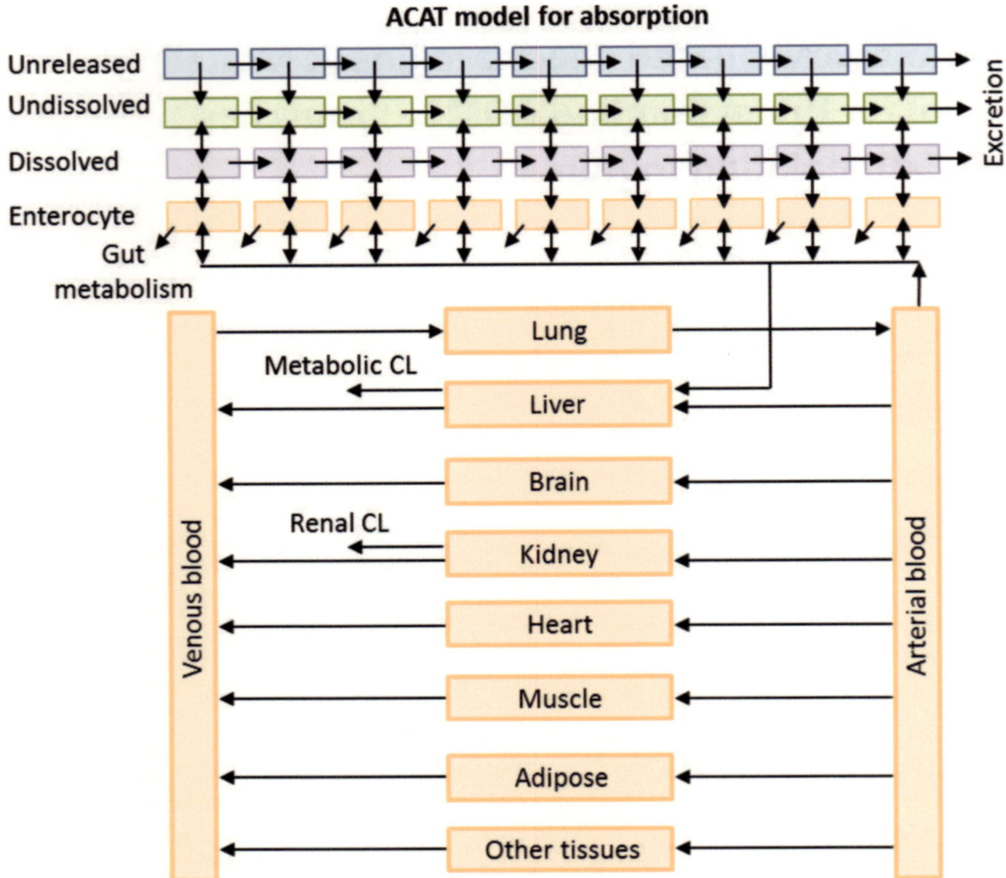

Figure 1. A schematic diagram of a PBPK model.

PBPK approaches have several advantages over other PK modeling approaches: (1) creating models from physiological, biochemical and anatomical information, entirely separate from collection of detailed concentration time-course curves; (2) evaluating mechanisms by which biological processes govern disposition of a wide range of compounds by comparison of PK results with model predictions; (3) using compounds as probes of the biological processes to gain more general information on the way biochemical characteristics govern the importance of various transport pathways in the body; (4) applying the models in safety assessments; and (5) using annotation of a modeling data-base as a repository of information on PK properties, toxicity and kinetics of specific compounds [6]. These attributes have led to widespread development of PBPK models in recent years [7], with acceleration in publication of PBPK modeling papers pertaining to drugs particularly over the last 10 years.

Here, we describe the historical development of the PBPK approach. Also, we discuss the emerging role of PBPK modeling in the pharmaceutical industry throughout drug development. Finally, we provide our thoughts on potential applications that have not yet been widely explored. Although advances have been made in applying PBPK modeling for biotherapeutics, this review focuses on small molecules.

2. Historical perspective

Interest in PK modeling in pharmacology and toxicology arises from the need to relate internal concentrations of active compounds at their target sites with the dose administered to an animal or human subject. The reason, of course, is a fundamental tenet in pharmacology or toxicology that both beneficial and adverse responses to a compound are related to the free concentration of active compound at the target tissue rather than the amount of compound at the site of absorption. The relationship between tissue dose and administered dose can be complex (Figure 2). PK models are valuable tools to assess internal dosimetry at target tissues for a wide range of exposure situations.

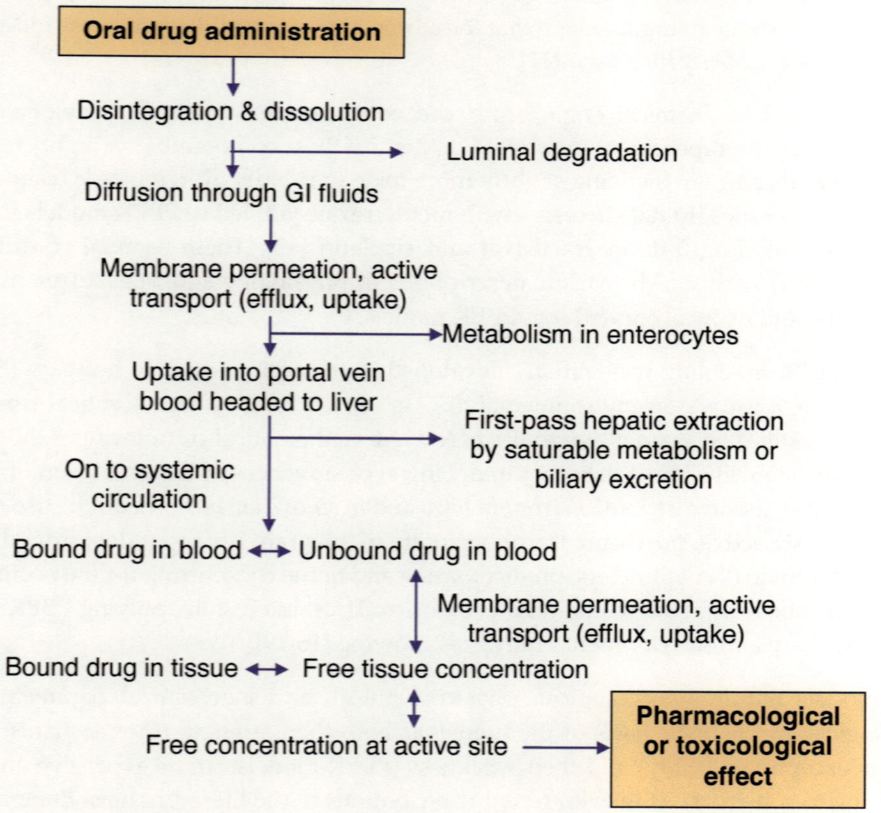

Figure 2. A schematic diagram of the processes impacting the free concentration of drug at the target. Modified from [8].

In the 1930's, Teorell [9-10] provided the first physiological model for drug distribution in a set of equations for uptake, distribution, and elimination of drugs from the body. However, computational methods were not available to solve the sets of equations at this time. Exact mathematical solutions could only be obtained for simplified models in which the body was reduced to a small number of compartments that did not have direct physiological correspondence. Over the next 30 years, PK modeling focused on simpler descriptions with exact solutions rather than on models concordant with the structure and content of the biological system. These approaches are sometimes referred to as 'data-based' compartmental modeling since the work generally took the form of a detailed collection of time-course blood/excreta concentrations at various doses. Time-course curves were analyzed by assuming particular model structures and estimating a small number of model parameters by curve-fitting.

In early models, all processes for metabolism, distribution, and elimination were treated as first-order (i.e., rates changed in direct proportion to drug concentration). Two issues that particularly affected data-based PK models arose in the 1960's and early 1970's. First, increased understanding of saturation of elimination pathways led to models that were not first-order, making it difficult to derive exact solutions to the sets of equations. Second, it was realized that blood flow rather than metabolic capacity of an organ might limit clearance; blood flow-limited metabolism in an organ meant that the elimination rate could not increase indefinitely as the metabolic capacity increased [11].

Scientists trained in chemical engineering and computational methods developed PBPK models for chemotherapeutic compounds [12]. Many of these compounds are highly toxic and have therapeutic efficacy by being slightly more toxic to rapidly growing cells (cancer cells) than to normal tissues. Initial successes with methotrexate [13] led to PBPK models for other compounds, including 5-fluorouracil [14] and cisplatin [15]. These seminal contributions showed the ease with which realistic descriptions of physiology and relevant pathways of metabolism could be incorporated into PBPK models.

Although PBPK modeling was initially developed in the pharmaceutical industry [6], until recently its major use was in environmental risk assessment. In the pharmaceutical area, PBPK model use was limited mainly due to the perceived mathematical complexity of the models and the labor-intensive input data required. However, advances in the prediction of hepatic metabolism and tissue distribution from *in vitro* and *in silico* data have made the use of these models more attractive, providing the opportunity to integrate key input data from different sources to estimate PK parameters, predict plasma and tissue concentration-time profiles, and gain mechanistic insight into compound properties. Thus, interest in applying PBPK models for the discovery and development of drugs is growing [16-19].

PBPK models require physiological, physicochemical, and biochemical parameters. The physiological, mechanistic basis of the models is both their strength (the mechanistic basis provides exceptional utility) and their weakness (PBPK models can be expensive and time-consuming to construct). However, recent contributions to the literature have demonstrated the effective application of "generic" PBPK models using the ADME data normally generated during preclinical development [5,20-22]. Since the development of the generic PBPK modeling approach incorporating typical ADMET data, PBPK modeling has seen increased application in the pharmaceutical industry.

The past 10 years have seen tremendous advances in the capabilities of generic PBPK models that can simulate PK for humans or preclinical species based on a combination of physicochemical properties and *in vitro* data. Such generic PBPK models can be constructed using programming packages such as MATLAB®, acslX, or Berkeley Madonna. Also powerful commercial PBPK simulation tools, which incorporate useful physiologically-based absorption models in the traditional PBPK model, are now available. Such packages include, e.g., GastroPlus™ (Simulations Plus Inc., www.simulations-plus.com), SimCyp (Simcyp, www.simcyp.com/), and PK-Sim® (Bayer Technology Services, www.pksim.com). These tools allow easy incorporation of preclinical ADMET data into a PBPK model for preclinical species and humans. The availability of such tools simplifies the technical use of PBPK models; however, a good understanding of the models and underlying equations is still mandatory in order to guarantee good interpretation of output.

Instead of taking a month or a day to construct a PBPK model, these generic models can be used to construct and validate models in a few hours, depending on the expertise of the user and the time required to gather the data. The generic PBPK model is an increasingly important tool in assessing DMPK properties in preclinical development [21-24]. PBPK models can incorporate the many complex processes that impact PK (Figure 2) in a mechanistically meaningful way (Figure 1).

3. Current applications of PBPK modeling in drug development

Increased application of PBPK in the pharmaceutical industry was characterized by Rowland et al., who quantified the number of scientific publications per year containing the phrase "physiologically-based pharmacokinetics" and pertaining to drugs in Web of Knowledge (Thomson Reuters); the number of publications meeting these criteria appears to be increasing exponentially over time [19]. While the extent of PBPK modeling in industry is difficult to quantify, and depends on the company, clearly PBPK modeling is increasingly used and useful, as we will illustrate in the following sections. PBPK modeling can be used from early preclinical development throughout the development process (Table 1). Drug discovery is increasingly "data rich" with high throughput chemistry generating numerous compounds that are rapidly screened for pharmacological and PK properties. Much of the typically generated preclinical ADMET data can be used in PBPK model development.

3.1. Lead identification and optimization stages

The first information generated includes *in silico* parameters (e.g., pKa, solubility, Peff, and logP values are calculated). Metabolic stability studies (e.g., in microsomes or hepatocytes) are often considered critical to determine if hepatic metabolism is a major route of elimination and if first pass metabolism might result in unacceptably low bioavailability [35,36]. Screens for permeability and solubility are often implemented early in the process. Plasma protein binding

Model application	Impact	Example
	Lead optimization	
Determining key in vitro data impacting absorption and PK	Providing guidance to chemists and providing basis for screening cascade	[24]
Predicting PK with in silico and in vitro data as inputs	Verifying that the PK properties of a chemical series are understood, prioritizing compounds for additional in vivo experimentation	[21-23]
Understanding mechanisms impacting PK	Comparing the PBPK model to in vivo PK data to identify potential reasons for mismatch and to guide additional experimentation	[25-27]
	Clinical candidate selection	
Absorption modeling	Predicting whether a compound will exhibit a significant food effect	[28]
Comparing exposure window for lead candidates	Linking human PK to PK/PD models for pharmacological and toxicological effects improves basis for choosing best candidate	[20]
Identifying key uncertainties	Allows targeted experimentation	[24]
	Entry into human	
Predicting human PK and efficacious dose	Determining whether a compound will be efficacious in the clinic	[5]
Understanding key sources of variability	Provides important information for clinical trial design	[29]
Simulate clinical trial results	Use the PBPK model simulation to optimize clinical trial design	[30-31]
	Clinical development	
PBPK/PD modeling	Increased understanding of dose of active compound delivered to target tissues and its relationship to toxicological and efficacious effects	[32]
Predicting PK for patient population	Incorporating physiological changes from a disease state allows prediction of PK in the patient population	[33]
Predicting PK for population of different age	Incorporating age-specific physiological differences allows prediction of PK for a specific age group, e.g., children or the elderly	[34]

Table 1. Role of PBPK modeling at various stages in preclinical and clinical development.

might be measured to determine if a compound will have a sufficient free concentration for therapeutic efficacy [37]. The blood-to-plasma ratio might be measured aid in interpreting PK data [38]. PBPK models can be used to determine the key data that should be generated. For example, absorption modeling can be used to determine if solubility or permeability is likely to limit the compound's bioavailability, i.e., to determine if a solubility or permeability assay would be a useful addition to a screening cascade.

Determination of *in vivo* PK is more costly and slower than *in vitro* screening, and so using simulations to prioritize compounds for in vivo experimentation can optimize resource expenditure. PBPK can be used at an early stage to determine which compounds should go on for further experimentation [21-23]. In a study applying generic PBPK modeling to predict rat PK following iv or po administration of test compound [23], it was determined that differences in PK parameters of more than twofold could be determined based upon minimal in vitro data. But to apply the method for new series, the use of the model should be verified for several compounds before it is generally applied.

For promising compounds, a rodent PK study might be performed to determine if a compound has drug-like PK properties and adequate bioavailability. Later studies might include PK studies in a nonrodent species. Hepatocyte or microsomal clearance data can be scaled to estimate the *in vivo* metabolic clearance in preclinical species and humans [39-40]. The scaled clearance in preclinical species can be compared to clearance in PK studies to determine if hepatic metabolism is a major route of elimination in preclinical species. If the clearance seen in PK studies is higher than the clearance scaled from hepatocyte or microsome data, urine and/or bile might be collected in PK studies to provide additional information on mechanisms of clearance.

Because of the mechanistic basis of PBPK models, when they do not adequately describe animal PK data, this means that a biological phenomenon affecting PK has not been included in the model and is not represented by the assays used to screen the compounds. Therefore, if a PK issue for a promising compound becomes apparent, PBPK modeling allows you to determine which mechanisms are consistent with the observed data. This information can be used to guide further experimentation to arrive more rapidly at the desired information. For example, Peters [25-26] proposed a method for assessing "lineshape" mismatch between simulated and observed oral profiles to gain mechanistic insights into processes impacting absorption and PK (e.g., saturable metabolism, enterohepatic cycling, transporter involvement in absorption from the gut, and regional variation in gut absorption). In related work, Peters and Hultin [27] used a similar approach to identify drug-induced delays in gastric emptying.

Preclinical ADMET studies provide pharmaceutical scientists with quantitative information on the PK in preclinical species and qualitative information on the potential human PK behavior of a compound. Using PBPK modeling, the results of the various preclinical assays can be integrated to provide a quantitative prediction of human PK [5,41]. Once the PBPK model exists, it can be used to determine which compounds have the largest impact on PK, providing chemists with additional clear information for the development of improved compounds.

During preclinical development, ADMET data is constantly being generated. A PBPK model can act as a repository of current information, and is easily updated when new PK or PD data become available. But adequate data are necessary to apply PBPK, which can be a limitation. For example, if a company does not generate hepatocyte or microsome data that can be scaled for a reasonably accurate estimate of metabolic clearance, the utility of PBPK is reduced.

3.2. Clinical candidate selection

Once PO PK data and detailed pharmaceutical data are available, physiologically based absorption modeling can be useful to verify that factors impacting oral absorption are understood and to help guide formulation development. Data on solubility, dissolution, precipitation, membrane permeation, whether a compound is a transporter substrate, and metabolic stability (particularly for CYP3A4, but other enzymes are also expressed in enterocytes [42]) are all important for predicting absorption [43]. PBPK models incorporate physiological information on the GI tract (e.g., transit times, pH values and transit times in the various regions). However, it can be important to carefully consider whether typical physiological conditions are appropriate for a given absorption simulation. For example, in typical dogs administered a solution, the stomach pH might be over 7, but in pentagastrin-pretreated dogs the stomach pH might be less than 3 for a period of time [44].

Absorption modeling can be very useful at later stages, e.g., for predicting whether PK will be different when a compound is administered with food. Jones et al. [28] developed GastroPlus human oral absorption models for six compounds. Food effects were predicted for a range of doses and compared to the results from human food effect studies. In general, the models were able to predict whether a food effect would be major (i.e., for two compounds) or minor (i.e., for four compounds).

PBPK can assist with clinical candidate selection where numerous factors must be considered and data related to the PK and PD of a compound need to be combined and compared in a rational way. Parrott et al. [20] demonstrated the use of PBPK modeling to select the best compound from among five candidates for the clinical lead. The preclinical data for each candidate was integrated and the efficacious human doses and associated plasma exposures were estimated. The PBPK models were linked to an Emax PD model so that the dose resulting in a 90% effect could be identified. This example showed that the PBPK approach facilitates a sound decision on the selection of the optimal molecule to be progressed by integrating the available information and focusing the attention onto the expected properties in human. Importantly, the method can include estimates of variability and uncertainty in the predictions to verify that decisions are based on significant differences between compounds.

3.3. Supporting entry into humans

After a clinical candidate has been selected, the first-in-human (FIH) dose must be selected. One method for selecting the FIH dose is to use a human PK model (developed based on preclinical ADMET data) to determine the dose that will result in a systemic exposure identified as therapeutic based on preclinical pharmacology data [45]. Determining the exposure required for efficacy requires a good understanding of the PK/PD relationship and what is driving the PD, be it Cmin, Cmax, AUC, or time above a threshold concentration.

Regardless of what is driving the PD, a human PBPK model can be used to determine the dose and regimen that can meet the efficacy requirement.

Luttringer et al. [41] examined the ability of PBPK modeling to predict human PK using epiroprim as a test compound due to significant species differences in its PK properties. By incorporating information on species differences in PK properties from in vitro studies (e.g., in protein binding, the blood-to-plasma ratio, and intrinsic clearance in hepatocytes), PBPK modeling was able to reduce the uncertainty inherent in interspecies extrapolation and to provide a better prediction of human PK than allometric scaling or by direct scaling of hepatocyte data.

Recently, Jones et al. [5] reported a method for predicting human PK based on preclinical data by separately predicting absorption, distribution and elimination from a physiological perspective. Human PK of 19 compounds that had entered into humans was predicted using Dedrick plot analysis (i.e., a type of allometric scaling of concentration-time profiles) and PBPK modeling. The ability of PBPK modeling to predict PK in preclinical species was tested, and the human PK was only predicted if the model could predict PK in preclinical species. Based on this criterion, for 70% of the 19 compounds included in the study a human PK prediction could be made. The prediction accuracy using PBPK was good for oral clearance, volume of distribution, terminal elimination half-life, Cmax, AUC, and tmax. The human PK data were more accurately predicted by the PBPK modeling approach than by the empirical approach. The strategy proposed by Jones et al. [5] can guide the strategy for gathering the data necessary for a complete understanding of likely human PK behavior.

Poor predictions with PBPK models are often a result of incomplete knowledge resulting in processes not correctly incorporated into the model (e.g., for biliary clearance and enterohepatic recirculation there are limited options for quantitatively predicting the effects on human PK). For such situations, an alternative method of performing the human PK extrapolation (e.g., allometric scaling) might seem attractive. However, allometric scaling is based on the assumption that clearance is proportional to $BW^{0.75}$ and that steady-state volume of distribution is proportional to BW^1 due to physiological properties (i.e., the same physiological properties that are incorporated in PBPK models). If PBPK modeling does not appear to be a good method for a compound, there is no reason to believe that allometric scaling or other empirical methods will work either. Additionally, developing methods for including increasingly complex PK mechanisms (e.g., first-pass metabolism and transporters in the gut, EH cycling, biliary excretion, impact of transporters on tissue concentration and elimination, and multiple pathways of elimination) is an active area of research, and methods for predicting human PK even with PK complications is increasingly possible.

In cases where uncertainty is high, the PBPK model can be a valuable tool for determining appropriate experiments and simulating "what-if" scenarios. Uncertainty can be illustrated by presenting a range of results (e.g., AUC, Cmax, Cmin, or complete time-course concentrations) for a range of values of a key parameter that is not known with great certainty. If uncertainty is too great, additional experiments can be designed to aid in narrowing the possible values of key parameters. PBPK modeling can be used as a tool to understand the quantitative impact of uncertainty from key knowledge gaps, and also helps to minimize uncertainty due to species differences in PK properties.

3.4. Clinical development

Population PK approaches and nonlinear mixed effect modeling are the techniques most used for analysis of clinical data. The Bayesian population PK approach can also be applied with PBPK models [46-47]. But this alternative has not been adopted by the pharmaceutical industry. Although several useful clinical applications of PBPK models have been demonstrated in the literature including the following examples, there are many potentially valuable applications that remain to be exploited [48].

PBPK simulations can be used to optimize clinical design. Chenel et al. [30] recently demonstrated selecting time points for an optimized sparse sampling design for a DDI clinical trial using Monte Carlo simulations for the victim midazolam and the CYP3A4 inhibitor that was the test compound. The PBPK models were parameterized using only in vitro data. The PBPK predictions of PK for both compounds were good using the PBPK model, but for the test compound variability was overestimated somewhat [32]. Regardless, data from the optimized trial design resulted in similar CL/F estimates and the same conclusion as the full empirical design upon analysis using a population PK approach.

Blesch et al. [32] demonstrated how PBPK modeling could fit into a clinical modeling strategy for capecitabine, a triple prodrug of 5-fluorouracil. For capecitabine, the modeling strategy included nonlinear mixed-effect modeling and PK/PD modeling for safety and efficacy to analyze clinical data. Nevertheless, a simple PBPK model incorporating the GI tract, blood, liver, tumor, and non-eliminating tissues compartments describing the PK of capecitabine and three metabolites including 5-fluorouracil was still useful for drug development. This approach allowed mechanistic knowledge gained preclinically to be leveraged. The PBPK model provided a tool for understanding the relationship between the dose of the triple prodrug capecitabine and the delivery of active compound to the tumor.

Because of the heterogeneity of the human population, it is expected that there will be a broad range of responses to biological effects of drugs. This heterogeneity is produced by interindividual variations in physiology, biochemistry, and molecular biology, reflecting both genetic and environmental factors, and results in differences among individuals in PK and PD. Because the parameters in a PBPK model have a direct biological correspondence, they provide a useful framework for determining the impact of observed variations in physiological and biochemical factors on the population variability in dosimetry. Willman et al. [49] demonstrated an approach for generically incorporating interindividual differences in physiological parameters using PK-Sim and showed that for two drugs, ciproflaxin and paclitaxel, the predicted variability was close to that observed clinically. Predicting variability in PK from factors including genetics (e.g., polymorphisms in enzymes that metabolize drugs), disease state (e.g., hepatic impairment or impaired renal function), and age from pediatric to elderly patients is a useful application of PBPK [19].

http://dx.doi.org/10.5772/54965

Recently there has been considerable work ongoing to predict PK of drugs in the pediatric population using PBPK modeling. For such simulations, the PBPK model must incorporate age-specific differences in body weight, organ weights, blood flows to tissue compartments, compartment volumes, plasma protein binding, renal function, and hepatic P450 expression levels, among other factors [50-51]. A recent study demonstrated successfully predicting PK in children for acetaminophen, alfentanil, morphine, theophylline, and levofloxacin, based on existing PBPK models for adults verified and/or calibrated using adult PK data [34]. This approach has utility in designing clinical trials for the first time dosing in children [50]. PBPK modeling can also be applied to predict PK in infants and neonates, e.g., as was done for oseltamivir [52]. PBPK modeling has been proposed as a useful tool benefitting the learn-and-confirm paradigm in pediatric trials and improving pediatric drug development programs [53].

The mechanistic basis of PBPK modeling also allows the modification of physiological parameters to describe disease state. For example, the physiological changes with cirrhosis of the liver include alterations in hepatic P450 expression and liver size, albumin and α-1 acid glycoprotein, blood flows, and renal function [54]. These physiological differences can be specifically incorporated in the PBPK model, allowing the prediction of PK in the population of people suffering from cirrhosis of the liver. The ability to predict PK for lidocaine and alfentanil for patients with differing degrees of cirrhosis was recently demonstrated by Edginton and Willmann [33] with promising results.

3.5. Support for regulatory decision making

Recent publications and regulatory guidance documents indicate that PBPK modeling is becoming increasingly useful from a regulatory perspective. The EMA has indicated that PBPK modeling can be a useful tool for the clinical investigation of hepatic impairment on pharmacokinetics [55]. Both the FDA and EMA in their drug-drug interaction (DDI) guidance documents mention PBPK modeling as a useful tool, e.g., for supporting DDI understanding and for designing DDI studies, and potentially for supporting labeling [56-57]. The FDA experience with applications of PBPK modeling during regulatory review [58-59] and pediatric drug trials [53] have been described. Clinical pharmacology reviewers at the FDA have done PBPK modeling to address PK and/or DDI issues in cases where the sponsor did not [58].

Guidance on best practices for PBPK modeling in addressing regulatory questions has been offered [60]. The successful application of PBPK modeling requires sufficient data and understanding of key processes impacting PK. For example, for using PBPK modeling to understand and simulate DDIs, information is needed on the mechanism of elimination and the fraction of compound metabolized through various pathways (e.g., mediated by different P450s). It has been recommended that a human, in vivo mass balance study be completed for the greatest confidence in DDI simulations [58]. To use PBPK modeling to address a regulatory issue, not only must sufficient data be available, but the effect of physiology on PK for a given issue must be understood. Potential data gaps such as a lack of understanding of development-related and disease-related effects on physiology and PK can limit application of PBPK in certain situations.

An early example of the application of PBPK in regulatory decision making is the case of a safety assessment for retinoic acid [61]. In the early 1990s all-trans retinoic acid (ATRA) was being considered for marketing approval by the Food and Drug Administration (FDA) for the indication of photo-damaged skin (wrinkles). The director of the FDA Center for Drug Evaluation and Research (CDER) requested the sponsor to evaluate, using PBPK simulation, the potential fetal exposure to ATRA applied topically in women of reproductive age. Aware that ATRA, like its isomer 13-cis retinoic acid, is highly teratogenic and that up to 10% of a topically applied dosage is absorbed systemically, FDA sought reassurance that significant fetal exposure and teratogenic effect potential would not result during clinical use. PBPK simulation was considered the only rational and ethical method of risk assessment available. The sponsor supported a PBPK analysis [4] that provided the necessary assurance to the FDA during its review and subsequent approval. FDA encourages sponsors to adopt PBPK, when appropriate and depending on the questions, during drug development with the aim to facilitate and enhance the capability to make better predictions, improve understanding, and provide improved regulatory decision making [61].

4. Future directions

4.1. Interindividual variability

As described in a previous section, investigators have begun using PBPK to understand variability from several sources: (1) variations across a population of healthy adults from physiological differences (e.g., body weight or sex) [62] or genetic polymorphisms [63]; (2) variations across a population from age differences, e.g., infants or the elderly [64-65]; and (3) variations from health status (e.g., from differences in protein or enzyme expression, tissue blood flow, or tissue compartment volumes or function altered by disease state) [33]. To the extent that the variation in physiological and biochemical parameters across these population dimensions can be elucidated, PBPK models can be used together with Monte Carlo uncertainty analysis to integrate their effects on the *in vivo* kinetics of a compound and predict the resulting impact on the distribution of PK across the population. The use of Monte Carlo uncertainty analysis has been described for drugs [66-67], but the ability of this powerful approach to evaluate the impact of interindividual variability on clinical trials outcomes is not yet fully utilized in the pharmaceutical industry.

There has been a tendency in drug development to use information on the variability of a specific parameter, such as the *in vitro* activity of a particular enzyme, as the basis for expectations regarding the variability in dosimetry for *in vivo* exposures. However, whether or not the variation in a particular physiological or biochemical parameter will have a significant impact on *in vivo* dosimetry is a complex function of interacting factors. In particular, the structures of physiological and biochemical systems frequently involve parallel processes (e.g., blood flows, metabolic pathways, excretion processes), leading to compensation for the variation in a single factor. Moreover, physiological constraints may limit the *in vivo* impact of variability observed *in vitro*. For instance, high affinity intrinsic clearance can result in essentially complete metabolism of all the compound reaching the liver in the blood; under these conditions, variability in amount metabolized *in vivo* would be more a function of variability in liver blood flow than variability in metabolism *in vitro*. Thus it is often true that the whole (the *in vivo* variability in dosimetry) is less than the sum of its parts (the variability in each of the PK factors). Due to the complex interactions among factors impacting PK, speculation regarding the extent of population variability on the basis of the observed variation in a single factor can be highly misleading. This possibility has been illustrated in the case of the impact of the CYP2C9 polymorphism on warfarin kinetics [63].

4.2. Modeling of pharmacodynamics

The growing popularity of the PBPK modeling approach represents a movement from simpler kinetic models toward more biologically realistic descriptions of the determinants that regulate disposition of drugs in the body. To a large extent, the application of these PBPK models to study the time courses of compounds in the body is simply an integrated systems approach to understanding the biological processes that regulate the delivery of drugs to target sites. Many PBPK models integrate information across multiple levels of organization, especially when describing interactions of compounds with molecular targets, such as reversible binding of ligands to specific receptors, as in the case of methotrexate binding to dihydrofolate reductase [13,68]. In such cases, the PBPK models integrate molecular, cellular, organ level, and organism-level processes to account for the time courses of compounds, metabolites, and bound complexes within organs and tissues in the body.

While the goal in applying a PBPK model is to predict plasma and tissue concentrations of a drug, the overall goal of using PBPK modeling in efficacy and safety assessment with drugs is broader. PBPK models once developed are extensible. The goal in the larger context is to understand the relationship between dose administered, the dose reaching the active site, and the resulting biological response. The specific steps that lead from these dose metrics to tissue, organ and organism-level responses, have usually been considered part of the PD process. In general, PD models used in drug evaluation have been more empirical, utilizing simple effect compartments correlated with blood or tissue concentrations of active compound. Inexorably, the systems approach will advance into the PBPK/PD and physiologically based pharmacodynamics (PBPD) arena, i.e., into a systems biology approach for describing perturbations of biological systems by compounds and the exposure/dose conditions under which these perturbations become sufficiently large to pose significant health risks or to achieve specific therapeutic outcomes. In fact, PBPK/PD models of toxic effects have been demonstrated to be useful for risk assessment purposes, as in the case of a PBPK/PD model linking chloroform metabolism, reparable cell damage, cell death, and regenerative cellular proliferation [69].

The systems biology approach focuses on normal biological function and the perturbations associated with exposure to compounds. Perturbations of biological processes by compounds lead to either adverse responses (toxicity) or restoration of normal function to a compromised tissue (efficacy). The effects of compounds, whether for good or ill, can best be described by PBPK approaches linked through PBPD models of responses of cellular signaling networks. Toxicity and efficacy are then defined by an intersection of compound action with the biological system. Toxicology and pharmacology are disciplines at the interface of chemistry/pharmacokinetics and biology/pharmacodynamics. Clearly, the main differences in the next generation of systems approaches in PK and PD modeling will be the increasingly detailed descriptions of biology afforded by new technologies and the expansion of modeling tools available for describing the effects of compounds on biological signaling processes.

Of particular importance, in using a PBPK model the pharmacodynamic effects of a drug can be investigated more directly, relating the effects to free concentration in the tissue (e.g., the brain) where the compound interacts with the biological system, rather than attempting to elucidate a potentially indirect relationship with plasma concentrations. By obtaining quantitative information on the dose-responses for both the efficacy and toxicity of the compound, the PBPK model can be exercised to evaluate the potential to increase the efficacy/toxicity ratio of the drug through manipulation of dose and route using novel drug delivery systems. These and other attributes of PBPK models for organizing and interpreting diverse data sets, with the specific goals of understanding efficacy and toxicity, are reviving interest in applying these tools in drug development and evaluation [32].

The rapid development of computational chemistry [70], genomics [71], and high-throughput screening [72] has brought increasing attention to the discovery phase of drug development, including growing interest in "discovery toxicology" [73]. PBPK modeling can play a complementary role to two other technologies that are finding increasing use in drug discovery: QSAR analysis and genomics. QSAR can be used to estimate compound-specific parameters for the PBPK model, while genomic data can provide mode of action insights that drive model structure decisions such as the selection of the appropriate dose metric and its linkage to pharmacodynamic elements. The PBPK model provides a quantitative biological framework for integrating the physicochemical characteristics of the drug candidate, together with *in vitro* data on its ADME and toxicity, within the constraints of the fundamental physiological and biochemical processes governing compound behavior *in vivo*. This approach is particularly effective when used consistently during drug development, because the information gained from modeling of previous candidate compounds can greatly facilitate model development for new compounds with similar structures or properties.

5. Conclusions

PBPK modeling has been identified as a technology that can be used by the pharmaceutical industry to accelerate the drug development process [17,62,74-75]. Conveniently, ADMET data typically generated during preclinical development can be used to develop PBPK models. PBPK models allow better use of these data by serving as a structured repository for quantitative information on the compound, a conceptual framework for hypothesis testing, and a quantitative platform for prediction. The power of PBPK modeling for understanding properties underlying PK and for allowing uncertainty and variability analysis make this tool valuable to the pharmaceutical industry.

http://dx.doi.org/10.5772/54965

Author details

Micaela B. Reddy[1], Harvey J. Clewell III[2], Thierry Lave[3] and Melvin E. Andersen[2]

*Address all correspondence to: HClewell@theHamner.org

1 Hoffmann-La Roche Inc., Nutley, New Jersey, USA

2 The Hamner Institutes for Health Sciences, Research Triangle Park, North Carolina, USA

3 Hoffmann-La Roche Inc., Basel, Switzerland

References

[1] Clewell HJ III, Reddy MB, Lave T, Andersen ME. Physiologically Based Pharmacokinetic Modeling. In: Gad SC. (ed.) Preclinical Drug Development Handbook. Hoboken: John Wiley & Sons; 2008. p. 1167-1227.

[2] Aarons L. Editors' view. Physiologically based pharmacokinetic modeling: a sound mechanistic basis is needed. British J Clin Pharm 2005;60(6) 581-583.

[3] Dedrick RL, Bischoff KB. Species similarities in pharmacokinetics. Fed Proc 1980;39: 54-59.

[4] Clewell HJ, Andersen ME, Wills RJ, Latriano L. A physiologically based pharmacokinetic model for retinoic acid and its metabolites. J Am Acad Dermatol 1997;36: S77-85.

[5] Jones HM, Parrott N, Jorga K, Lave T. A novel strategy for physiologically based predictions of human pharmacokinetics. Clin Pharmacokinet 2006;45: 511-542.

[6] Andersen ME, Yang RSH, Clewell HJ, Reddy MB. Introduction: A Historical Perspective of the Development and Application of PBPK Models. In: Reddy MB, Yang RSH, Clewell HJ III, Andersen ME. (eds.) Physiologically Based Pharmacokinetic Modeling: Science and Applications. Hoboken: John Wiley & Sons; 2005. p. 1-18.

[7] Reddy MB, Yang RSH, Clewell HJ III, Andersen ME, editors. Physiologically Based Pharmacokinetic Modeling: Science and Applications. Hoboken: John Wiley & Sons; 2005.

[8] Martinez MN, Amidon GL. A mechanistic approach to understanding the factors affecting drug absorption: A review of fundamentals. J Clin Pharmacol 2002;42: 620-643.

[9] Teorell T. Kinetics of distribution of substances administered to the body. I. The extravascular mode of administration. Arch Int Pharmacodyn 1937;57: 205-225.

[10] Teorell T. Kinetics of distribution of substances administered to the body. I. The intravascular mode of administration. Arch Int Pharmacodyn 1937;57: 226-240.

[11] Andersen ME. Saturable metabolism and its relation to toxicity. Crit Rev Toxicol 1981;9:105-150.

[12] Bischoff KB, Brown RG. Drug distribution in mammals. Chem Eng Prog Symp Ser 1966;62(66): 33-45.

[13] Bischoff KB, Dedrick RL, Zaharko DS, Longstreth, JA. Methotrexate pharmacokinetics. J Pharm Sci 1971;60: 1128-1133.

[14] Collins JM, Dedrick RL, Flessner MF, Guarino AM. Concentration dependent disappearance of fluorouracil from peritoneal fluid in the rat: Experimental observations and distributed modeling. J Pharm Sci 1982;71: 735-738.

[15] Farris FF, Dedrick RL, King FG. Cisplatin pharmacokinetics: Applications of a physiological model. Toxicol Lett 1988;43, 117-137.

[16] Lupfert C, Reichel A. Development and application of physiologically based pharmacokinetic-modeling tools to support drug discovery. Chem & Biodiversity 2005;2: 1462-1486.

[17] Nestorov I. Whole body pharmacokinetic models. Clin Pharmacokinet 2003;42: 883-908.

[18] Lave T, Parrott N, Grimm HP, Fleury A, Reddy M. Challenges and opportunities with modelling and simulation in drug discovery and drug development. Xenobiotica 2007;37(10-11): 1295-1310.

[19] Rowland M, Peck C, Tucker G. (2011). Physiologically-based pharmacokinetics in drug development and regulatory science. Cho AK (ed.). Book series, Annual Review of Pharmacology and Toxicology, vol 51, pp. 45-73.

[20] Parrott N, Jones H, Paquereau N, Lave T. Application of full physiological models for pharmaceutical drug candidate selection and extrapolation of pharmacokinetics to man. Basic & Clin Pharmacol & Toxicol 2005;96: 193–199.

[21] Brightman FA, Leahy DE, Searle GE, Thomas, S. Application of a generic physiologically based pharmacokinetic model to the estimation of xenobiotic levels in rat plasma. Drug Metab Disposition 2006;34: 84-93.

[22] Brightman FA, Leahy DE, Searle GE, Thomas S. Application of a generic physiologically based pharmacokinetic model to the estimation of xenobiotic levels in human plasma. Drug Metab Disposition 2006;34: 94-101.

[23] Parrott N, Paquereau N, Coassolo P, Lave T. An evaluation of the utility of physiologically based models of pharmacokinetics in early drug discovery. J Pharm Sci 2005;94: 2327-2343.

[24] Berry P, Parrott N, Reddy M, David-Pierson P, Lavé T. Putting it all together. Faller B, Urban L. (eds.) In: Hit and Lead Profiling: Identification and Optimization of Drug-like Molecules. In book series, Methods and Principles in Medicinal Chemistry. Series edited by R Mannhold, H Kubinyi and G Folkers. Hoboken: John Wiley & Sons; 2010. p. 221-242.

[25] Peters S. Evaluation of a generic physiologically based pharmacokinetic model for lineshape analysis. Clin Pharmacokinet 2008;47: 261-275.

[26] Peters SA. Identification of intestinal loss of a drug through physiologically based pharmacokinetic simulation of plasma concentration-time profiles. Clin Pharmacokinet 2008;47(4): 245-259.

[27] Peters SA, Hultin L. Early identification of drug-induced impairment of gastric emptying through physiologically based pharmacokinetic (PBPK) simulation of plasma concentration-time profiles in rat. J Pharmacokinet Pharmacodynam 2008;35(1): 1-30.

[28] Jones HM, Parrott N, Ohlenbusch G, Lavé T. Predicting pharmacokinetic food effects using biorelevant solubility media and physiologically based modelling. Clin Pharmacokinet 2006;45: 1213-1226.

[29] Jamei M, Dickinson GL, Rostami-Hodjegan A. A framework for assessing inter-individual variability in pharmacokinetics using virtual human populations and integrating general knowledge of physical chemistry, biology, anatomy, physiology and genetics: A tale of 'bottom-up' vs 'top-down' recognition of covariates. Drug Metab Pharmacokinet 2009;24(1): 53-75.

[30] Chenel M, Bouzom F, Aarons L, Ogungbenro K. Drug-drug interaction predictions with PBPK models and optimal multiresponse sampling time designs: application to midazolam and a phase I compound. Part 1: comparison of uniresponse and multiresponse designs using PopDes. J Pharmacokinet Pharmacodynam 2008;35(6): 635-659.

[31] Chenel M, Bouzom F, Cazade F, Ogungbenro K, Aarons L, Mentre F. Drug-drug interaction predictions with PBPK models and optimal multiresponse sampling time designs: application to midazolam and a phase I compound. Part 2: clinical trial results. J Pharmacokinet Pharmacodynam 2008;35(6): 661-681.

[32] Blesch KS, Gieschke R, Tsukamoto Y, Reigner BG, Burger HU, Steimer JL. Clinical pharmacokinetic/pharmacodynamic and physiologically based pharmacokinetic modeling in new drug development: the capecitabine experience. Invest New Drugs 2003;21(2): 195-223.

[33] Edginton AN, Willmann S. Physiology-based simulations of a pathological condition prediction of pharmacokinetics in patients with liver cirrhosis. Clin Pharmacokin 2008;47(11): 743-752.

[34] Edginton AN, Schmitt W, Willmann S. Development and evaluation of a generic physiologically based pharmacokinetic model for children. Clin Pharmacokin 2006;45(10): 1013-1034.

[35] Lave T, Dupin S, Schmitt C, Valles B, Ubeaud G, Chou RC, Jaeck D, Coassolo P. The use of human hepatocytes to select compounds based on their expected hepatic extraction ratios in humans. Pharm Res 1997;14: 152-155.

[36] Thompson,TN. Early ADME in support of drug discovery: The role of metabolic stability studies. Current Drug Metabolism 2000;1: 215-241.

[37] Poggesi I. Predicting human pharmacokinetics from preclinical data. Current Opinion in Drug Discovery & Development 2004;7: 100-111.

[38] Hinderling PH. Red blood cells: A neglected compartment in pharmacokinetics and pharmacodynamics. Pharmacol Rev 1997;49: 279-295.

[39] Riley RJ, McGinnity DF, Austin RP. A unified model for predicting human hepatic, metabolic clearance from *in vitro* intrinsic clearance data in hepatocytes and microsomes. Drug Metab Disposition 2005;33: 1304-1311.

[40] Obach RS. Prediction of human clearance of twenty-nine drugs from hepatic microsomal intrinsic clearance data: An examination of *in vitro* half-life approach and nonspecific binding to microsomes. Drug Metab Disposition 1999;27: 1350-1359.

[41] Luttringer O, Theil F-P, Poulin P, Schmitt-Hoffmann AH, Guentert TW, Lave T. Physiologically based pharmacokinetic (PBPK) modeling of disposition of epiroprim in humans. J Pharm Sci 2003;92: 1990–2007.

[42] Yang JS, Jamei M, Yeo KR, Tucker GT, Rostami-Hodjegan A. Prediction of intestinal first-pass drug metabolism. Curr Drug Metab 2007;8(7): 676-684.

[43] Sugano K. Introduction to computational oral absorption simulation. Expert Opinion Drug Metab & Toxicol 2009;5(3): 259-293.

[44] Akimoto M, Nagahata N, Furuya A, Fukushima K, Higuchi S, Suwa T. Gastric pH profiles of beagle dogs and their use as an alternative to human testing. Eur J Pharmaceutics Biopharm 2000;49(2): 99-102.

[45] Reigner BG, Blesch KS. Estimating the starting dose for entry into humans: Principles and practice. Eur J Clin Pharmacol 2002;57: 835-845.

[46] Gueorguieva I, Aarons L, Rowland M. Diazepam pharamacokinetics from preclinical to phase I using a Bayesian population physiologically based pharmacokinetic model with informative prior distributions in WinBUGS. J Pharmacokinet Pharmacodyn 2006;33(5): 571-594.

[47] Langdon G, Gueorguieva I, Aarons L, Karlsson M. Linking preclinical and clinical whole-body physiologically based pharmacokinetic models with prior distributions in NONMEM. Eur J Clin Pharmacol 2007;63(5): 485-498.

[48] Edginton AN, Theil FP, Schmitt W, Willmann S. Whole body physiologically-based pharmacokinetic models: their use in clinical drug development. Exp Opin Drug Metab Toxicol 2008;4(9): 1143-1152.

[49] Willmann S, Hohn K, Edginton A, Sevestre M, Solodenko J, Weiss W, Lippert J, Schmitt W. Development of a physiology-based whole-body population model for assessing the influence of individual variability on the pharmacokinetics of drugs. J Pharmacokin Pharmacodyn 2007;34(3): 401-431.

[50] Bouzom F, Walther B. Pharmacokinetic predictions in children by using the physiologically based pharmacokinetic modeling. Fundamental Clin Pharmacol 2008;22(6): 579-587.

[51] Ginsberg G, Hattis D, Sonawane B. Incorporating pharmacokinetic differences between children and adults in assessing children's risks to environmental toxicants. Toxicol Appl Pharmacol 2004;198(2): 164-183.

[52] Parrott N, Davies B, Hoffmann G, Koerner A, Lave T, Prinssen E, Theogaraj E, Singer T. Development of a physiologically based model for oseltamivir and simulation of pharmacokinetics in neonates and infants. Clin Pharmacokinet 2011;50(9): 613-623.

[53] Leong R, Vieira MLT, Zhao P, Mulugeta Y, Lee CS, Huang SM, Burckart GJ. Regulatory experience with physiologically based pharmacokinetic modeling for pediatric drug trials. Clin Pharmacol & Ther 2012;91: 926-931.

[54] Johnson TN, Boussery K, Rowland-Yeo K, Tucker GT, Rostami-Hodjegan A. A semi-mechanistic model to predict the effects of liver cirrhosis on drug clearance. Clin Pharmacokinet 2010;49 (3): 189-206.

[55] European Medicines Agency. (2005). Guideline on the Evaluation of the Pharmacokinetics of Medicinal Products in Patients with Impaired Hepatic Function. Committee for Human Medicinal Products (CHMP), London, United Kingdom. 17 Feb 2005. http://www.ema.europa.eu/docs/en_GB/document_library/Scientific_guideline/2009/09/WC500003122.pdf.

[56] European Medicines Agency. (2012). Guideline on the Investigation of Drug Interactions. Committee for Human Medicinal Products (CHMP), London, United Kingdom. Final guideline, 21 June 2012. http://www.ema.europa.eu/docs/en_GB/document_library/Scientific_guideline/2012/07/WC500129606.pdf. Accessed 10 Sept 2012.

[57] Food and Drug Administration. (2012). Guidance for Industry. Drug Interaction Studies— Study Design, Data Analysis, Implications for Dosing, and Labeling Recommendations. Draft Guidance, February 2012. U.S. Department of Health and Human Services, Food and Drug Administration, Center for Drug Evaluation and Research (CDER), Silver Spring, Maryland. http://www.fda.gov/downloads/Drugs/GuidanceComplianceRegulatoryInformation/Guidances/ucm292362.pdf. Accessed 10 Sept 2012.

[58] Zhao P, Zhang L, Grillo JA, Liu Q, Bullock JM, Moon YJ, Song P, Brar SS, Madabushi R, Wu TC, Booth BP, Rahman NA, Reynolds KS, Berglund EG, Lesko LJ, Huang SM. Applications of physiologically based pharmacokinetic (PBPK) modeling and simulation during regulatory review. Clin Pharmacol & Ther 2011;89: 259-267.

[59] Huang S-M, Rowland M. The role of physiologically based pharmacokinetic modeling in regulatory review. Clin Pharmacol & Ther 2012;91: 542-549.

[60] Zhao P, Rowland M, Huang S-M. Best practice in the use of physiologically based pharmacokinetic modeling and simulation to address clinical pharmacology regulatory questions. Clin Pharmacol & Ther 2012;92: 17-20.

[61] Rowland M, Balant L, Peck C. Physiologically based pharmacokinetics in drug development and regulatory science: a workshop report (Georgetown University, Washington, DC, May 29-30, 2002). AAPS PharmSci 2004;6(1): E6.

[62] Price PS, Conolly RB, Chaisson CF, Gross EA, Young JS, Mathis ET, Tedder DR. Modeling interindividual variation in physiological factors used in PBPK models of humans. Crit Rev Toxicol 2003;33(5): 469-503.

[63] Gentry PR, Hack CE, Haber L, Maier A, Clewell III, HJ. An Approach for the Quantitative Consideration of Genetic Polymorphism Data in Chemical Risk Assessment: Examples with Warfarin and Parathion. Toxicol Sci 2002;70: 120-139.

[64] Clewell HJ, Gentry PR, Covington TR, Sarangapani R, Teeguarden JG. Evaluation of the potential impact of age- and gender-specific pharmacokinetic differences on tissue dosimetry. Toxicol Sci 2004;79: 381-393.

[65] Clewell HJ, Teeguarden J, McDonald T, Sarangapani R, Lawrence G, Covington T, Gentry PR, Shipp AM. Review and evaluation of the potential impact of age and gender-specific pharmacokinetic differences on tissue dosimetry. Crit Rev Toxicol 2002;32(5): 329-389.

[66] Gueorguieva I, Nestorov IA, Aarons L, Rowland M. Uncertainty analysis in pharmacokinetics and pharmacodynamics: application to naratriptan. Pharm Res 2005;22(10): 1614-1626.

[67] Gueorguieva II, Nestorov IA, Rowland M. Fuzzy simulation of pharmacokinetic models: case study of whole body physiologically based model of diazepam. J Pharmacokinet Pharmacodyn 2004;31(3): 185-213.

[68] Dedrick RL. Pharmacokinetic and pharmacodynamic considerations for chronic hemodialysis. Kidney Int 1975;7(Suppl 2), S7-S15.

[69] Liao KH, Tan YM, Conolly RB, Borghoff SJ, Gargas ML, Andersen ME, Clewell HJ. Bayesian estimation of pharmacokinetic and pharmacodynamic parameters in a mode-of-action-based cancer risk assessment for chloroform. Risk Anal 2007;27(6): 1535-1551.

[70] Jorgensen WL. The many roles of computation in drug discovery. Science 2004;303(5665): 1813-1818.

[71] Ricke DO, Wang S, Cai R, Cohen D. Genomic approaches to drug discovery. Curr Opin Chem Biol 2006;10(4): 303-308.

[72] Lahoz A, Gombau L, Donato MT, Castell JV, Gomez-Lechon MJ. In vitro ADME medium/high-throughput screening in drug preclinical development. Mini Rev Med Chem 2006;6(9): 1053-1062.

[73] van de Waterbeemd H, Gifford E. ADMET in silico modelling: towards prediction paradise? Nat Rev Drug Discov 2003;2(3): 192-204.

[74] Peck CC, Barr WH, Benet LZ, Collins J, Desjardins RE, Furst DE, Harter JG, Levy G, Ludden T, Rodman JH, et al. Opportunities for integration of pharmacokinetics, pharmacodynamics, and toxicokinetics in rational drug development. J Pharm Sci 1992;81(6): 605-10.

[75] Charnick SB, Kawai R, Nedelman JR, Lemaire M, Niederberger W, Sato H. Perspectives in pharmacokinetics. Physiologically based pharmacokinetic modeling as a tool for drug development. J Pharmacokinet Biopharm 1995;23: 217-229.

Chapter 10

Plasma Methadone Level Monitoring in Methadone Maintenance Therapy: A Personalised Methadone Therapy

Nasir Mohamad, Roslanuddin Mohd Salehuddin, Basyirah Ghazali, Nor Hidayah Abu Bakar, Nurfadhlina Musa, Muslih Abdulkarim Ibrahim, Liyana Hazwani Mohd Adnan, Ahmad Rashidi and Rusli Ismail

Additional information is available at the end of the chapter

http://dx.doi.org/10.5772/54850

1. Introduction

1.1. Opioid substitution therapy

Substitution therapy for opiate abusers reduces dependencies on illicit drugs by utilizing opioid agonists that bind to opioid receptors in the brain. Apart from the physical benefits of reducing cravings and withdrawal symptoms, it also plays a role in reducing other problems associated with opioid abuse. Their longer duration of action means they do not require frequent administration and hence enables patients to carry out activities of daily living without disruption. The spread of infectious blood borne diseases is also curbed by the fact that they are usually administered orally [1].

Methadone and buprenorphine are the two most commonly prescribed and effective opioid agonists for substitution maintenance therapy in Malaysia as their oral preparation can avoid injecting behaviour among opiate users. Hence, the harm reduction promotion will be further strengthen as injecting related behaviour among opiate users are the main contributor to HIV transmission in Malaysia. Methadone Maintenance Therapy (MMT) was started in 2005 through harm reduction programme and is getting a strong foothold since then. Therefore we are seeing a lot of opioid abuser on methadone in Emergency Department with potential overdose or withdrawal symptoms. A lot of these opiate abuser drafted into the program also frequently have whole hosts of other health problems such HIV, Hepatitis B and C or Tuberculosis which may complicate diagnosis and treatment.

MMT adds importantly to our ability to deal with the ever increasing menace of illicit drug use. Methadone is a long-acting drug. It occupies the opioid receptors at a slow pace and this creates a steady level of opioid in the blood. This characteristic avoids the "high and low" levels that generally occur with short-acting opioid administrations.

1.2. Methadone Pharmacokinetics (PK)

The efficacy of methadone is determined by the stability of methadone concentration in blood, and therefore in the action site located in the brain. Maximum concentration of methadone is reached around two to four hours after dose administration and gradually falls until the moment of next dose administration. As Methadone is extensively metabolized in the liver, its metabolic clearance is shown by the elimination rate of methadone. The clearance rate of methadone from the body was found to be 158 ml/ min and 129 ml/ min for (R)-methadone and (S)-methadone respectively. Main metabolite of methadone, which is 2-ethylidene-1, 5-dimethyl-3, 3-diphenylpyrrolidine is inactive. The apparent volumes of distribution were varies with mean values 3.9 l/kg [2]. Methadone is administered single daily as in methadone maintenance treatment, the average half-life of methadone is around 24 hours. This means that at the end of the 24th hour after dose administration, the concentration of methadone should have fallen to half its peak value. Most of us would consider the increasing methadone concentration in the blood is associated with the increasing dose. However, this general rules is not necessarily expected as we can see in the patients with methadone doses as high as 70–170 mg per day, have blood concentrations similar to those of patients whose doses are as low as 25 mg per day. It is note that the blood concentrations of methadone act as an indicator of its concentration in the action sites than the dose taken. Because of this, methadone plasma concentrations measured after 24 hours have repeatedly been proposed as a parameter for the evaluation of the adequacy of treatment. The necessary level of plasma methadone concentration is found between 150 and 600 ng/ml to counter for the craving effect of opioid addicts [3]. However, plasma concentration differs in different individuals and in single person under different conditions. The determinant factor for this variability include genetic factor, physiological, pathological, and pharmacological factor. Methadone is metabolized in the body by the enzymes of P450 cytochrome system . Polymorphism in cytochrome CYP450 can affect a higher or lower level of its activity and responsible for a more rapid or a slower elimination of methadone, with a consequent shortening or lengthening of methadone's half-life and a rise or fall in its levels in plasma. Concentration of methadone in blood is influenced by various steps of absorption, plasma protein binding, metabolism and excretion processes. Interference at the level of the P450 microsomal system also can cause an induction of the methadone metabolism, with a consequent fall in its levels in plasma, or an inhibition of its metabolism, with a rise in methadone levels in plasma. Less than 200 ng/ml is associated with poor compliance and higher than 700 ng/ml is associated with toxicity, ranges from excessive sedation with small pupils, respiratory depression and fatal tachyarrhythmia such as torsade de pointes (TdP) [4]. Based on the methadone concentration in plasma, inter-individual and intra-individual varieties persist in response to methadone. By studying plasma concentration, probably the optimum dose of methadone can be achieved faster and minimized unwanted side effect, therefore the patient will remain in the MMT programme [5]. Other special feature of methadone is it undergoes extended reversible absorption into tissues particularly the liver and hence steady-state concentrations can be achieved after multiple administrations. Methadone is usually administered orally and as such is rapidly absorbed. There are two processes involved in metabolizing methadone, primarily in the liver namely demethylation and cyclization. The cyclization process produces 2-Ethylidene-1, 5-dimethyl-3,3-diphenylpyrrolidine (EDDP) distinct from its parent molecule. Methadone and metabolites are primarily excreted in the feces. Unmetabolized methadone excretion in the urine accounts for less than 11% of the administered dose. It is excreted unchanged and as its metabolite in the urine. The excretion of methadone is markedly enhanced by the acidification of the urine

1.3. Methadone: AUC

Major measurements in pharmacokinetic study are plasma and urine. Plasma concentration data provides an important data in PK study. The AUC (the area under curve) can be presented graphically as the area under the plasma concentration versus time curve. AUC is an important parameter in PK analysis as it often used to measure the drug exposure. AUC plays many important roles in pharmacokinetics. AUC provides a measure how much and how long a drug stays in a body. [6] In other words, AUC shows an overall amount of drug in the bloodstream after a dose administration. Studying AUC probably is the best way to understand how people handle a drug. The plasma concentration of the drug measured by AUC can be useful for clinicians or doctors to optimize the drug dosage. Each person who takes methadone has differences in the way their body handles the drug in terms of absorption, distribution, metabolism and/or elimination processes. Therefore, a patient can have a high or low methadone blood levels after taking the same dose just because of the way they handle the drug. The PK of drug also changed by certain factors. For example, the blood levels of methadone can be increased or lowered by not following the food requirements with dosing, taking antacids with the drugs, or taking certain other drugs or herbals that can cause big inhibition or induction interactions in drug metabolism. Thus, it is important to find the dose requirements out so that patients know how best to take the drugs. Finally, the level of drug concentration in the body affect how well the drug works and whether the drug might cause side-effects, particularly in a case of high drug levels. Low levels of drug also can result in poor efficacy of the methadone maintenance treatments. In case of "therapeutic drug monitoring" (TDM), a doctor may think to measure methadone blood levels as a best idea to adjust the dose. Based on the results, the doses may be adjusted and then re-check the blood levels of drug to try and get them right where they want them [7]. Much information can be obtained on drug absorption, disposition of drug molecules between blood and tissues and drug elimination by measuring the amounts or the concentrations of drugs in blood, urines or other fluids or tissues at different times after the administration. AUC is a parameter that is dependent on the drug amount that enter into the systemic circulation and on the ability that the system has to eliminate the drug (clearance). Therefore it can be used to measure the drug amount absorbed or the efficiency of patient's physiological processes that characterize the drug elimination. Accurate estimation of the AUC can be achieved by applying "trapezoidal rule" [8]. AUC can be calculated by two PK models, which are linear PK models and non-linear PK models. Linear PK models are conducted without specifying any mathematical models (noncompartmental methods). It is helpful to use linear models as a guide in therapeutic decision making [9].

1.4. Volume of distribution (Vd)

The amount of drug in the body calculated from measurement of plasma concentration is assessed using a parameter called Volume of Distribution (Vd). The clinical importance of Vd is for computing a loading dose (eg. the first dose of a multiple dosage regimen) to reach the target therapeutic plasma concentration [10]. For example, if 1000 mg of a drug is given and the subsequent plasma concentration is 10 mg/L, that 1000 mg seems to be distributed in 100 L (dose/volume = concentration; 1000 mg/x L = 10 mg/L; therefore, x = 1000 mg/10 mg/L = 100 L). Vd is not the actual volume of the body or it's fluid compartment, but it is the distribution of a drug in the body. For the drug that is highly-bounded by a tissue, the dose that remains in the circulation is low, hence plasma concentration will be low and Vd will be high [11]. Methadone is a lipophilic drug and exhibits tissue distribution [12]. Methadone is also widely distributed to brain, kidney, gut, liver, muscle and lung with their specific plasma partition coefficients [13]. Vd of methadone is reported to be high in humans [14]. The apparent volume of distribution at steady-state (Vss) studied by other authors is much higher than actual physiological volume, indicating that methadone is predominantly tissue-bounded compared to plasma proteins binding. In opiate addicts, Vss of methadone ranged from 4.2 – 9.2 l/kg and in patient with chronic pain, the Vss is from 1.71 – 5.34 l/kg [15]. Methadone is highly bound to plasma protein by 86% and it is similar as reported in rats [16], [17]. Because of basic properties of methadone, it binds predominantly to α_1-acid glycoprotein (AAG) [18, 19]. AAG is an acute-phase serum protein that exhibits different concentration in plasma levels based on physiological or pathological conditions. In stress condition, AAG will increase and this will result in lower free fraction (*fu*) of methadone in plasma of cancer patients and opiate addicts compared in healthy volunteers [20,21]. Hence, after rapid administration of methadone, *fu* will decrease in early period and total plasma drug concentration (C_p) will increase as Vss is proportional to *fu*, but unbound plasma drug concentration (C_u) remains unchanged. A study on methadone distribution should pay attention on demographics features like weight and sex and AAG. About 33% Interindividual variability in Vss is due to sex and weight. Female exhibit higher Vss than male and this is related to weight. Meanwhile, a decrease in Vss is associated in time-dependent increase in AAG. [22]

1.5. Metabolism of methadone

Methadone is used clinically as a racemate, although R-enantiomers are responsible for the activation of opioid activity. The major pathway in methadone metabolism is *N*-demethylation to inactive 2-ethylidine-1,5- dimethyl-3,3-diphenylpyrrolidine (EDDP). This activity is mediated by cytochrome P450 CYP3A4 and CYP2B6 and somewhat by CYP2C19 in vitro which was less active [23]. In vitro, CYP2B6 is regarded as a predomi-

http://dx.doi.org/10.5772/54850

nant catalyst of stereo-selective methadone metabolism and may be a major determinant of methadone metabolism and disposition in vivo. In addition, CYP2B6 activity and stereo-selective metabolic interactions may confer variability in methadone disposition. CYP3A4 is the most abundant CYP form in the liver. No genetic polymorphism is observed in this enzyme. However, interindividual variability in the expression of this enzyme had been noted. CYP3A4 is inducible and this might be the reason for the induction of the methadone metabolism at the beginning of a maintenance treatment. Thus, a pattern of decrease in steady-state plasma levels of methadone is observed during maintenance treatment with racemic methadone [24]. Meanwhile, CYP2B6 gene is reported to be highly polymorphic. It is noted that CYP2B6 has a couple of variant alleles that are associated with lower expression/activity. Among of those alleles are CYP2B6*6, CYP2B6*16 and CYP2B6*18 in particular [25, 26, 27]. CYP2B6*6 is rather common in several different populations (20–30% frequency), whereas both CYP2B6*16 and CYP2B6*18 are common in Black subjects where the allele frequency is relatively high, about 7–9% [26, 27]. To a smaller extent CYP1A2 enzymes which is found in the kidney may also has influence on methadone metabolism. Knowledge from genotype analyses is importance in clinical use. It is an explanation for us to understand the therapeutic problem or a failure in question based from three major population phenotype, and these are poor metabolisers (PM), lack of functional enzyme due to defective or deleted genes, the extensive metabolizers (EM), carrying 2 functional genes; and the ultra-rapid metabolizers (UM), with more than 2 active genes encoding a certain P450 [27]. This genotyping analyses definitely will be a valuable aspect to contribute to a more efficient and safer drug therapy in the psychiatric clinic possible.

1.6. Dose of methadone

The believe that zero drug is best has similarly also led to frequent premature cessation of MMT, even though evidence suggests that maintenance therapy for at least two years is required for the maximum probability of success. Ironically the reason to discontinue MMT quite often comes from care providers working in maintenance programs. They often do not try to adequately address the reasons why patient was taking opioid was taken in the first place or the existence of coexisting psychiatric illnesses. This frequently results in increasing anxiety among patients that may explain their needs for other mood-altering drugs, such as the benzodiazepines. A lot of physicians who are directly involved in MMT programs in Malaysia or indeed worldwide are quite reluctant to increase dose to a required level due to the lack of understanding of methadone Adverse Drug Reactions (ADR). Although its efficacy and safety are well documented worldwide throughout the world, the bad perception of opioid is hard to shake off. A serious side effect like hypoventilation, respiratory depression, arrhythmia and prolonged QT interval were rare and normally occurs with other concomitant drugs such as benzodiazepine [28]. Most guidelines advises gradual increase in methadone dose to achieve sufficient tolerance so that an injection of any amount of street opioid will not be able to produce euphoria, thus eliminating the reward for injecting drugs. A high dose of methadone is usually required to achieve this effect and it averages 80 - 100 mg per day.

Typically when these principles are followed, MMT is effective with a tolerable adverse drug reaction (ADR), and the individual and society can gains from it.

It is however unfortunate that these principles are rarely followed. Consequently, although current knowledge supports a daily dose of at least 80 mg to 100 mg to abolish further craving for opioids, a big majority, including in Malaysia, are maintained on much lower doses [5, 28-31]. To ascertain optimal dosing for MMT in clinical settings is very challenging. As explained before, higher doses (> 80mg) had been postulated to have serious adverse drug reactions (ADR) while low dose encourage defaulter and illicit drug seeking behaviour. It has been observed that physicians are too afraid to maximize methadone dosage to a required level mainly due to misconception about its side effects. This study hopes to clarify this misconception and encourage physician to optimize personalized methadone dosing. In view of the heavy burden of opioids addiction to society generally and healthcare specifically, we choose to study about methadone substitution therapy and its implementation in details. Our focus is to compare the different of ADR between high dose methadone and low dose methadone. We hope that the results from our study will be able to highlights the main side effects in different methadone groups, its safety profile and ultimately encourage a higher dose MMT regime. An increasing importance of methadone as an effective substitution therapy, as well as its potential in treating chronic pain as in outpatient settings warranted further evaluation of its safety and efficacy [32-34]. Though we are likely producing results that have already been studied, we feel it is still important as these have never been shown in our local setting. Local data such as these is extremely important in trying to convince the authorities in adopting new and bold measures to combat the drug abuse menace and the rise of HIV in Malaysia.

By determining the relationship between clinical dose of methadone and its plasma level, the methadone prescribers would probably able to determine the relationship between clinical dose of methadone with its plasma level for a better optimum dose for the best effect and response. This would further helping physician in determining and evaluate the different withdrawal effects in opioid dependant subjects with different doses of methadone. The end point measurement of this would probably keep opioid dependent patients remain in the MMT programme for a better monitoring and curbing the spread of HIV infection through the intravenous routes.

2. Methods and material

This was a comparative prospective cross sectional study, in which the sample size will be selected from MMT clinic run by government institution (HUSM Psychiatric Department) and from the authorized private MMT centre (Klinik Sahabat, Kota Bharu).

The patients selected were already enrolled into MMT programme in these clinics. During recruitment phase, we will ensure that the subjects were already receiving daily methadone therapy for 6 month, hence minimize early adverse symptoms during induction phase. During

http://dx.doi.org/10.5772/54850

recruitment phase, baseline ECG from the clinics will be studied. If these pre-induction baseline ECGs shows corrected QT interval more than 450ms in male, they will be excluded from the study. This will filter out the subjects with the prolong QT interval caused by other condition such as long QT syndrome.

After recruitment the researcher will be blinded to the treatment regimes and methadone dosage. Recruited subjects then subsequently will be tested on urine drug test, electrolyte levels and questioned about concomitant drug used. If urine drug test was positive or electrolyte levels were abnormal or subjects were found to take medication that can alter Methadone level, they will be excluded from study. However they can still be included in the study during the next follow up.

Validated questionnaire will be used to grade the symptoms frequency according to the scale (0 = never, 1 = seldom, 2 = frequent). Vitals signs, pupil size measurement, and ECG will be taken using standardized equipment. Height, weight and other demographic data will be taken from patient file in the clinic. Then blood samples will be taken for plasma level measurement and genetic screening.

3. Results

3.1. Socio-demography

Forty nine subjects were enrolled into this study. All of our sample were Malay male, age between 19 – 50 years old (mean age 35.14 ± 6.66), weight ranged between 46kg to 73kg (mean weight 61.41± 6.53) and with a mean height of 167.76±5.21 cm, ranged between 154cm to 181cm, table 1. Mean value for heart rate, mean arterial pressure (MAP), respiratory rate, SPo2 and pupil size were 85 beat per min, 89.13 mmHg, 9 breath per min, 98% saturation and 3mm pupil size respectively (table 2).

Majority of patient had secondary education level (81.63%), 14.29% patients had education of high school level, and 2.04% had education level of degree. Majority of them were single (51%) while 34.7% were married and 7 or 14.3% of them were divorced.

Twenty patient or 40.8% was given less than 80mg oral methadone. Mean methadone dose was 85.51mg ± 29.85sd while mean plasma level of methadone was 235.26 (±153.27). Mean corrected QT interval was 442.49 (±20.42), table 3.

Variables (n= 49)	Minimum	Maximum	Mean	Std. Deviation
Height (cm)	154	181	167.76	5.206
Weight (kg)	46	73	61.41	6.529
Age(years)	19	50	35.14	6.658

Table 1. Descriptive statistics of height, weight and age of subjects

Variables (n = 49)	Minimum	Maximum	Mean	Std. Deviation
spo2 (%)	95	100	98.00	1.646
mean arterial pressure (mmHg)	69.33	113.33	89.92	12.363
pulse rate (/min)	62	117	85.45	14.348
respiratory rate (breath/min)	6	16	9.18	1.976
pupil size (mm)	1	3	2.61	0.571

Table 2. Descriptive statistics of vital signs of the study subjects

Variables (n = 49)	Minimum	Maximum	Mean	Std. Deviation
methadone dose (mg)	30	160	85.51	29.85
plasma methadone level (ng/ml)	26.90	708.50	235.26	153.27
QTc interval (ms)	409	500	442.49	20.42

Table 3. Descriptive Statistics of methadone dose, plasma methadone level and corrected QT interval

3.2. Methadone dose and its relationship with plasma methadone level

Methadone dosage in this study ranged between 30mg to 160mg with mean methadone dosage of 85.51±29.85mg. Mean plasma methadone was 235.56 mg (minimum 26.90mg and maximum of 708.50mg). Histogram for methadone dosage showed normal unimodal distribution curve (figure 1) which signify normal paramateric distribution. Table 4 showed the association between methadone dosage with its plasma level and other numerical variables. Using Simple Linear Regression analysis, only plasma methadone level and corrected QT interval were found to be statistically significant (p < 0.001 and CI didn't cross 0). However R^2 value (coefficient of determination) was only 'fair' for plasma methadone level and QTc interval (between 0.26 – 0.50). Therefore in summary, results from simple linear regression analysis had shown that there were 'fair' linear relationships between methadone dose and plasma level. For every increase in 1mg of methadone, there was an increase of 2.685 ng/ml of plasma methadone level (p<0.001, b=2.685, 95% CI 1.436, 3.934) However only 28.5% of individual can be explained by this regression model (R^2 0.285). Scatter plot (figure 2) is showing the relationship between plasma methadone and methadone dosage. Thus, relationship between Methadone dosage and Plasma Methadone can be summarised with the equation:

$$\textit{Plasma Methadone}\ (ng/ml) = \mathbf{4.641} + \mathbf{2.685}(\textit{Methadone Dose in mg})$$

QTc interval also had a fairly significant linear regression with the methadone dose (p <0.001, b = 0.287 (95%CI 0.147, 0.426), R^2=0.267).

http://dx.doi.org/10.5772/54850

Variable (n=49)	Parameter vector, b[a] (95% C I)	R^2(regression coefficient)	p value
Plasma methadone (mg)	2.685 (1.436 , 3.934)	0.285	0.001*
QTc (msec)	0.287 (0.147, 0.426)	0.267	0.001*
Pulse rate (/min)	0.17 (0.038,0.302)	0.125	0.103
Respiratory Rate (/min)	0.007 (-0.012 ,0.270)	0.013	0.439
MAP (mmHg)	0.06 (-0.153,0.09)	0.006	0.605
SpO2 (%)	-0.006 (- 0.022 , 0.01)	0.011	0.477
Pupil size (mm)	-0.004 (-0.010 , 0.001)	0.049	0.128
Height (m)	0.008 (-0.044 , 0.059)	0.002	0.765
Weight (kg)	0.032 (- 0.088 , 0.930)	0.000	0.930

a = simple linear regression

* = statistically significance

All assumptions are met in statistically significant group

Table 4. Relationship between methadone dose with plasma methadone and other numerical variables

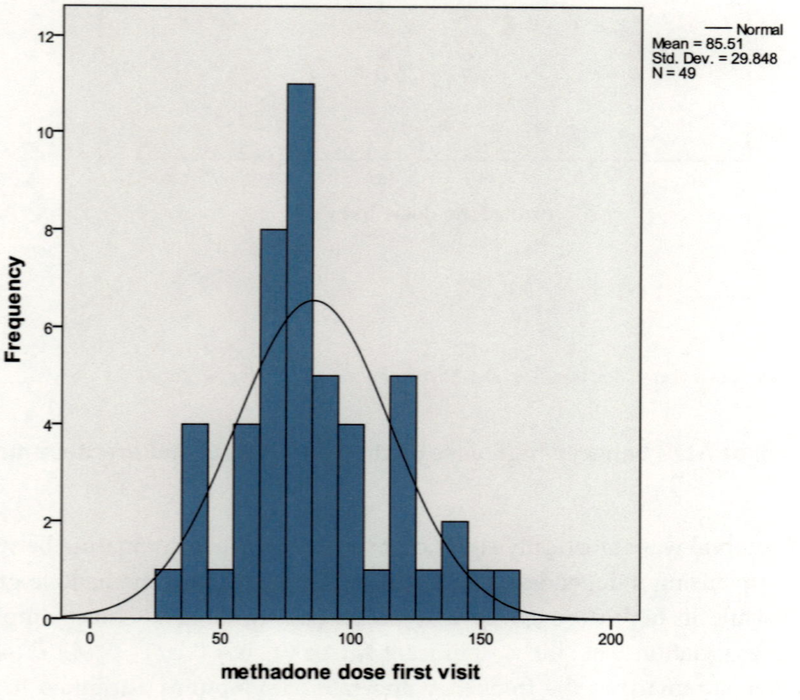

Figure 1. Histogram shows unimodal distribution of methadone dose

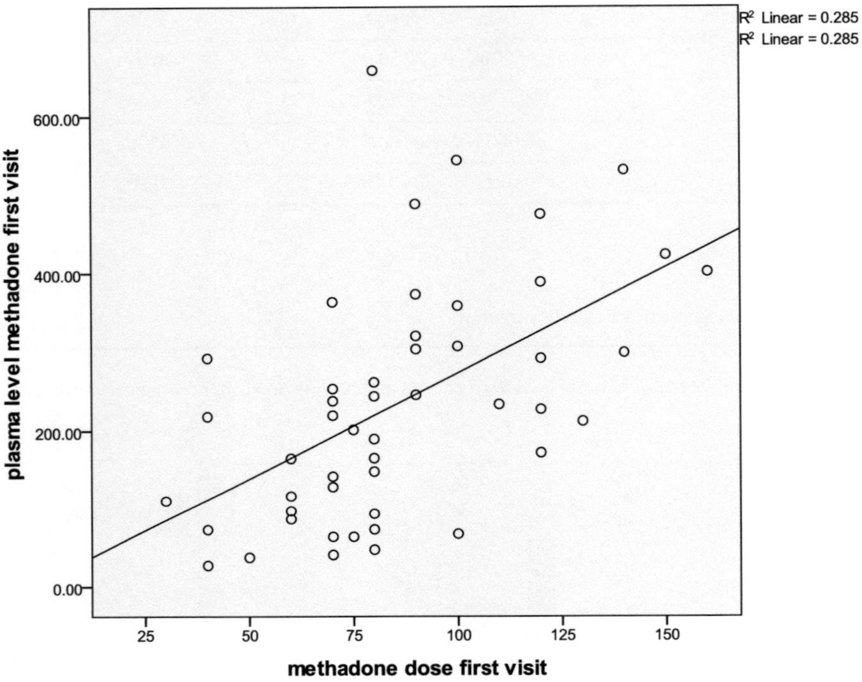

Figure 2. Scatter plot shows correlation between plasma methadone and methadone dose

3.3. Comparison of ADR between high dose methadone (≥80mg) and low dose methadone (<80mg)

Corrected QT interval was statistically significant (p = 0.025) when comparing between both methadone groups using independent-t test. Mean QTc in low dose methadone group was 434.70 (13.79) while in high dose group was 447.86 (22.64), table 5. Using Simple Linear regression, the association was fairly significant (p <0.001, b = 0.287 (95%CI 0.147, 0.426), $R^{2=}$0.267). Table 6 summarized the frequency and rate of symptoms attributed to different groups of methadone maintenance therapy (MMT). Overall, side effects with statistically significant p value (constipation, corrected QT interval, stomach upset, including nausea, vomiting, wind, diarrhoea, headache, lightheadedness and dizziness, chronic fatigue, sleepiness and exhaustion, drowsiness and sleepiness) showed strong positive association between methadone dose and the frequency and severity of the side effects. In other words, with increasing dose of methadone, there was high occurrence of more severe and frequent symptoms. Between the two groups of methadone, constipation and stomach upset (including nausea, vomiting, wind and diarrhea) were most significant symptoms (p = 0.001 and *p = 0.003*). Majority of subjects suffered from constipation in high dose methadone group (n = 27) albeit with minimal frequency (seldom, n = 21 out of 29).

Constitutional symptoms such as stomach upset including nausea, vomiting, wind and diarrhea were very common occurrence in patient taking methadone. Thirty seven of 49 patients in this study experienced one of these symptoms. In higher group of methadone, the situation is more pronounced (27 out of 29 patients) but less bothersome (seldom, n = 21). Using Chi square test/ Fischer exact test, problems with erection or ejaculation, was the main hormonal side effect with a *p* value of 0.005. There were 16 patients (seldom 11 and frequent 5) or more than 50% of patient from methadone ≥80mg is having problems with erection or orgasm. This was in contrast with low dose Methadone group who has only 2 patients having infrequent symptoms (10%). Headache, lightheadedness and dizziness were a common occurrence in both groups of methadone (29 out of 49 subjects). Although it was more common in high dose group (21 out of 29), it was mainly tolerable to subjects (seldom, n=21). Chronic fatigue, sleepiness and exhaustion were also common with a significant $p<0.021$. In higher methadone group (>80mg), there was at least one episodes of fatigue, sleepiness and exhaustion compared to low dose (n = 4 in low dose methadone group while n=15 in high dose group). Patient who suffered frequent symptoms also was higher in high dose group compared to low dose group with n =5 and n= 4 respectively. Nineteen out of 29 patients were suffering from drowsiness and sleepiness, with 15 of them were having infrequent episodes in high dose methadone group. Only 6 patients were having similar symptoms in low dose methadone group, with all have them having mild symptoms.

Other potential life threatening symptoms such as shallow breathing, hypoventilation, breathlessness and palpitation was not statistically significant when comparing between both methadone groups. In that respect, both methadone groups had experienced almost similar rate of symptoms.

Variables	Mean(SD) Methadone< 80mg (n= 20)	Mean (SD) Methadone≥80mg (n=29)	*p* value (95% CI)
QT_C (ms)	434.70(13.79)	447.86(22.64)	*0.025(1.73,24.60)

* statistically significant,

analysed by independent – t test

Table 5. Comparison of corrected QT interval between high dose methadone and low dose methadone

Variables	**Methadone <80mg (n=20)**	**Methadone ≥80mg (n= 29)**	***p value***
Constipation			
Never	10	2	
Seldom	10	21	*0.001[a]
Frequent	0	6	
Stomach upset, including nausea, vomiting, wind, diarrhoea			
Never	9	2	
Seldom	11	22	*0.003[a]
Frequent	0	5	
Problems with erection and ejaculation			
Never	18	13	
Seldom	2	11	*0.005[a]
Frequent	0	5	
Headache, lightheadedness, dizziness			
Never	11	8	
Seldom	7	21	*0.017[a]
Frequent	2	0	
Chronic fatigue, sleepiness and exhaustion			
Never	12	9	
Seldom	4	15	*0.021[a]
Frequent	4	5	
Drowsiness, sleepiness			
Never	14	10	
Seldom	6	15	*0.029[a]
Frequent	0	4	
Breathlessness			
Never	18	20	
Seldom	1	8	0.133[a]
Frequent	1	1	
Coughing			
Never	18	18	
Seldom	1	10	0.052[a]
Frequent	1	1	
Shallow breathing			
Never	19	20	
Seldom	1	8	0.083[a]
Frequent	0	1	
Palpitation			
Never	19	20	
Seldom	0	6	0.062[a]
Frequent	1	3	

Variables	Methadone <80mg (n=20)	Methadone ≥80mg (n= 29)	*p value*
Dry mouth			
Never	8	25	
Seldom	1	4	0.124[a]
Frequent	1	0	
Hallucination			
Never	20	26	
Seldom	0	3	0.138[b]
Frequent	0	0	
Euphoria, elated mood			
Never	18	25	
Seldom	2	3	0.710[a]
Frequent	0	1	
Sad, depression, hopelessness			
Never	17	29	
Seldom	3	0	0.062[b]
Frequent	0	0	
Weight gain			
Never	12	10	
Seldom	7	15	0.187[a]
Frequent	1	4	
Rash			
Never	20	22	
Seldom	0	6	0.060[a]
Frequent	0	1	
Galactorrhoea	No data		
Seizure, athetosis, abnormal movement	No data		

a = Chi Square test

b = Fischer exact test

* statistically significant, p<0.05

Table 6. Comparison of ADR between high dose methadone and low dose methadone (categorical variables)

3.4. Comparison of withdrawal or mixed side effects between low dose methadone (<80mg) and high dose methadone (≥80mg)

Table 7 Illustrates a comparison of main withdrawal or mixed side effects between the two groups of methadone. Using either Chi square test or Fischer exact test, itchiness was the most significant (p =0.001) withdrawal side effect in this study. Eighteen out of 20 patients in low dose methadone had at least 1 episodes of skin itchiness, although majority of them (n = 15) was not frequent. High dose methadone group had only 8 mild skin itchiness cases and 1 frequent case. It indicates that higher dose methadone group has less withdrawal side effect including itchiness. Increase sweating had a second lowest *p* value at 0.005. Eight patients or 40% from lower methadone dose group have experienced increase sweating at some point of time, but 7 of them experienced infrequent symptoms. Only 1 patient from higher methadone group suffers from the same symptoms (3.5%).

Variables	Methadone <80mg (n=20)	Methadone ≥80mg (n=29)	*p value*
Itchiness			
Never	2	22	
Seldom	15	8	*0.001[a]
Frequent	3	1	
Increase sweating			
Never	12	28	
Seldom	7	1	*0.005[a]
Frequent	1	0	
Insomnia, lack of sleep			
Never	12	26	
Seldom	6	2	*0.033[a]
Frequent	2	0	
Flushing			
Never	11	26	
Seldom	8	3	*0.019[a]
Frequent	1	0	
Poor weight gain, anorexia			
Never	18	21	
Seldom	2	6	0.263[a]
Frequent	0	1	
Difficulty urination			
Never	20	28	
Seldom	0	1	1.000[b]
Frequent	0	0	
Aggressive, agitation			
Never	20	27	
Seldom	2	0	0.357[b]
Frequent	0	0	
Swelling of hand and feet	No data		

a = Chi Square test, b = Fisher Exact test

* statistically significant

Table 7. Comparison of main withdrawal side effects between high dose methadone and low dose methadone.

http://dx.doi.org/10.5772/54850

Withdrawal patients also reported having flushing symptoms. Comparing the 2 groups of methadone, there was a significant statistical significant (p = 0.019). Nine patients having flushing symptoms in low dose group compared to 3 in high dose group.

Eight out of 20 patients were having insomnia or lack of sleep in low dose methadone group (p = 0.033). However, majority (6 out of 8) were having only infrequent symptoms. In high dose group, only 2 patients suffered from infrequent insomnia or lack of sleep (6.8%). Other variables were not statistically significant.

4. Discussion

Some centre for methadone maintenance treatment (MMT) programs prescribe inadequate daily methadone doses. Patients complain of withdrawal symptoms and continue illicit opioid use, yet practitioners are reluctant to increase doses above certain arbitrary thresholds. Plasma methadone levels (PMLs) may guide practitioners' dosing decisions, especially for those patients who have low PMLs despite higher methadone doses. To date, methadone dosing is still an issue of debate and controversy among clinicians who are involved in methadone maintenance programs. One meta analysis [35] which studied 24 articles suggest to have a goal for methadone dosing in the range of 60 to 100 mg daily However newer research suggests that doses ranging from 100 mg/d to more than 700 mg/d, with correspondingly higher PMLs, may be optimal for many patients [36-39].There does not appear to be a maximum daily dose limit when determining what is adequately "enough" methadone. In this study, there were 49 subjects taking daily methadone in the range of 30mg to 160mg. Mean methadone dosage was 85.51mg whereas methadone plasma levels ranged between 26.90 and 708.50 ng/ml with a mean of 234.24 ng/ml. Results from this study showed there was a positive, fair and significant correlation between methadone doses with its plasma level. (Pearson R = 0.36, Regression coefficient, R^2 =0.285, parameter vector b = 2.685, p = 0.001) and can be summarised into an equation:

$$\textit{Plasma methadone}\ (ng/ml) = \mathbf{4.641} + \mathbf{2.685}\ (\textit{methadone dose in mg})$$

Thus, according to the formula, every increase in 1mg of methadone, there was an increase of 2.685 ng/ml of plasma methadone level plus a constant (b=2.685, 95% CI 1.436, 3.934, $p<0.001$) However only 28.5% of individual can be explained by this regression model (R^2 0.285). Result from our study is well replicated in other publication. Adelson et al. in 2007, had studied 151 MMT patient in Israel and found a significant correlation between methadone dosage and plasma level (Pearson R = 0.36, $P<0.005$). The study also noted a stronger correlation in patient who do not have illicit drugs [38]. Eap et al. reported on use of high methadone doses, as well as methadone levels in the plasma; they evaluated 211 MMT patients (including 31 patients who were undergoing dose reduction to stop treatment), all of whom were receiving the same methadone dose for at least 5 days. [40]

The mean methadone dose in the 211 patients was 100 ± 58 mg/day, range 5-350 mg/days, and their mean methadone level in plasma was 281 ± 169 ng/ml, range 16-976 ng/ml. They found a significant correlation between methadone levels in plasma and methadone doses expressed as mg/kg body weight; the highest correlation was in patients with no co-medications (benzodiazepines and antidepressants) or drug abuse, and with the active enantiomer R-methadone (R = 0.65). The correlation with the racemic methadone solution was R = 0.50. However, no scatter-plot was published. Results from this study and those highlighted here shows that although the plasma methadone level was fairly correlated (R between 0.26 – 0.5), true significant linear associations is impossible. This is because the plasma level depends on the dose that the patient is actually taken, which can be subjected to cheating. It is well known that some patients may abuse methadone. High blood levels of methadone may occur for several reasons:

1. Up to 75% of the patients with high-methadone serum levels indeed were receiving high methadone doses, above 70mg/day;
2. Some patients may obtain illicitly additional methadone or other illicit drugs outside the clinic on any day;
3. Some patients, especially those who have take-home privileges, may not consume their entire doses and may have sold some of the methadone.

There are several other factors that relate to inter-subject variability among patients' serum methadone level. Specific cytochrome P-450 gene polymorphisms which Eap et al. hypothesized might produce "slow metabolizers," "rapid metabolizers," and "ultra-rapid metabolizers". Chen et al. in 2011, studies the effect CYP450 polymorphism in relation to withdrawal symptoms and side effects. In this cross sectional study, the average methadone dose was 55 mg/day among 366 methadone maintenance patients whose average steady-state plasma methadone concentrations were 193 and 142 ng/ml for R- and S-methadone enantiomers. It found out a polymorphism of the CYP3A4 is associated with opioid withdrawal symptoms (permutation, $p < 0.0097$), especially the symptom of heart rate, which was assessed as an item within 11 items of the clinical opioid withdrawal scale total score.CYP3A4 polymorphism also is associated with methadone side effects specifically the sedation side effects. The metabolism of methadone is carried out through the CYP3A4, CYP2B6, CYP2C19 and CYP2D6 isoenzymes of the CYP system in the liver [41,42]. Through the metabolic process, it produces an inactive metabolite 2-ethylidene-1, 5-dimethyl-3, 3-diphenylpyrrolidine (EDDP). It has been estimated that approximately 50% of all clinical therapeutic drugs are metabolized by CYP3A4. The subfamily of CYP3A enzymes is responsible for the other 30% of drug metabolism in adults, hence its activity and regulatory mechanism may have an impact on methadone disposition and variability [43]. Apart from polymorphism from CYP450 system, variation in acute α-glycoprotein (AAG) in plasma may play a significant role in its inter-individual variability. Methadone binds to plasma protein to a high degree of 86 percent, predominantly to acute α-glycoprotein (AAG) [44]. AAG is an acute phase protein that exhibits significant variations in its plasma levels according to the physiological and or pathological situation of the patient [45-47]. AAG levels are significantly increased in stress, leading to very low concentrations in the free fraction of methadone in cancer patients compared to healthy participants [48,49].

http://dx.doi.org/10.5772/54850

Other factors that may contribute to variability include: age and sex. It has been suggested that these factors may explain about 33 percent of the inter-individual variations in steady state level [50]. From the study, females and increase in weight was found to have a positive linear relationship. However, we could not replicate the findings in our study most probably due to small sample size and "all male" subjects of our samples (for age, linear correlation, $p = 0.77$).

In summary this study has concurred with the current view (r =0.36) of fairly strong relationship between methadone dosage and plasma methadone in patient currently subscribed into MMT. The correlation is higher when the patient has a complete abstinence from illicit drug. Nevertheless only 28.5% (R^2 0.285) of correlations can be explained by the correlation equation, or in other words, the inter-variability between patient is huge. Factors such as polymorphism of cytochrome P450 system especially CYP, variation in weight and gender, unpredictable relationship between AAG and stress level and also patient factor is the main contributor for this variation. Regardless of the route of administration, opioids can produce a wide spectrum of unwanted side effects, especially during the early days of treatment when daily dose is being stabilised. Some of these are distressing but generally not dangerous such as constipation, sedation, itchiness, sweating, nausea and vomiting; whereas others are more serious and even life-threatening like respiratory depression, severe hypotension and abnormal QT interval (potentiates episodes of Torsade de Pointes (TdP). TdD is polymorphic ventricular tachycardia (VT) characterized by a gradual change in the amplitude and twisting of the QRS complexes around the isoelectric line. Often, Tdp is associated with a prolonged QT interval usually terminates spontaneously but frequently recurs and may degenerate into ventricular fibrillation. The ventricular rate can range from 150 beats per minute (bpm) to 250 bpm. The QT interval requires to be increased markedly (600 msec or greater). Therefore, a prolonged QT interval signifies a higher risk of arrhythmias especially TdP, which can deteriorates into sudden cardiac failure and sudden death. In vitro studies of levomethadyl, methadone, and buprenorphine have each demonstrated considerable blockade of the human ether-a-go-go-related–gene (*hERG*) channel activity, a property that is strongly associated with prolongation of the QT interval and the induction of torsade de pointes ventricular tachycardia (TdP) [51].

Mean and SD for corrected QT interval was 434.70(13.79) ms for low dose methadone group and 447.86(22.64) for high dose methadone group. Independent t- test showed statistically significant different between these two groups (t =2.316, mean difference = 13.16, p value = 0.025, CI = 1.73, 24.6) (table 3).

In addition, simple linear regression showed there is fair association between methadone dose and corrected QT (R=0.404, $b = 0.287$, CI = 0.147, 0.426, $R^2 = 0.267$, $p = 0.001$). Although this result proved there is an association between methadone dose and QTc, only 26.7% of the patient can be predicted by the result (R2 = 0.267) (table 2).

Results from this study are in line with dozens other findings in proving the association between methadone dose and prolongation of QTc. [52-55]. As with most QT interval prolonging drugs, the effects of methadone on cardiac repolarization are dose dependent, as evident in case reports as well as cross-sectional and prospective studies. Methadone dosages exceeding 100 mg/d have frequently been noted in published cases of torsade de pointes, and some case reports [56-58] highlight QTc interval normalization after methadone discontinuation or dose reduction. Furthermore, many studies, including those of oral and intravenous methadone, demonstrate a positive correlation between doses and delayed cardiac repolarization [59-63] among both addiction treatment and pain management cohorts. In Peles and colleagues' study [61], the correlation achieved statistical significance in the subset of patients abusing cocaine, which is consistent with a synergistic effect of methadone and cocaine on hERG channel blockade. In Fanoe and colleagues' study, the QTc interval increased by 10 ms for every 50-mg increase in methadone dose, which corresponded to a higher risk for syncope (odds ratio, 1.2 [CI, 1.1 to 1.4]). Cruciani et al. found the correlation between methadone doses with QTc in "all male" subjects similar to this study. With regard to serum levels, Martell and colleagues prospectively demonstrated that the increase in QTc interval from baseline to 12 months after methadone initiation correlated with both trough and peak serum concentrations. Wedam and colleagues observed similar relationships with the methadone derivative levacetylmethadol. This creates a safety– efficacy paradox, because higher doses of methadone may reduce illicit opioid use (or diminish chronic pain) yet place patients at greater arrhythmia risk. It is important for clinicians to recognize that sudden cardiac death associated with methadone has been described at dosages as low as 29 mg/day, which suggests that arrhythmia can occur across a wide therapeutic range that includes dosages commonly used in both chronic pain and addiction treatment. This in turn suggests that methadone dosage is just one consideration with regard to limiting arrhythmia risk.

In view of the overwhelming evidence which associate methadone dose with prolonged QTc and subsequent Torsades de Pointes, a clinical guidelines in QTc interval screening in methadone therapy was proposed by Krantz et al. (2009) [64].

Respiratory depression, the hallmark of serious opioid overdose, is only seen in about 50% of patients with CNS depression and should not to be confused with [65]. It is also synonymous with drowsiness and lethargy which may confuse the observer. Methadone can reduces or eliminates the normal drive to recommence respiration or increase the rate once it diminished in the body. Overdose-induced adult respiratory distress syndrome (ARDS) has also been described for methadone toxicity [66].

Methadone overdose can follow an unpredictable course in non-tolerant patients who are at risk of death. When methadone is consumed, the effect on the breathing pattern depends on the plasma concentration of the drug. At low concentrations there is a decrease in tidal volume (normal volume of air breathed in and out), but no change in respiratory rate; at higher concentrations both tidal volume and rate are depressed [67]. Preclinical studies indicate that at very high concentrations, there may be some additional disruption to respiration as a result of NMDA (N-methyl-D-Aspartate) antagonism [68] and possible serotonergic (re-uptake inhibition) and catecholaminergic activity [69].

Generally, opioid activates the mesolimbic reward system in the midbrain. Subsequently, the system generates signals in the ventral tegmental area. As a result, dopamine neurotransmitter is released from the nucleus accumbens result in feelings of pleasure. Other areas of the brain create a lasting memory that associates these good feelings with the circumstances and environment in which they occur. These memories, called conditioned associations, often lead to the craving for drugs. Beside relieving craving and withdrawal, methadone on the other

http://dx.doi.org/10.5772/54850

hand, through G-protein–coupled mechanisms also directly affect cation channel function in the postsynaptic membrane. Methadone as an agonist at both mu and delta receptors acts to increase potassium channel opening (reducing production of cAMP through inhibition of adenylate cyclase activity) and decrease the opening of voltage-operated calcium channels (inhibiting inward Ca 2+ currents). Consequent reduction in neuronal membrane excitability (depolarizing effect) exerts an inhibitory effect upon respiratory systems to diminish sensitivity to changes in O2 and CO2 outside normal concentration ranges [70]. Mu and delta receptor activity contribute in an additive way to respiratory depression. Several studies have investigated the control of respiration during chronic dosing (MMT) with the drug. Usually, while PaO_2 in blood is normal, dopamine is released inhibiting chemoreceptors in the carotid and aortic bodies. Hypoxia reduces the release of this dopamine and in doing so releases chemoreceptors, which stimulate the respiratory centre. Santiago et al. [72] found at the start (< 2 months) of MMT, ventilation was reduced and arterial blood gas altered, along with decreased sensitivity of CNS chemoreceptors to both CO_2 and hypoxia. However, after more than 8 months in MMT these indices had returned to normal except for the persistent reduction in sensitivity of the CNS receptors to hypoxia.

Durstellar et al. in 2010, had compared multiple symptoms of methadone to heroin in opioid dependence [72]. Breathing difficulties were encountered more in methadone group at 25.4% out of 63 patients compared to heroin group (11.1% out of 54 patients; $p < 0.05$).

Our samples showed similar rate in both methadone group; breathlessness (11 patient out of 49 or 22.45%, where 9 in high dose group, 2 in low dose group), shallow breathing (10 patients out of 49 or 20.41%, where 9 were in high dose group and coughing (13 out of 49 patients or 26.5%). However when comparing between low dose methadone and high dose methadone groups, none were statistically significant.

Looking at the respiratory symptoms pattern, up to 20-25% of the patient had experienced some degree of respiratory symptoms attributable to methadone or indeed other opioids. However, life threatening respiratory compromise remains rare as evidence from mortality review worldwide [73-75]. Like early research by Santiago et al. which has been stated above, Marks and Goldring [76] found hypercapnia uniformly developed in the early phases of methadone treatment persisting for up to 8 months and which was consistently associated with alteration in the central control of ventilation.

Although results from this study were comparable with previous study, more refined research with better methodology especially in detecting respiratory depression in induction phase (first 6 month) is warranted to study the dose-dependent respiratory depression.

5. Conclusion

In summary this study has concurred with the current view (r =0.36) of fairly strong relationship between methadone dosage and plasma methadone in patient currently subscribed into MMT. The correlation is higher when the patient has a complete abstinence from illicit drug.

Nevertheless only 28.5% (R^2 0.285) of correlations can be explained by the correlation equation, or in other words, the inter-variability between patient is huge. Factors such as polymorphism of cytochrome P450 system especially CYP, variation in weight and gender, unpredictable relationship between AAG and stress level and also patient factor is the main contributor for this variation

Acknowledgements

We would like to acknowledge the Research University Grant of Universiti Sains Malaysia, Kubang Kerian, 16150, Kelantan, Malaysia: 1001/PPSP/812056 for supporting this research.

Author details

Nasir Mohamad[1,2], Roslanuddin Mohd Salehuddin[1], Basyirah Ghazali[2], Nor Hidayah Abu Bakar[3], Nurfadhlina Musa[2], Muslih Abdulkarim Ibrahim[2], Liyana Hazwani Mohd Adnan[3], Ahmad Rashidi[2] and Rusli Ismail[2]

1 Department of Emergency Medicine, School of Medical Sciences, Universiti Sains Malaysia, K.Kerian, Kelantan, Malaysia

2 Pharmacogenetic Research Group, Institute for Research in Molecular Medicine, Universiti Sains Malaysia, K.Kerian, Kelanta, Malaysia

3 Department of Pathology, Hospital Raja Perempuan Zainab II, Kota Bharu, Kelantan, Malaysia

References

[1] Who (2004) Who/Unodc/Unaids Position Paper Substitution Maintenance Therapy In The Management Of Opioid Dependence And Hiv/Aids Prevention

[2] K. Wolff, A.W.M. Hay, D. Raistrick, and R. Calvert (1993). Steady-state pharmacokinetics of methadone in opioid addicts. *Eur J Clin Pharmacol* 44: 189- 194

[3] Maremmani I., Metteo P., Pier P.P. (2011). Basics on Addiction. A Training Package for Medical Practitioners or Psychiatrists who Treat Opioid Dependence. Heroin Addict Rel Clin Probl; 13(2):5-40.

[4] Stewart B. Leavitt (2003). Addiction Treatment Forum. Methadone dosing and safety in the treatment of opioid addiction. Clinco Communications, Inc.

[5] Mohamad, N., Nor Hidayah A.B., , Nurfadhlina M., , Nazila T. & , Rusli I. (2010) Better Retention Of Malaysian Opiate Dependents Treated With High Dose Methadone In Methadone Maintenance Therapy. Harm Reduction Journal, 7, 30.

[6] John He, Duramed Inc., Bala-Cynwyd, PA (2008). SAS Programming to Calculate AUC in Pharmacokinetic Studies —Comparison of Four Methods in Concentration Data. Paper SP06-2008.

[7] Peter L. Anderson (2005). The ABCs of Pharmacokinetics, The Body, The Complete HIV/AIDS resources.

[8] R. Urso, P. Blardi, G. Giorgi (2002). A short introduction to pharmacokinetics. European Review for Medical and Pharmacological Sciences 6: 33-44.

[9] Principles of Pharmacokinetics, NCBI. Bookshelf ID: NBK12815

[10] Toutain, P. L., Bousquet-Me´lou A (2004). Volumes of distribution. J. vet. Pharmacol. Therap. 27: 441–453.

[11] Drug Distribution to Tissues. The Merck Manual.

[12] Säwe, J. (1986). High-dose morphine and methadone in cancer patients: clinical pharmacokinetic considerations of oral treatment. Clin Pharmacokinet 11, 87–106.

[13] Gabrielsson, J. L., Johansson, P., Bondesson, U., & Paalzow, L. K. (1985). Analysis of methadone disposition in the pregnant rat by means of physiological flow model. J Pharmacokinet Biopharm 13, 355–372.

[14] M.J. Garrido, I.F. Trocóniz (1999) Methadone: a review of its pharmacokinetic/pharmacodynamic properties. J Pharmacol Toxicol 42: 61–66

[15] Wolff, K., Hay, A. W. M., Raistrick, D., & Calvert, R. (1993). Steady-state pharmacokinetics of methadone in opioid addicts. Eur J Clin Pharmacol 44, 189–194.

[16] Inturrisi, C. E., Colburn, W. A., Kaiko, R. F., Houde, R. W., & Foley, K.M. (1987). Pharmacokinetics and pharmacodynamics of methadone in patients with chronic pain. Clin Pharmacol Ther 41, 392–401.

[17] Garrido, M. J., Jiménez, R., Gómez, E., & Calvo, R. (1996). Influence of plasma protein binding on analgesic effect on methadone in rats with spontaneous withdrawal. J Pharm Pharmacol 48, 281–284.

[18] Romanch, M. K., Piafsky, K. M., Abel, J. G., Khouw, V., & Sellers, E. M. (1981). Methadone binding to orosomucoid (α1-acid glycoprotein): determinant of free fraction in plasma. Clin Pharmacol Ther 29, 211–217

[19] Wilkins, J. N., Ashofteh, A., Setoda, D., Wheatley, W. S., Huigen, H., & Ling, W. (1997). Ultrafiltration using the Amicon MPS-1 for assessing methadone plasma protein binding. Ther Drug Monit 19, 83–87

[20] Abramson, F. P. (1982). Methadone plasma protein binding: alterations in cancer and displacement from α1-acid glycoprotein. Clin Pharmacol Ther 32, 652–658.

[21] Calvo, R., Aguirre, C., Troconiz, I. F., López, J., & Garrido, M. J. (1996). Alpha1-acid glycoprotein and serum protein binding of methadone in heroin addicts during withdrawal. Proceedings of the Sixth World Congress on Clinical Pharmacology and Therapeutics, Buenos Aires, Argentina, p. 174.

[22] Rostami-Hodjegan, A., Wolff, W., Hay, A. W. M., Raistrick, D., & Calvert, R. (1999). Population pharmacokinetics of methadone in opiate users: characterization on time-dependent changes. Br J Clin Pharmacol 48, 43–52

[23] R.A. Totah, K.E. Allen, P. Sheffels, D. Whittington, and ED. Kharasch (2007). Enantiomeric Metabolic Interactions and Stereoselective Human Methadone Metabolism. The journal of pharmacology and experimental therapeutics 321:389–399.

[24] Chin B. Eap, Jean-Jacques Déglon, Pierre Baumann (1999). Pharmacokinetics and Pharmacogenetics of Methadone: Clinical Relevance. *Heroin Add & Rel Clin Probl* 1 (1): 19 34

[25] Tsuchiya K, Gatanaga H, Tachikawa N et. al (2004). Homozygous CYP2B6 *6 (Q172H and K262R) correlates with high plasma efavirenz concentrations in HIV-1 patients treated with standard efavirenz-containing regimens. Biochemical and Biophysical Research Communications 319: 1322–1326

[26] Wang J, Sönnerborg A, Rane A, et. al (2006). Identification of a novel specific CYP2B6 allele in Africans causing impaired metabolism of the HIV drug efavirenz. Pharmacogenet Genomics. Mar;16(3):191-8.

[27] Rotger M, Tegude H, Colombo S. Predictive value of known and novel alleles of CYP2B6 for efavirenz plasma concentrations in HIV-infected individuals. Clin Pharmacol Ther. 2007 Apr;81(4):557-66. Epub. Jan 18.

[28] M. Ingelman-Sundberg, S. C. Sim, A. Gomez, C.Rodriguez-Antona (2007). Influence of cytochrome P450 polymorphisms on drug therapies: Pharmacogenetic, pharmacoepigenetic and clinical aspects. Pharmacology & Therapeutics 116 496–526

[29] Jesjeet Singh Gill, A. H. S., Mohd Hussain Habil (2007). The First Methadone Programme In Malaysia: Overcoming Obstacles And Achieving The Impossible. Asean Journal of Psychiatry;8 (2):54-70.

[30] Lin, C. & Detels, R. A. Qualitative Study Exploring The Reason For Low Dosage Of Methadone Prescribed In The Mmt Clinics In China. Drug & Alcohol Dependence, 117, 45 49.

[31] Noordin, N. M., Merican, M. I., Rahman, H. A., Lee, S. S. & Ramly, R. (2008) Substitution Treatment In Malaysia. Lancet, 372, 1149-1150

[32] Mazlan, M., Schottenfeld, R. S. & Chawarski, M. C. (2006). New Challenges And Opportunities In Managing Substance Abuse In Malaysia. Drug And Alcohol Review, 25, 473-478.

[33] Stewart B. Leavitt, P. E., At Forum (2003). Methadone Dosing & Safety In The Treatment Of Opioid Addiction. Addiction Treatment Forum.

[34] Ballantyne, J. C. & Mao, J. (2003). Opioid Therapy For Chronic Pain. New England Journal Of Medicine, 349, 1943-1953

[35] Rowley, D., Mclean, S., O'gorman, A., Ryan, K. & Mcquillan, R. Review Of Cancer Pain Management In Patients Receiving Maintenance Methadone Therapy. The American Journal Of Hospice & Palliative Care, 28, 183-187

[36] Fareed, A., Casarella, J., Amar, R., Vayalapalli, S. & Drexler, K. Methadone Maintenance Dosing Guideline For Opioid Dependence, A Literature Review. Journal Of Addictive Diseases, 29, 1-14.

[37] Adelson, M., Peles, E., Bodner, G. & Kreek, M. J. (2007). Correlation Between High Methadone Doses And Methadone Serum Levels In Methadone Maintenance Treatment (MMT) Patients. Journal Of Addictive Diseases, 26, 15-26

[38] Peles, E., Kreek, M. J., Kellogg, S. & Adelson, M. (2006) High Methadone Dose Significantly Reduces Cocaine Use In Methadone Maintenance Treatment (Mmt) Patients. Journal Of Addictive Diseases, 25, 43-50.

[39] Maxwell S, S. M. (1999) Optimizing Response To Mmt: Use Of Higher Dose Methadone. Journal Of Psychoactive Drugs, 31, 95-102.

[40] Eap, C. B., Bourquin, M., Martin, J., Spagnoli, J., Livoti, S., Powell, K., Baumann, P. & Dã©Glon, J. (2000) Plasma Concentrations Of The Enantiomers Of Methadone And Therapeutic Response In Methadone Maintenance Treatment. Drug And Alcohol Dependence, 61, 47-54.

[41] Donny Ec, B., Bigelow Ge, Stitzer Ml, Walsh Sl, (2005). Methadone Doses Of More Than 100mg Or Greater Are More Effective Than Lower Doses At At Suppressing Heroin Self Administration In Opiod Dependent Individuals. Addiction, 100, 1496-509.

[42] Chang, Y., Fang, W. B., Lin, S.-N. & Moody, D. E. Stereo-Selective Metabolism Of Methadone By Human Liver Microsomes And Cdna-Expressed Cytochrome P450s: A Reconciliation. Basic & Clinical Pharmacology & Toxicology, 108, 55-62.

[43] Chen, C.-H., Wang, S.-C. et. al. Genetic Polymorphisms In Cyp3A4 Are Associated With Withdrawal Symptoms And Adverse Reactions In Methadone Maintenance Patients. Pharmacogenomics, 12, 1397-1406.

[44] Shiran, M.-R., Lennard, M. S., Iqbal, M.-Z., Lagundoye, O., Seivewright, N., Tucker, G. T. & Rostami-Hodjegan, A. (2009) Contribution Of The Activities Of Cyp3A, Cyp2D6, Cyp1A2 And Other Potential Covariates To The Disposition Of Methadone In Patients Undergoing Methadone Maintenance Treatment. British Journal Of Clinical Pharmacology, 67, 29-37.

[45] Romach, M. K., Piafsky, K. M., Abel, J. G., Khouw, V. & Sellers, E. M. (1981) Methadone Binding To Orosomucoid (Alpha 1-Acid Glycoprotein): Determinant Of Free Fraction In Plasma. Clin Pharmaco Ther, 29, 211-7.

[46] Fournier, T., Medjoubi-N, N. & Porquet, D. (2000) Alpha-1-Acid Glycoprotein. Biochimica Et Biophysica Acta (Bba) - Protein Structure And Molecular Enzymology, 1482, 157-171.

[47] Mestriner, F. L. A. C., Spiller, F., Laure, H. J., Souto, F. O., Tavares-Murta, B. M., Rosa, J. C., Basile-Filho, A., Ferreira, S. H., Greene, L. J. & Cunha, F. Q. (2007) Acute-Phase Protein A-1-Acid Glycoprotein Mediates Neutrophil Migration Failure In Sepsis By A Nitric Oxide-Dependent Mechanism. Proceedings Of The National Academy Of Sciences, 104, 19595-19600.

[48] Yang, Y., Wan, C., Li, H., Zhu, H., La, Y., Xi, Z., Chen, Y., Jiang, L., Feng, G. & He, L. (2006) Altered Levels Of Acute Phase Proteins In The Plasma Of Patients With Schizophrenia. Analytical Chemistry, 78, 3571-3576.

[49] Gómez, E., Martinez-Jordá, R., Suárez, E., Garrido, M. J. & Calvo, R. (1995) Altered Methadone Analgesia Due To Changes In Plasma Protein Binding: Role Of The Route Of Administration. General Pharmacology: The Vascular System, 26, 1273-1276.

[50] Wolff, K., Rostami-Hodjegan, A., Hay, A. W. M., Raistrick, D. & Tucker, G. (2000) Population-Based Pharmacokinetic Approach For Methadone Monitoring Of Opiate Addicts: Potential Clinical Utility. Addiction, 95, 1771-1783

[51] Eap, C. B., Crettol, S., Rougier, J. S., Schlapfer, J., Sintra Grilo, L., Deglon, J. J., Besson, J., Croquette-Krokar, M., Carrupt, P. A. & Abriel, H. (2007) Stereoselective Block Of Herg Channel By (S)-Methadone And Qt Interval Prolongation In Cyp2b6 Slow Metabolizers. Clin Pharmacol Ther, 81, 719-28.

[52] Byrne, A. & Stimmel, B. (2007) Methadone And Qtc Prolongation. Lancet, 369, 366; Author Reply 366-7.

[53] Schmittner, J. & Krantz, M. J. (2006) High-Dose Methadone And Qtc Prolongation: Strategies To Optimize Safety. J Opioid Manag, 2, 49-55.

[54] Krantz, M. J., Martin, J., Stimmel, B., Mehta, D. & Haigney, M. C. (2009) Qtc Interval Screening In Methadone Treatment. Ann Intern Med, 150, 387-95.

[55] Wolff, K. (2002) Characterization Of Methadone Overdose: Clinical Consideration And The Scientific Evidences. J Therapeutic Drug Monitoring, 24, 457-470.

[56] Drudi, F. M., Poggi, R., Trenta, F., Manganaro, F. & Iannicelli, E. (1997) [A Case Of The Adult Respiratory Distress Syndrome Induced By A Methadone Overdose]. Radiol Med, 94, 393-6.

[57] Santiago, T. V., Pugliese, A. C. & Edelman, N. H. (1977) Control Of Breathing During Methadone Addiction. Am J Med, 62, 347-54.

[58] Lalley, P. M. (2003) Mu-Opioid Receptor Agonist Effects On Medullary Respiratory Neurons In The Cat: Evidence For Involvement In Certain Types Of Ventilatory Disturbances. Am J Physiol Regul Integr Comp Physiol, 285, R1287-304.

[59] Codd, E. E., Shank, R. P., Schupsky, J. J. & Raffa, R. B. (1995) Serotonin And Norepinephrine Uptake Inhibiting Activity Of Centrally Acting Analgesics: Structural Determinants And Role In Antinociception. J Pharmacol Exp Ther, 274, 1263-70.

[60] White, J. M. & Irvine, R. J. (1999) Mechanisms Of Fatal Opioid Overdose. Addiction, 94, 961-72.

[61] Fanoe, S., Hvidt, C., Ege, P. & Jensen, G. B. (2007) Syncope And Qt Prolongation Among Patients Treated With Methadone For Heroin Dependence In The City Of Copenhagen. Heart, 93, 1051-5.

[62] Cruciani, R. A., Sekine, R., Homel, P., Lussier, D., Yap, Y., Suzuki, Y., Schweitzer, P., Yancovitz, S. R., Lapin, J. A., Shaiova, L., Sheu, R. G. & Portenoy, R. K. (2005) Measurement Of Qtc In Patients Receiving Chronic Methadone Therapy. J Pain Symptom Manage, 29, 385-91.

[63] Latowsky, M. (2006) Methadone Death, Dosage And Torsade De Pointes: Risk-Benefit Policy Implications. J Psychoactive Drugs, 38, 513-9.

[64] Krantz, M. J., Martin, J., Stimmel, B., Mehta, D. & Haigney, M. C. (2009) Qtc Interval Screening In Methadone Treatment. Ann Intern Med, 150, 387-95.

[65] Pirnay, S., Borron, S. W., Giudicelli, C. P., Tourneau, J., Baud, F. J. & Ricordel, I. (2004) A Critical Review Of The Causes Of Death Among Post-Mortem Toxicological Investigations: Analysis Of 34 Buprenorphine-Associated And 35 Methadone-Associated Deaths. Addiction, 99, 978-88

[66] Marks, C. E., Jr. & Goldring, R. M. (1973) Chronic Hypercapnia During Methadone Maintenance. Am Rev Respir Dis, 108, 1088-93.

[67] Lalley, P. M. (2003) Mu-Opioid Receptor Agonist Effects On Medullary Respiratory Neurons In The Cat: Evidence For Involvement In Certain Types Of Ventilatory Disturbances. Am J Physiol Regul Integr Comp Physiol, 285, R1287-304.

[68] Codd, E. E., Shank, R. P., Schupsky, J. J. & Raffa, R. B. (1995) Serotonin And Norepinephrine Uptake Inhibiting Activity Of Centrally Acting Analgesics: Structural Determinants And Role In Antinociception. J Pharmacol Exp Ther, 274, 1263-70.

[69] White, J. M. & Irvine, R. J. (1999) Mechanisms Of Fatal Opioid Overdose. Addiction, 94, 961-72.

[70] Codd, E. E., Shank, R. P., Schupsky, J. J. & Raffa, R. B. (1995) Serotonin And Norepinephrine Uptake Inhibiting Activity Of Centrally Acting Analgesics: Structural Determinants And Role In Antinociception. J Pharmacol Exp Ther, 274, 1263-70.

[71] Santiago, T. V., Goldblatt, K., Winters, K., Pugliese, A. C. & Edelman, N. H. (1980) Respiratory Consequences Of Methadone: The Response To Added Resistance To Breathing. Am Rev Respir Dis, 122, 623-8.

[72] Dürsteler-Macfarland, K. M., Fischer, D. A., Mueller, S., Schmid, O., Moldovanyi, A. & Wiesbeck, G. A. Symptom Complaints Of Patients Prescribed Either Oral Methadone Or Injectable Heroin. Journal Of Substance Abuse Treatment, 38, 328-337.

[73] Vormfelde, S. V. & Poser, W. (2001) Death Attributed To Methadone. Pharmacopsychiatry, 34, 217-22.

[74] Pirnay, S., Borron, S. W., Giudicelli, C. P., Tourneau, J., Baud, F. J. & Ricordel, I. (2004) A Critical Review Of The Causes Of Death Among Post-Mortem Toxicological Investigations: Analysis Of 34 Buprenorphine-Associated And 35 Methadone-Associated Deaths. Addiction, 99, 978-88

[75] Vormfelde, S. V. & Poser, W. (2001) Death Attributed To Methadone. Pharmacopsychiatry, 34, 217-22.

[76] Marks, C. E., Jr. & Goldring, R. M. (1973) Chronic Hypercapnia During Methadone Maintenance. Am Rev Respir Dis, 108, 1088-93.